McCANCE & WIDDOWSON

A Scientific Partnership
of 60 years

McCance & Widdowson

A Scientific Partnership of 60 Years
1933 to 1993

A commemorative volume prepared as a tribute to the 60-year scientific partnership between Robert Alexander McCance CBE, FRS and Elsie May Widdowson CBE, FRS.

'Two are better than one: because they have a good reward for their labour'   Ecclesiastes 4:9

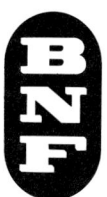

Edited by Margaret Ashwell

Published by the
British Nutrition Foundation

Published by:
The British Nutrition Foundation
52-54 High Holborn House
High Holborn
London WC1V 6RQ
Tel : 071-404-6504 Fax : 071-404-6747
First edition 1993

© 1993 The British Nutrition Foundation
       All rights reserved

Apart from any fair dealing for the purposes of research or private study, or criticism or review, as permitted under the UK Copyright Designs and Patents Act, 1988, this publication may not be reproduced, stored, or transmitted, in any form or by any means, without the prior permission in writing of the publishers, or in the case of reprographic reproduction only in accordance with the terms of the licences issued by the Copyright Licensing Agency in the UK, or in accordance with the terms of the licences issued by the appropriate Reproduction Rights Organization outside the UK. Enquiries concerning reproduction outside the terms stated here should be sent to the publishers at the London address printed on this page.

The publisher makes no representation, express or implied, with regard to the accuracy of the information contained in this book and cannot accept any legal responsibility or liability for any errors or omissions that may be made.

ISBN Number: 0 907667 07 4

- Design by Colin Barker (Whaddon, Cambs)
- Sub-editing by Sandra Carey (London)
- Typesetting by Impact Origination (Baldock, Herts)
- Printing and binding by Streets Printers (Baldock, Herts)

The fascimile reproductions of some of McCance and Widdowson's publications are reproduced by kind permission from the publishers of the *Proceedings of the Royal Society of Medicine*, the *Lancet*, the *British Medical Journal* and *Nutrition Reviews*.

The photographs are from the private collections of Professor McCance, Dr Widdowson and other contributors to this volume. The Editor wishes to record her gratitude to all those who have lent photographs.

Contents

	Page
Acknowledgements	7
Contributors	9
Illustrations	12
Foreword by HRH The Princess Royal	13
Editor's Introduction	15
A 60-year partnership in several locations	17

The autobiographies of McCance and Widdowson	18
Selected publications of McCance and Widdowson	45
Citation facts about McCance and Widdowson publications	53
Twenty questions and their answers from McCance and Widdowson	57
Advice to a young scientist from McCance and Widdowson	63
The scientific achievements of McCance and Widdowson	67

The composition of foods *David Southgate*	69
Mineral metabolism *Douglas Black*	79
Body composition *John Dickerson*	87
The physiology of the newborn *Brian Wharton*	99
Normal and retarded growth *David Lister*	111
Third World nutrition *Roger Whitehead*	121

Day-to-day recollections of life with McCance and Widdowson	133
Monica Verdon-Roe	134
David Whitteridge	136
James Robinson	138
Andrew Huxley	143
Jan Jonxis	146
Barbara Alington	148

Amicia Melland	149
Romaine Hervey	151
Douglas Black	156
Maureen Young	158
Christine Walsham	161
Betty Wilkinson	163
Lois Thrussell	164
Dorothy Rosenbaum	168
Eric Glaser	170
Daphne Learmouth	172
Marion Harrison	174
Terry Cowen	176
Ashton B Morrison	178
John Dickerson	182
Peter John	184
J Russell Elkinton	186
Vernon Pickles	189
Jana Pařísková	191
John Cowley	193
Hamad Elneil	198
Kelvin McCracken	200
Alison Paul	201
Joy Dauncey	203
Michael Gurr	206
Marta Fiorotto	208
Olav Oftedal	209

Selected lectures 213

a) The Practice of Experimental Medicine. *RA McCance* (1950). 215
b) Food, Growth, and Time. *RA McCance* (1962). 221
c) Harmony of Growth. *EM Widdowson* (1970). 237
d) Animals in the Service of Human Nutrition.
   EM Widdowson (1986). 251

Honours 257

Index 259

Acknowledgements

This is a book about science but, even more importantly, it is a book about people. It has always been my intention that it was to be priced so that individuals could afford it, as well as libraries. This would not have been possible without the generous financial assistance provided by the Ministry of Agriculture, Fisheries and Food, the Department of Health, the Medical Research Council and Sidney Sussex College, Cambridge.

I am indebted to many people for their help and encouragement in its writing and publishing. My good friend, Dr Janet Kirtland, helped in the early days when the book was just a 'twinkle' in my eye. Dr David Conning, Director-General of the British Nutrition Foundation (BNF) and the Council of the Foundation then encouraged me to convert the 'twinkle' into a reality.

My wonderful Personal Assistant, Sandra Rodrigues, has been responsible for cheerfully 'processing' every word and other members of the BNF Science Group, namely Liz Heatherington and Hilary Groom, have assisted me with selected aspects of the book. Anne Halliday has helped in no small way by taking responsibility for other projects, allowing me to devote more time to this book.

Much of the book has been researched during weekends and holidays and written in the wee small hours of the morning and I would like to thank my husband, Allan, for his tolerance and understanding when I have had to work unsocial hours. I am also most grateful to my teenage daughters, Alexandra and Lynsey for their interest and for allowing me to use 'their' telephone for business purposes and 'their' bath for relaxation on occasions!

Last, but in no way least, I would like to thank all the contributors to the book; I have enjoyed talking to them, corresponding with them and reliving their memories. I have been very lucky not only to have consolidated some existing friendships but also to have made many new friends through our mutual admiration for two great people—McCance and Widdowson.

Margaret Ashwell
January 1993

The Contributors

Dr Margaret Ashwell
The Old Forge
36 Kingsland Way
Ashwell, Baldock
N Herts SG7 5PZ

Sir Douglas Black
The Old Forge
Duchess Close
Whitchurch-on-Thames
Near Reading
Berks RG8 7EN

Mrs Barbara Cassels
(was Barbara Alington)
Little Stonnards
Wimbish Green
Saffron Walden
Essex CB10 2XJ

Mr Terry Cowen
Whateley Hall Hotel
7 Florence Road
Boscombe
Bournemouth
Dorset SH5 1HH

Professor John Cowley
4 Park Street
Old Hatfield
Herts AL9 5AX

Dr M Joy Dauncey
Department of Molecular
& Cellular Physiology
AFRC Institute of Animal
Physiology & Genetics Research
Babraham, Cambridge CB2 4AT

Professor John Dickerson
Aston, Woodlands Close
Cranleigh
Surrey GU6 7HP

Professor J Russell Elkinton
4 Andover Court
Bedford, Massachusetts
MA 01730
USA

Mrs JS Ellis
(was Monica Verdon-Roe)
3 Otterbourne House Gardens
Otterbourne
Winchester
Hampshire SO21 2ER

Dr Hamad Elneil
21 Fenners Lawn
Gresham Road
Cambridge CB1 2EH

Dr Marta Fiorotto
Children's Nutrition Research
Center
1100 Bates Street
Houston, Texas 77030 2600 USA

Dr Eric Glaser
Bratach Ban
Ballachulish
Argyll PA39 4JX
(sadly, Eric died in
December 1992)

Professor Michael Gurr
Vale View Cottage
Maypole, St Mary's
Isles of Scilly TR21 0NU

Professor Romaine Hervey
Garth House
Beryl Lane, Wells
Somerset BA5 2XQ

Sir Andrew Huxley
Trinity College
Trinity Street
Cambridge CB2 1TQ

Mr Peter John
161 Sturton Street
Cambridge CB1 2QH

Professor Jan Jonxis
Rijksstraatweg 65
9752 AC Haren, Groningen
The Netherlands

Dr David Lister
Meadow Cottage
Fountain Lane, Sidcot,
Winscombe, Avon BS25 1LS

Professor Robert McCance
Shelford Lodge
144 Cambridge Road
Great Shelford
Cambridge CB2 5JU
(sadly, Professor McCance died on 5th March 1993)

Dr Kelvin McCracken
Food & Agricultural
Chemistry Research Division
The Queen's University of
Belfast
Newforge Lane
Belfast BT9 5PX

Professor Ashton B Morrison
Professor of Pathology
UMDNJ/Robert Wood Johnson
Medical School
University of Medicine
and Dentistry of New Jersey
401 Haddon Avenue
Camden, New Jersey 08103-1505
USA

Dr Olav Oftedal
5320 Olney Laytonsville Road
Olney, Maryland 20832 USA

Dr Jana Pařízková
Biomedicinské Centrum
Fakulta Tělesné Vychovy a
Sportu (FTVS)
University Karlovy
J Martiho 31
162 52 Praha 6
Czech Republic

Miss Alison Paul
MRC Dunn Nutrition Centre
Downhams Lane
Milton Road
Cambridge CB4 1XJ

Dr Vernon Pickles
65 Yarnells Hill
Oxford OX2 9BE

Professor James Robinson
42 Prestwick Street
Maori Hill
Dunedin
New Zealand

Professor Marion Robinson
(was Marion Harrison)
42 Prestwick Street
Maori Hill, Dunedin
New Zealand

Dr Dorothy Rosenbaum
Erichstrasse 2
5600 Wuppertal 2
Germany

Professor David Southgate
8 Penryn Close
Norwich NR4 7LY

Mrs Christine Spray
(was Christine Walsham)
Windhover
Manton Down lane
Marlborough
Wilts SN8 1RP

Mrs Lois Strangeways
(was Lois Thrussell)
59 Rock Road
Cambridge CB1 4UG

Mrs Daphne Tabor (was Daphne Learmouth and McDermott)
5 Kestrel Close
Beacon Hill
Burnham Market
Kings Lynn
Norfolk PE31 8EF

Dr Elizabeth Tayler
(was Betty Wilkinson)
Merlebanks
Church Hill
Merstham
Surrey RH1 3BJ

Dr Brian Wharton
Old Rectory
Belbroughton
Worcs DY9 9TF

Dr Roger Whitehead
MRC Dunn Nutrition Centre
Downhams Lane
Milton Road
Cambridge CB4 1XJ

Professor David Whitteridge
Winterslow
Boars Hill
Oxford OX1 5DZ

Dr Elsie Widdowson
Orchard House
9 Boot Lane
Barrington
Cambridge CB2 5RA

Dr Amicia Young
(was Amicia Melland)
21 Southwood Court
Bigwood Road
London NW11 6SR

Professor Maureen Young
4 Preston Close
Millers Road
Toft
Cambridgeshire
CB3 7RU

Illustrations

I	Professor McCance and Dr Widdowson—a 60-year partnership.
II	King's College Hospital, London, 1934 to 1938.
III	The English Lake District, January 1940—the testing ground for physical fitness during the Experimental Study of Rationing.
IV	The bread experiments, Cambridge 1938 to 1945.
V (and front cover)	Professor McCance and Dr Widdowson in the English Lake District, January 1940.
VI	The Food Tables (British and American).
VII	The Food Tables (British and Japanese).
VIII	Studies in Germany, 1946 to 1949.
IX	Staff of the Department of Experimental Medicine, 1966.
X	People and places, 1949 to 1966.
XI	Activities in the Department of Experimental Medicine, Cambridge 1957.
XII	People and places, 1966 to 1973.
XIII	Awards and Honours, 1973 to 1993.
XIV	Awards and Honours, 1973 to 1993.
XV	A 60-year partnership in several locations.
XVI	Research for this commemorative volume, 1990 to 1993.

Foreword by HRH The Princess Royal

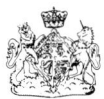

BUCKINGHAM PALACE

Professor McCance and Dr Widdowson first met in 1933. Since then they have become household names, not only for students of medicine, physiology and nutrition, but for anyone with a professional interest in food and the human diet. Sixty years later their collaborative partnership continues to thrive – no longer at a laboratory bench, but very much so in terms of intellectual discussion and their lively interest in topical nutritional matters.

McCance and Widdowson have given their names over many years to successive editions of what is acknowledged as a standard international work of reference on the composition of foods and they have contributed greatly to our understanding of mineral metabolism, body composition, neonatal physiology, determinants of growth and Third World nutrition. Their unique contribution to science will be remembered and perpetuated by the results of their work for many years to come. It is wholly appropriate therefore that their colleagues from all over the world should have collaborated to produce this commemorative volume as a tribute to mark the Sixtieth Anniversary of this remarkable partnership.

Readers will find a rich and rewarding feast of recollections concerning the work of two dedicated pioneers in a field of scientific research where great progress has been made, but much still remains to be done. Those seeking inspiration will draw strength and encouragement from this record of McCance and Widdowson's outstanding achievements.

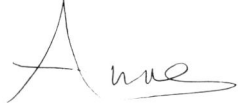

Editor's Introduction

'Walk up Sussex Street until you come to an aneurysm in the road. The door to my flat is on your right hand side.' Thus was I directed to Professor RA McCance's flat belonging to Sidney Sussex College, Cambridge in 1970—the first and last time I have ever had to consult a medical dictionary as well as a road map to find my way!

After that, I met both Professor McCance and Dr Widdowson several times, but it was not until the mid-1980s that I began to take a particular interest in the story behind their remarkable scientific achievements. I was working at the Dunn Nutrition Centre in Cambridge. Guinea pigs were my experimental model because Dr Widdowson had emphasised, on many occasions, that they could be likened to the human baby in that the fat content of the two species at birth was roughly similar. What I hadn't realised was that my friendly animal technician, Terry Cowen, had been one of the animal technicians trained and cherished by McCance and Widdowson. Terry and I would sit for hours taking measurements at ten-minute intervals. Now ten minutes is an awkward time—it's too short to go off to do anything else and it's too long to remain silent. So that is how Terry and I got talking about his many years as part of the Department, and it was Terry who first told me some of the remarkable stories that are related on these pages.

I was fascinated, but did not take things any further. However, on joining the British Nutrition Foundation in 1988, my meetings with Dr Widdowson became more frequent. She has been an extremely diligent President of the Foundation since 1986 and attends all our meetings. Gradually the idea began to form in my mind—everyone knows the *Food Tables* as 'McCance and Widdowson'—so why not write a book about McCance and Widdowson?

I approached Dr Widdowson with a certain amount of trepidation; I felt that I might be yet another in a long line of people who had asked the same question. 'Has anyone ever approached you and the Professor to write a book about your work together?' 'Oh no', she said, 'Whoever would want to read a book about us?'

Once they had both agreed, they put together what they called their 'Christmas card list'. This consisted of the names and addresses of all the people who had worked in the Department of Experimental Medicine with whom they were still in touch. I was amazed how many

INTRODUCTION

of these people I already knew. Anyone who was anyone in nutrition seemed to be a 'graduate' of the McCance and Widdowson school! I vowed I would try to visit and talk to as many as I could, rather than rely on their written recollections and I'm pleased that this has been possible in most cases.

Gradually, I was able to piece together some of the stories to get a flavour of life with McCance and Widdowson. I still had the problem of *how* to write what I originally saw as a biography. How could I possibly write anything that could compete with their own inimitable style of writing? When two people pay special attention to detail and to writing style, a biographer has a tough time.

I expressed my despondency to Alison Paul who showed me the book about Sir Frederick Gowland Hopkins that was published as a tribute to him after he retired as Professor of Biochemistry at Cambridge University. Eureka! I would gather together material for a commemorative volume rather than attempt a biography. In this way, you can enjoy reading about McCance and Widdowson in their own words and the words of others who have known them.

It seems somewhat ridiculous for an Editor of a tribute such as this to say that the book could not have been written without the two main subjects—but the tremendously active participation of both Dr Widdowson and Professor McCance must be acknowledged. Not only have they pointed me in the right direction—the right people to see and the right scientific publications to read—but they have insisted, in their usual manner, on total accuracy throughout and have read and checked every word.

During the last few years, I have come to know Professor McCance, and Dr Widdowson in particular, very well. I have witnessed, first-hand, some of the characteristics that are described so well by other contributors. The one which will remain in my memory above all others is their complete mastery of the understatement. Dr Widdowson asked me to accompany her to Washington DC when she was given the Edna and Robert Langholz Prize International Nutrition Award in October 1992. Mr Langholz read out her long list of achievements but Dr Widdowson's immediate response was to tell an incredulous audience to take all that he had said 'with a pinch of salt'!

I have thoroughly enjoyed researching and editing this book. Once I told Professor McCance that I felt deeply honoured to have been trusted to do it. 'Well', he said, 'You must be very easily honoured!' Somehow, I don't think I am.

Margaret Ashwell
January 1993

A sixty year partnership in several locations

	McCANCE	McCANCE and WIDDOWSON	WIDDOWSON	
1933		Biochemical Department, King's College Hospital, London		*1933*
1938				1938
		Department of Medicine, University of Cambridge (Housed in Pathology Building)		
1946	Wuppertal, Germany		Wuppertal, Germany	1946
1949		Department of Experimental Medicine, University of Cambridge		1949
1955				1955
1958		Peterhouse Huts, Tennis Court Road, Cambridge / 5 Shaftesbury Road, Cambridge		1958
	Infantile Malnutrition Research Unit, Kampala, Uganda			
1966				1966
1968			Infant Nutrition Research Division (Dunn Nutrition Unit)	1968
1973				1973
	Active Retirement in Cambridge	Continual Collaboration	Department of Investigative Medicine, Addenbrooke's Hospital, Cambridge	
1988				1988
			Active Retirement, Barrington, Cambridgeshire	
1993				*1993*

AUTOBIOGRAPHIES

The autobiographies of McCance and Widdowson

Professor McCance and Dr Widdowson have already published several short autobiographies and I have drawn on these to put together two longer ones, giving the reader a clear idea of the work that they have done together in approximately chronological order. So much of the work has been done jointly that I had some difficulty in deciding in which autobiography the details should be described. I have however been guided by the demarcations that Professor McCance and Dr Widdowson themselves have used.

I am exceedingly grateful to CAB International, The Nutrition Society and to Sidney Sussex College for giving me permission to reproduce extracts from these articles:

The Nutrition Society 1941-1991. Presidents and Honorary Members: Their stories and recollections. Compiled by Elsie M Widdowson. CAB International, Wallingford, Oxon. 1991; 79-86 and 111-118.

Adventures in nutrition over half a century. Elsie M Widdowson. Proc Nutr Soc 1980; 39:293-306.

Reminiscences. RA McCance. Sidney Sussex College, Cambridge 1987.

MA

Reference numbers in these autobiographies refer to the selected publications of McCance and Widdowson which are to be found on pages 45 to 52.

Professor RA McCance

I was born in the north of Ireland in 1898 in what was then real country north west of Belfast. I went to school at St Bees, Cumbria, as my two brothers had done. I then joined the RNAS (Royal Naval Air Service) and served as a pilot in the latter part of the 1914-1918 war. I had been trained to fly 'Camels', which were single-seater fighter machines, but found myself flying two-seater 'observation' aircraft off one of the midship turrets of the *Indomitable,* one of the second Battle Cruiser squadron of the Grand Fleet.

After the war I thought of going into the Department of Agriculture in Ireland. On the advice of those in charge of it I went up to Cambridge, intending to take a Diploma in Agriculture. So 1919 found me working at the County Farm near Antrim for six months, a valuable experience which has stood me in good stead ever since. I went up to Sidney Sussex College, Cambridge, in October. There I took both parts of the Natural Sciences Tripos instead of the Diploma in Agriculture because, during those three years, there had been a 'rebellion' in Ireland, and no one could offer me anything with any certainty.

Towards the end of this time I was appointed supervisor in physiology at several colleges in Cambridge, and the money I earned enabled me to marry Mary Lindsay MacGregor in 1922. I worked under Professor FG Hopkins for three years, where I learned something about Biochemistry and what research it might involve. I obtained my PhD on the strength of the work I had done.

I went to King's College Hospital, London, in 1926 to complete my qualifications in Medicine. I had a grant of £30 per annum to assist Dr RD Lawrence (RDL) in the Biochemical and Diabetic Department. I worked there in my spare time and made some analyses for RDL on the carbohydrate content of cooked fruit and vegetables, a matter of great importance to diabetics in those days. I introduced a new dimension to this work by separating the available carbohydrates, sugars, dextrins and starch from the polysaccharides that are always present in vegetables and fruits, and which are now known as dietary fibre. The results of the work were published as a Medical Research Council Special Report (1). This Report contained not only values for the available carbohydrates in fruit and vegetables but also a long review on the food value of vegetable carbohydrates, available and unavailable.

Professor Cathcart of Glasgow looked with favour on these efforts of mine to study the composition of cooked foods. He was studying the foods eaten by the poor, and wanted information about the composition of cooked foods, particularly meat and fish; he suggested that I should undertake this work and apply to the Medical Research Council for a grant to cover the cost of an assistant and a technician. So HL Shipp joined me at King's College Hospital in 1930 and a detailed study of the composition of meat and fish began. The results of this study were published in 1933 (4).

I used to go to the hospital kitchen in the basement to get the big joints cooked in the hospital ovens. There I encountered Elsie Widdowson, a momentous meeting, for we have now remained together for 60 years.

A highly productive period followed. Diabetics, and particularly those in coma, provided me with many problems, one being that their urine contained no chloride (7). This observation led on to my experimental and quantitative study on salt deficiency in man, which involved making a number of subjects, male and female, salt deficient. This was really rather a herculean task, for it involved persuading healthy young men and women to eat a salt-free diet and to lie and sweat in a hot-air bath for two hours a day for 14 days.

The subjects lay on a macintosh sheet inside the warmed-up apparatus for two hours every afternoon, keeping their temperatures between 100° and 101°F. The amount of salt they lost was measured by washing them down, and the macintosh sheet as well of course, with a jet of distilled water after each session, and analysing the washings; their water loss was measured by their loss of weight. Then, when they were salt-deficient, they had to submit to a variety of tests, in particular of their renal function (10).

Dr Widdowson was roped in to help with these experiments and they added considerable light relief to the food analysis and dietary calculations. This work gave us an insight into experiments on man, not only their interest and importance, but also their potential danger; on two occasions we had very alarming experiences but, fortunately, not utter disaster.

The first occasion was when I wondered whether I could take the salt experiment a step further and, by overbreathing, produce urine that was without sodium. This was a technique I had learned from JBS Haldane. I sat in a chair and leaned over a sink with the hot water tap running to keep my throat moist. Then I breathed in and out as deeply and as rapidly as I could for 45 minutes until the relative lack of carbon dioxide in my body made my blood more alkaline than normal.

As a safety precaution, Elsie stood by while I was overbreathing, but when I had finished and was sitting comfortably in a chair, she went out for a moment. Suddenly, something went wrong. My body had become so alkaline from the loss of the carbon dioxide that no signal was being sent to the respiratory centre in my brain to stimulate breathing. When Elsie returned, she found me blue because I had just passed out. She ran for expert help and when she got back, I was just recovering. The first thing I said apparently was 'Give me my bottle', so that I could donate a sample of urine (15).

I had been unconscious for several minutes and remained weak for several hours thereafter. I was lucky because I could have suffered permanent damage to my brain or other organs.

These experiments helped doctors appreciate the important role of fluids and sodium. Today, maintaining fluid and chemical balance is a standard part of the treatment of patients with diabetic coma, kidney disorders and heart attacks, and of those who experience episodes of severe vomiting and fever, as well as the treatment of patients after surgery.

Somewhere about 1934, I was allowed some beds for my patients in King's College Hospital and began admitting those referred to me who presented problems. One in particular I remember with polycythemia rubra vera. This lady, although she never knew it, played a large part in the future of three members of the Department. I treated her with acetyl phenylhydrazine, and by so doing broke down enough red cells to liberate 5g of iron in her body. To our intense surprise none of it was excreted, in spite of all I had been taught (12). We then injected iron intravenously into ourselves and colleagues, and we did not excrete the iron either (18). This led us to suggest that the amount of iron in the body must be regulated, not by excretion, but by controlled absorption (14).

The publication of this led to an invitation from Professor JA Ryle, Regius Professor of Physic, to come to Cambridge as Reader in Medicine, with a Fellowship in my old College. I accepted and the Medical Research Council agreed to my taking Elsie and our technician, Alec Haynes, with me, so our joint work was little interrupted.

Some time before this, however, my house physician at King's College Hospital, Winifred Young, who was there while the salt-deficiency experiments were going on, had gone to the Children's Hospital in Birmingham under Sir Leonard Parsons. One of her jobs was to test the babies' urine for albumen and sugar. Partly from habit, she tested some for chlorides and to her surprise found they contained none. This led to many investigations on renal function in infancy and indeed to interest in infant physiology as a whole.

The renal function of full-term infants, and even more so of premature infants, was immature compared with that of adults, whether the basis of comparison was surface area or body-weight (22,23,56). Infants had hypotonic urines, low urea clearances and glomerular filtration rates and low excretion of sodium and chloride (35,50). Newborn rats, kittens, puppies and pigs were used for subsequent investigations, and the story was always the same. The renal function of the newborn appeared to be very inefficient compared with that of the adult (57,58,63,64,79).

It puzzled us that, in spite of the failure of the newborn to excrete nitrogen and electrolytes like an adult, the serum chemistry remained normal. It became clearer and clearer as time went on that growth was by far the most important influence in maintaining a normal internal environment. Inefficient though the kidneys were by adult standards, they were quite capable of maintaining homeostasis, provided the infants and animals were growing while being fed on food of exactly the right composition—that is the milk of the mother. Newborn rabbits, puppies and pigs for example retain 90% of the nitrogen in their food for purposes of growth, so the kidneys are never required to excrete an amount of nitrogen equivalent to more than 10% of the intake, and this they are perfectly capable of doing (64,65,76,81).

As soon as we realised the importance of growth, rather than the kidneys, in maintaining a stable volume and composition of the body fluids, everything fell into place.

We had a slight accident during our first year in Cambridge when we were studying the absorption and excretion of strontium, one of the so-called 'trace elements', chemicals that exist in minute amounts in the body. It resembles calcium, but while a considerable amount was known about calcium's role in the body, very little was known about the role of strontium. The element had been used medicinally for a long time for a variety of disorders, but although an understanding of how it is excreted is fundamental to its proper use in medicine, few studies had been made. We designed an experiment to determine how the element was excreted from the body. We would inject strontium into each other's veins each day for a week and then measure the amount in our stools and urine. Again we encountered the kind of unpredictable accident that can occur in any human experiment.

We started on a Monday with my injecting strontium lactate into a vein in Elsie's arm. Nothing happened after 24 hours, so we decided to double the dose to 47 milligrams. On Tuesday, I took my first dose. For the next five days, we carried out our scheme without problems. But by Friday, we had used up the entire original batch and had to sterilise some more strontium lactate from the original solution.

At eleven on Saturday morning, the sixth day of the experiment, we injected the prescribed dose into each other's arms. We had become overconfident, one of the biggest hazards of self-experimentation. During the week, someone had always stood by, but because nothing had happened, we carried out this extension of the experiment alone. Less than an hour later we began to feel ill. We suffered intense headaches and teeth-chattering rigours. Our backs and thighs hurt. We felt dreadful and did not know what had gone wrong, and were apprehensive.

Fortunately, someone came by and called John Ryle, the Regius Professor, who rushed to the laboratory. After realising that our lives were not in immediate danger, Ryle took us home with him, where he and his wife could look after us. By this time about four hours had passed, and both of us had developed fevers of about 102°F. Despite feeling ill, we still managed to collect the samples we needed. Later analysis showed that substances known as pyrogens, also called endotoxins, due to bacterial contamination, were present in the second batch of strontium. We had suffered a pyrogen reaction, which occurred much more commonly then than now, because purification techniques were cruder.

We recovered quickly, but gave ourselves no further injections of strontium. The results of this experiment showed that the body rids itself of strontium slowly and that about 90% of the excretion is through the kidney—not the bowel (20).

As soon as the Second World War began, Elsie and I started an 'experimental study of rationing' to see how far food produced in Britain could meet the needs of the population and enable them to fare well, and hence how much shipping could be saved. This was fun, and indeed all our work in the first years of the war was made interesting because the subjects of our experiments were such stimulating people: Colin Bertram, a zoologist who had worked in the Antarctic, and his wife Kate, also a zoologist, Douglas Black and Andrew Huxley, both later knighted and one of them a Nobel prize winner, and last but by no means least, Jimmy Robinson. He met his wife Marion in our Department and both later became Professors in Dunedin, New Zealand.

In our experimental study of rationing our allowances of milk, meat, eggs and other good things were so small that they were considered intolerable by our critics; we had wholemeal flour for bread and cooking purposes, and this was unrationed, as were potatoes. Our total allowances per person per week were four ounces of fat, five ounces of sugar, including sugar in jam and marmalade, one egg, four ounces of cheese and sixteen ounces of meat and fish combined. Six ounces of home-grown fruit a week was allowed, but wholemeal bread and vegetables, including potatoes, were unrationed. The milk ration, our main source of calcium, was 35 fluid ounces a week, or a quarter of a pint a day. We realised that even with four ounces of cheese a week, our calcium intakes were likely to be very low, so we took the precaution of adding chalk to the flour used for the bread in these and subsequent experiments.

After three months we felt so strong that we decided to go the Lake District to test our physical fitness. Just after Christmas, Jimmy Robinson and I started by cycling to Langdale against a northerly wind. We got there in two and a half days, the latter half of the distance over snowy roads. The rest of the party (Elsie Widdowson, Andrew Huxley and my son Colin) came up by car, bringing a lot of food, including the flour, with them. We got the bread baked locally. We made many expeditions. Andrew Huxley and I ascended Bow Fell by 'The Band' from the gate of Stool End Farm in 53 and 51 minutes respectively, and on another day climbed Coniston Old Man from the church in 81 minutes, with Andrew carrying 42lb of bricks in a rucksack and myself carrying 100 ft of rope, an ice axe etc. Conditions were good except for a little frozen snow. On another day Andrew Huxley and I set out at 6am from the cottage in Great Langdale where we were staying, carrying loads of 8.5lb each, crossed into Borrowdale by Stake Pass, and then over the Honister, Scarth Gap and Black Sail Passes to Wasdale Head by 11.45am. After a pause of 35 minutes we went over Eskdale Fell to Boot, where we stopped for ten minutes to telephone. We returned over Hardknott and Wrynose Passes, by Elterwater, to reach our base in Langdale at 5.45pm. There was some snow and ice on all the passes and we covered the distance of 36 miles and 7000 feet of climbing at an average speed of 3.2 miles per hour, including stops.

These were not records, but they were enough to show that we were fit, and that our rations had served us well (29).

After we had finished our experimental study of rationing we had come to the conclusion that the population of Great Britain would not get as much calcium as they needed if milk and cheese were to be severely rationed and people had to give up their beloved white bread and take to bread of higher extraction. We believed the wholemeal breads interfered to some extent with the absorption of calcium.

We decided to put this to the test and this led to a long series of balance experiments. In these we set out to measure all the calcium and other minerals that went into and came out of the body. For this sort of work great accuracy was needed because we were measuring a small difference (absorption) between two large numbers (intake and faecal excretion). Everything that one ate had to be weighed and measured separately and an exactly similar but smaller portion set aside for analysis and all excreta had to be collected. Sounds easy; but it was not, for if one wanted any lunch while one was at a meeting in London, this meant sandwiches prepared beforehand and duplicates taken for analysis; if one wanted anything to wash it down it meant having a bottle of distilled water or other liquid as well.

This was not the end, however, for one needed to take a bottle for urine if one was a man and a filter funnel as well if one was a woman. For anyone with regular habits staying a night away meant a bowl with a cover of some sort and there were no plastic wrappings in 1940!

With the financial support of the Medical Research Council ten of us took part in the experiment. Each experimental period lasted three or four weeks and the whole study with the ancillary experiments lasted nine months. In each experiment, 40 to 50% of the energy was provided by the flour under study at the time. The main conclusions were that there was something in brown i.e. high extraction flours which interfered with calcium absorption by the gut. This was not due to the laxative properties, although these were considerable, but to a phosphorus compound, phytic acid. Vitamin D did not improve the absorption, but fortifying the flour with calcium carbonate or phosphate did.

We recommended therefore that to every 100g of 69% extraction white flour, 65mg of calcium should be added; to every 100g of National, 85% wheatmeal flour 120mg calcium; to 100g of wholemeal flour of 92% extraction, 200mg of calcium (24).

On the basis of these experiments calcium was by law added to the 85% flour used for making bread at the time, but wholemeal, which most needed the calcium to ensure that we absorbed enough for our needs, was not fortified. This was in deference to the pure food enthusiasts. No sooner was the proposal made to add calcium that it was bitterly opposed. It was said to be causing stones in the kidneys and hardening of the arteries even before it had been added. A man called Isaac Harris, who wrote a booklet called 'The Calcium Bread Scandal', was particularly vociferous. However, the fortification became statutory and the fuss over it died down. When eventually in the early 1950s the loaf made from white flour came into being again, it was decided to continue to fortify it with calcium carbonate. Ever since, when the flour and bread regulations have come up for review, it has been decided to continue the fortification. Even as late as 1974, this was again the recommendation, but it was made in a rather less positive way, '…we therefore, do not recommend that chalk be no longer added to flour'. So, in accordance with the double negative, we still have calcium carbonate added to our flour, although all the reasons for adding it in the first place have gone and supplies of milk and cheese are unlimited.

As the War drew to a close we persuaded Sir Edward Mellanby (Secretary of the Medical Research Council) to sponsor a visit to Germany to see what effect the war and the rationing and shortages of food had had on the civilian population. Accordingly, in the spring of 1946 Elsie and I set out to see whether we could find somewhere we might set up a base for studies we wished to make. We visited Hannover, Hamburg, Kiel, Göttingen, Essen and Wuppertal. Only in the last place did we find a satisfactory hospital in which to work and a good laboratory (the I G Farben). Best of all we found a doctor, Dorothy Rosenbaum, who spoke both German and English, and who was anxious to help us.

Although we surmised that undernutrition must alter the composition of the 'lean body mass' we were anxious to find out why some people got oedema when they were undernourished and some did not (41). We wanted, therefore, to take samples of blood and compare the concentration of albumen in it in men with oedema and those without.

When we visited the gaol at Kiel we asked for three subjects with oedema and three without to be shown to us. The warders, feeling perhaps that they were a little unsure what oedema looked like, and that we had better be left to make our own selection, lined up eight men completely naked in front of us, thus leaving us to make our own decision as to which of them had or had not got oedema.

The policy we adopted at our base was to invite people experienced in the new subjects, which none of us felt competent to cover ourselves, to come and join the team. Sheila Sherlock examined the livers and Sheila Howarth the hearts; Philip Gell came to see if anything was wrong with the immune response. This put rather a strain on our admirable research nurse, Lois Thrussell, and indeed on myself too, because it was all very well to catheterize people with heart disease and puncture those with faulty livers, but normal people had to be examined to establish a base line. Tact was almost as necessary as catheters and puncturing needles, and we owe a great debt of gratitude to Dorothy Rosenbaum for all she did to help to overcome the problems.

Other 'working' visitors were Derek Russell Davis who looked sympathetically into patients' anxiety neuroses, and Mavis Gunther who studied breast milk production and tried to improve it. Dr Berridge—now alas dead—put all his radiological skill at our disposal. Patients' bones were X-rayed and also their gastrointestinal tracts. He found, for example, that wholemeal bread passed through more rapidly than white. I was one of the well-nourished controls, and Berridge found that my appendix had a lot of calcified lumps in it. This explains the grumbling appendicitis I had as a child reared on unpasteurized milk from a very few cows.

We had some distinguished visitors. Sir Edward and Lady Mellanby, Dame Harriette Chick and Dr Hume, and one I shall never forget was Sir James Spence. When he left we all went along in two cars to see him off at Köln station, only to find that the time had been advanced one hour, which none of us had remembered, and the train had left. The only thing to do was to beat the train to the Dutch frontier where we knew it would make a long stop for 'customs'. When we got to the frontier we were relieved to see that the train was still there!

Meanwhile I was getting involved in work on naval matters. During the War, I had been made Chairman of a joint Medical Research Council and Royal Naval Committee on Survival at Sea. Our work involved the problem of whether one should ever drink sea water when dehydrated after shipwreck. The answer was, one should not (28, 61)

Much of this work would have been impossible had it not been for two Cambridge graduates in physiology, Romaine Hervey and Bill Keatinge. Both joined the Navy for their National Service and were seconded to work on these problems in our Department. We made a useful discovery in this work by showing that 100g of glucose or cane sugar—or for that matter boiled sweets—were metabolised to 100g of water, all much easier than water to fit into a survivor's ration.

When Eric Glaser joined the Department, he pioneered some work of a different kind. One of his exploits was to plunge with two friends into the swimming pool in the Emmanuel College garden in the middle of winter to study the effects of sudden immersion in cold water. All three subjects were gasping for breath inside half a minute of entering the water and two of them had to leave the water within this time because they were too breathless to swim. The third, who was a much better swimmer than the first two, gradually got less breathless and was then able to go on swimming for nine minutes. The skin of all three was painful while they were in the water and became bright red when they left it. Eric Glaser also swam for half a minute at Tromsö when the water temperature was 3°C.

Bill Keatinge took this up in a much more scientific way and extended his observations to other aspects of the subject. He started by getting a tank with the following dimensions and fittings made for his experimental work on cold. The tank was 8 feet long, 4 feet wide and 4 feet deep. It was insulated with a layer of cork on the outside and the temperature of the water could be controlled closely between 0.5°C and 35°C. It was fitted with a good mechanical stirrer and a device for taking exercise.

Keatinge's tests were mostly made on 12 naval volunteers, but to a limited extent on himself and University personnel. The investigation was made difficult by the fact that there were considerable, but consistent, differences between individuals, and this has been confirmed by others. However, certain facts stood out. The first was, as might have been expected, that in cold water fat men maintained their body temperature better than thin ones. This was amply confirmed by two studies of Channel swimmers, but there were great individual differences and some men, even thin ones, have undoubtedly got much greater ability to live through long periods of immersion in cold water than others, and survive with their faculties intact.

When Bill Keatinge departed to the London Hospital, his tank was a little too big to be put into a dark cupboard. No one seemed to want this treasure, even as a present, till one day Elsie's sister, Eva, put in a bid for it. She had a cottage on the Dingle Peninsula in the South West of Ireland which had no piped water supply, in fact no water supply at all except for the rain which was plentiful and only needed a tank 8ft long, 4ft wide and 4ft deep to hold enough of it to do the family's washing—and there Bill Keatinge's tank is doing as good service as ever, even if not such a scientific one.

An important part of our task was to study the habitability and the boarding facilities of the new inflatable life rafts. Romaine Hervey played a very important part in this work. There were numerous trials at Portsmouth. Volunteers, some Wrens among them, jumped into the water from a height of 10-20ft and boarded the rafts waiting for them not far away. The habitability of rafts was tried out in the cold of Tromsö in January and later in the heat of Singapore. Motion sickness was a very real problem for soldiers in landing craft and in this Eric Glaser was at his best. We used the artificial waves in swimming baths for our trials and finally the naval ship tank. This always impressed me, for it was so long it had to conform to the curvature of the earth's surface. The only effective drug against sea sickness was 1. hyoscine, and in very small doses too.

We ended up with some Atlantic trials conducted from a small destroyer, the Carron. Our time was limited and the sea very rough. We took a battering on the way to our appointed spot. During the morning the weather eased a little and the rafts were prepared for launching. The Royal Navy raft, looked after by Surgeon Captain Baskerville, behaved splendidly, although we could only see it now and again when it was on the right side of the really monstrous waves.

The crew were re-embarked with the aid of helicopter straps. Glaser now set off in a round raft produced commercially, with a crew of volunteers. Within minutes all were sick and one would have been overboard had not Eric Glaser grasped him by the leg. Things began to get dangerous and flares were sent off. The *Carron* came alongside and the volunteers were all safely transferred to her.

As a follow-up to our work on undernutrition in Germany, we made comparable experiments on animals. My responsibility was the pigs. 'Large White' pigs grow very fast and should reach a weight of 250kg or more in the course of a year. They can, however, be made so severely undernourished that at the end of the year they weigh only 5-5.5kg (70). They grow well if rehabilitated, and become pregnant if they are served, and make good mothers, but they never attain the size of a pig that has not been held back by undernutrition. Elsie had the bright idea of keeping these pigs undernourished for longer periods, say for two or three years. At the end they will show a burst of growth if they are rehabilitated. The extent of this growth is more limited, however, the longer the period of undernutrition has been (91).

When we were in Germany, milk and even dried milk was in short supply. Rex Dean worked for some time on a soya bean preparation for rehabilitating undernourished infants. After we had returned to Cambridge, Sir Harold Himsworth suggested to Dean that he should go to Uganda to investigate the use of this preparation for malnourished children. A Unit was eventually established in Kampala, near Mulago Hospital, destined to become the medical and surgical centre for East Africa.

While working there Dean fell victim to a slowly ascending paralysis of his feet and legs which crippled him, but with great fortitude he struggled on till he was on the point of death and had to be invalided home. Roger Whitehead, who had joined Dean some years earlier, looked after the Unit for a time. When I retired from Cambridge in 1966, my wife had recently died and when Sir Harold asked me if I would look after the Unit for a year or so till a suitable young medically qualified doctor could be found to replace Dean, I was glad to go, recruited some staff and set out in 1966.

I soon found that the wards, even in Mulago Hospital, and more especially in the small ward we had in the Unit, were different from anything I had seen before. I did not expect to find the mothers lying about on the floor, for instance, and most of the children suffering from worms or horrid superficial ulcers on their hips and buttocks, sometimes with dangerous diphtheroid micro-organisms in them.

I was lucky in my staff, for Brian Wharton made some really first class observations, among others that the children were suffering from hypothermia during the night. Tom Hall, the son of our clergyman at Woodbourne near Belfast where I had spent my childhood, was one of the staff I had recruited. He had been a public health officer all his active life, and I had met him in Gibraltar during the war. He was my ally in retirement, as he had been as a boy.

For anyone like myself Kampala was a lovely place in which to live in the 1960s. The villages were a mass of bougainvillaeas, a tree in the garden grew avocado pears, and the geckos ran upside-down on the ceilings, not to speak of the bird life of which I identified about 200 different species. The game parks and reserves were rather fun, especially for visitors. If one rose early and went for a walk, one might always find an elephant taking the lid off one's dustbin to see what he could find in it to eat. A colleague, Keith McCullagh, was working on elephants, and I had the interesting experience of an aeroplane trip with him, flying low over a large area including the Murchison Falls, to locate a herd of elephants. Two men were with us who had been assigned the job of culling a large part of the elephant population because they were breaking into the Budongo forest and destroying all the young mahogany trees.

In 1968 I retired to Cambridge, and a few years later was knocked off my bicycle, on which I had cycled well over 200,000 miles, by a pedestrian on Midsummer Common. This fractured my femur, and after a few more minor mishaps, I fell down the stairs in my residence in Sussex Street and fractured my pelvis, which was very painful. I don't advise this accident, but it led to my finding a less risky home for myself.

January 1993

I am now in my nineties, and not able to be as active as I once was. However, I am able to think about times past and my friends and colleagues of long ago. Recently, I have been thinking particularly about several who came to my Department and whose investigations 30 or 40 years ago set the stage for their later research. Romaine Hervey came to us in 1942. He showed conclusively that shipwrecked persons who managed to scramble aboard lifeboats or rafts, and who had little or no fresh water, were better off if they drank nothing then if they drank sea water. After his naval service ended, Romaine stayed with us and embarked on a completely different investigation for his PhD on the effects that lesions of the hypothalamus of one of a pair of parabiotic rats had on the appetite and deposition of fat in the other. This aroused his interest in obesity, its causes and effects and led to his many later investigations

I have already described in some detail Bill Keatinge's contribution to all the work on survival at sea that were made in the 1950s. He later followed this up with studies on the maintenance of body temperature in long-distance swimmers, and survivors after shipwreck.

Archie Morrison was a pathologist, and his investigations on the renal function of partially nephrectomised rats made him realise what a useful model this was for studies on chronic renal disease in man. When he moved to the United States of America, he continued to use these operated rats for this purpose.

Three of the contributors to this book, John Dickerson, David Southgate and David Lister, describe how their later work on body composition, food composition and normal and retarded growth stemmed from their early investigations in our Department. There were many others, and it gives me great pleasure to think of the times I spent with each of them, discussing their problems and sharing in their discoveries. May they long continue.

Dr Elsie Widdowson

My schooldays were spent in South East London. I lived in Dulwich with my parents and sister and cycled each day to school in Sydenham. Zoology was my favourite subject in the sixth form, and I had the idea of taking it for a degree. However, we had a very good chemistry mistress, and she persuaded me to take chemistry instead. The tradition at the school was for the girls to go to one of the London colleges for women, usually Bedford College. Encouraged by three girls who were a year ahead of me, and who went to Imperial College, I decided to do the same. This was a man's world with three women in our year of about 100. I took the BSc examination after two years, but had to spend another year at the College before the degree was awarded. I spent this time in the small Biochemistry laboratory presided over by Professor SJ Schryver—Sammy Schryver as he was generally known.

Everybody in the laboratory was separating amino acids from various plant and animal materials. This was long before the days of chromatography, and we all worked on a vast scale, starting with bucketsful of material rather than beakers. We extracted the proteins from our various materials and converted them to amino acids, which we then precipitated as their copper salts. We made use of the fact that the copper salts have different solubilities in various solvents to separate them. Great was the excitement when, in 1928, one of the people in the laboratory, Bernard Town, discovered a hitherto unknown amino acid, which we now know as proline. I made no such discoveries.

Towards the end of the year an emissary from the Department of Plant Physiology, across the quadrangle from the Biochemistry laboratory, came over to find me. Rumour had reached them that I might be looking for a job. A grant was available in the Department, and if I was interested, would I go for an interview. I was interested, I went, and the result was that I worked there for over three years with Helen Archbold (later Helen Porter FRS) who was in charge of a long series of experiments for the Department of Scientific and Industrial Research on the chemistry and physiology of apples.

My part in the investigations was to separate and measure the changes in the individual carbohydrates in the fruit from the time it first set on the tree until it ripened, and then during storage. It was my responsibility to go by train every two weeks to Swanley in Kent, then walk about a mile to an orchard to pick fruit from specified Worcester Pearmain and Bramley's Seedling apple trees and bring them back to the laboratory for the various studies that were being made. I thoroughly enjoyed those outings, especially on lovely summer days. I developed a method for separating and measuring the starch, hemicelluloses, sucrose, fructose and glucose in the fruit, and the first paper I ever published on the determination of reducing sugars in the apple appeared in the *Biochemical Journal* in 1931 (2). I little realised how momentous this was going to be for the whole of my scientific life.

All this time I worked under the guidance of Helen Archbold, who was always available to help and advise me, and she initiated me into the art of writing up the results for publication (3). I owe a great deal to her, and she undoubtedly gave me my life-long love of research. I was able to use my work for a PhD.

At the end of the three and a half years the grant ran out and in any case, much as I enjoyed my time with the apples, I did not want to devote my life to plants. I was really more interested in animals and man. So in 1932 I went to the Courtauld Institute at the Middlesex Hospital for a year or so, under Professor EC Dodds, to get some experience in human biochemistry. One paper came out of that period, a comparative investigation of urine and serum proteins in nephritis (5). I was quite startled, but gratified, to see fairly recently this little effort of mine referred to as 'the pioneer work on the subject'.

In 1933 I was faced with finding a job, and research jobs were difficult to come by at that time. I went for several interviews but nobody wanted me. Professor Dodds told me that dietetics was an up-and-coming profession, and on his advice I enrolled for the first one year postgraduate diploma course in dietetics at King's College of Household and Social Science under Professor VH Mottram.

As a preliminary to this course I was sent to work in the main kitchen at King's College Hospital to learn something about large-scale cooking. While I was there I often saw Dr McCance come into the kitchen and bring joints of meat to be cooked. I was told that he was doing research on cooking. Naturally I was interested, and one day I plucked up courage and spoke to him. He invited me to visit his tiny laboratory, where he told me about the work he was doing on the composition of meat and fish and their losses on cooking (4), and about his previous study on the available carbohydrate of foods. This had been published in 1929 as an MRC *Green Report* (1). It contained information about the reducing sugars present after acid hydrolysis in fruits, vegetables and nuts. I at once realised, from my experience with apples, that the figures for carbohydrate in fruit were too low, for some of the fructose must have been destroyed during the acid hydrolysis. I told Dr McCance this, and the outcome was that he invited me to join him. He got me a grant from the Medical Research Council—it was easier to do this in those days than it is now—and we started another study on the composition of fruits, vegetables and nuts which included water, nitrogen, fat and inorganic constituents as well as carbohydrate. Where appropriate the foods were analysed cooked and raw (11).

I finished the Dietetics Diploma course, and that served me well in two ways. In the first place, it aroused my interest in nutrition. Secondly, as part of the course, I spent six weeks in the diet kitchen at St. Bartholomew's Hospital (Bart's) with Margery Abrahams. I should really have spent six months there, but those six weeks were long enough to convince me that we badly needed comprehensive tables showing the composition of British foods. The composition of patients' diets was being calculated from American tables which gave values only for raw foods, and in which the carbohydrate had not been determined directly but calculated 'by difference', that is what was left after deducting water, protein and fat from the total weight. It thus contained everything that we now know as 'dietary fibre'. Dr McCance knew all about the difficulties in using 'carbohydrate by difference' in prescribing diets for diabetics, and in fact, at that momentous first interview with him, he told me about his work on unavailable carbohydrate, the cellulose, hemicelluloses, pentosans, pectins etc. which he had separated from the available carbohydrate, the sugars and starch, in his original studies (1).

I thought a lot about the need for British food tables and one Saturday afternoon in 1934, while I was on a family outing to Box Hill, a beauty spot in Surrey, the idea came to me that meat, fish, fruit and vegetables would soon have been completely analysed, so there only remained cereal foods, dairy products and some miscellaneous items such as beverages and sweets. If these were also analysed we should have all the material available for making a practical set of tables showing the composition of British foods. I put the idea to Dr McCance the following Monday morning. He was willing, and this is how *The chemical composition of foods* came to be conceived and born. The first edition was published in 1940 (21). All the values were checked and rechecked many times over. There were about 15,000 separate values in the tables and it was almost impossible not to let a mistake slip in here and there. For example, the decimal point slipped in the figure for nitrogen in blackcurrants, so that it was ten times too high. We never heard the end of that. I sometimes think that of all the various aspects of nutrition I have dabbled in over the past 60 years my first venture, on the composition of foods, will be the longest lasting.

I kept in touch with Margery Abrahams after I left Bart's; and in fact we wrote a book together, *Modern Dietary Treatment*, first published in 1937. In 1936 she persuaded me to go to America where the profession of Dietetics had started and where she herself had been trained. So I crossed the Atlantic on the *Aquitania*, which was quite an adventure for me, and I travelled to Washington to visit Charlotte Chatfield and Georgian Adams at the United States Department of Agriculture (USDA) in Washington. They were responsible for the tables of food composition then in use in the United States and also in Britain, until our tables were published in 1940. I remember Miss Chatfield and I discussed whether it was better for compilers like herself to prepare tables from the published work of others, in this case that of Atwater, dating from 1900, or for people like myself, who had analysed the foods, to make the tables. I was in my 20s at the time and very much Miss Chatfield's junior. She was a rather forceful person and thought she had won the argument, but she did not convince me!

While I was at the USDA, I also saw Hazel Stiebeling, and the lesser-known Sybil Smith, to whom I owed a great deal. She arranged a tour for me so that I could visit some of the women nutritionists in charge of institutes and departments in the United States in the 1930s. I first went by train to Iowa City where I saw Genevieve Stearns, a paediatrician interested in the calcium metabolism of infants, and Kate Daum who was working on iron metabolism. I also saw Amy Daniels at the Iowa Child Welfare Research Station; she was concerned with the nutrition of pre-school children, particularly their mineral and vitamin requirements. Then I went to Ames, to the Iowa Agriculture Experiment Station to visit Precious Mabel Nelson and Pearl Swanson. They were studying mineral metabolism in rats and making dietary surveys on groups of the local population.

My next port of call was the Children's Fund of Michigan, to see Icie Macy, Helen Hunscher and their colleagues. This, was the largest group I visited, and their names are still well known for their work on nutritional requirements of children and of pregnant and lactating women, and on the composition of breast milk. Then I went on to visit Lydia Roberts at the University of Chicago; she also was making studies of nutrition and growth of children. Finally, last but not least, I went to see Mary Schwartz Rose at Teachers' College, Columbia University, New York whose main responsibility was to teach nutrition to large groups of students.

All these women were pioneers in the new science of nutrition nearly 60 years ago. I was just a beginner, but they treated me with great kindness and they made a deep impression on me.

Because Dr McCance and I had so much information about food composition, we were in a strong position to calculate the intakes of energy and nutrients by men, women and children. Up to the 1930s almost all dietary surveys had been made on families. The family was assigned a 'man-value', based on the sum of the supposed energy needs of each individual within it. The intake of the family was divided by the 'man-value', and this was then compared with the existing tables of requirements. This was obviously unsatisfactory, and in fact Professor Cathcart had written a review setting out some of the fallacies of this method of approach in the first number of *Nutrition Abstracts and Reviews*, published in 1931. We clearly needed information about the intakes of individuals, and I started my individual dietary surveys, first on 63 men and 63 women (8,9), and I followed this up with the help of Monica Verdon-Roe with the measurement of individual dietary intakes over a period of a week, of more than 1000 children between one and 18 years (30). These surveys brought out very clearly the large variation in the intake of energy and nutrients between one individual and another of the same sex and age.

Because of our knowledge about the composition of foods people came to us from time to time for help in sorting out results of dietary surveys they had made in various parts of the world. Among them was Dagmar Wilson. Dagmar was a most remarkable woman. She had worked with the Women's Medical Service in India for many years and, among her other activities, she had recorded the food intakes of various Indian communities having wheat or rice or millet as their staple cereal. She was particularly interested in the relation between diet, growth, and incidence of disease and she made a special study of the cause of the rickets and osteomalacia which were prevalent in some parts of India. Her results showed clearly, as Dame Harriette Chick's had done 20 years earlier, the vital importance of sunshine falling on a bare skin. Where diets were based on whole cereals, devoid of vitamin D and low in calcium, rickets did not occur if the women and children exposed their bodies to the sun; in areas where they shut themselves indoors and covered their bodies with clothing when they went out, rickets and osteomalacia were widespread (26).

Another visitor was Audrey Richards. She was an anthropologist working in what was then Northern Rhodesia, and among her investigations she had collected information about food intakes of people of the Bemba tribe. She also needed help, and again I managed to sort out her records so that we could calculate the nutrient intakes. Where we did not know the composition of an important food, samples were obtained and we analysed them. This was one of the first collaborations between an anthropologist and one who would nowadays be called a nutritionist (17).

In 1938, during the Munich crisis, we moved to Cambridge to the Department of Medicine. The first year was spent finishing the food tables and writing up the study on individual children's diets. Then the war started. We all felt we must do something to further the war effort. Professor McCance has described our experimental study of rationing (29) and our balance experiments with various sorts of bread (24). This occupied us fully during the first years of the War. Our work on the effect of high extraction flour on the absorption of calcium brought us a minor adventure during the war in the shape of a trip to Dublin. Due to a shortage of wheat, 100% wholemeal flour was being used for bread-making and the incidence of rickets started to increase in the cities in Eire. Somehow, Professor Jessop got to hear of our experiments and we were invited to Dublin to describe them to a group of doctors and politicians, including the Taoiseach, Mr De Valera. As a result it was decided to lower the extraction rate of the flour used for bread-making in Eire, and later to add calcium phosphate to it, and the incidence of rickets in children over one year decreased.

I next turned my attention to another use of the analytical experience we had gained during our years of food analysis, the composition of the human body. This was a more difficult problem than food analysis. I will not go into the difficulties we had in obtaining bodies or dealing with them once we had obtained them. We managed to overcome the difficulties, and we started the work. Then the War ended and we changed course completely; for in the spring of 1946 we went to Germany to study the effects of undernutrition on men, women and children.

Professor McCance has described some of our experiences during the first part of our time there. We intended to stay in Germany for six months, but in the end some of us stayed for nearly three years. This came about because in December 1946, while I was home on leave, Sir Edward Mellanby called a meeting to discuss the post-war loaf. Up to that time there was no question in the minds of nutritionists that high-extraction flour was more nutritious than white, but there was a question as to whether white flour could be made as nutritious as wholemeal by adding to it the B vitamins and iron. At the meeting Sir Edward Mellanby said to me 'There must be a lot of hungry children in Germany. You go and find out the truth about all this'.

I returned to Germany at the beginning of January, and Rex Dean and I drove about in deep snow looking for a suitable orphanage where we could feed children on different kinds of bread. We found one in Duisburg, about 30 miles from Wuppertal where we had our headquarters. The children, aged between 5 and 14, were underheight and underweight at the outset. They gained height and weight equally rapidly on bread made from all five types of flour, 100% (wholemeal), 85% and 72% extraction (white), and white enriched with B vitamins and iron to the amounts in 100% and 85% extraction flours. All the flours contained added calcium carbonate. Bread provided 75% of the energy and the diets contained only 8g of protein from animal sources a day. The experiment lasted for 18 months; the children improved physically and it was impossible for the outsider to tell which kind of bread the child was eating (51). During the latter part of the experiment the British Medical Association (BMA) held its annual conference in Cambridge and I brought five of the girls, one from each group, from Wuppertal to Cambridge, so that the audience could see for themselves the results

I was describing. The girls thought this was a tremendous adventure. We had several other investigations going on in Germany at the same time as the bread experiment. Rex Dean was busy feeding infants a food based on soya, wheat and barley. The children did not do very well at first, and I remember well Dr Lugg from Australia coming to visit us and telling us about the trypsin inhibitor recently discovered in soya flour; when steps were taken to remove this the children did much better.

We left Germany in January 1949, and I returned to the work I had begun four years earlier on the composition of the body. I approached this in two ways. The first was to study the effect of growth and development on body composition, and we analysed the bodies of 19 human fetuses and still-born babies (38), of one four year old boy, and of three men and one woman (39). The adult bodies were dissected by Dr Barrett, the hospital pathologist, which was a great help. We measured the amounts of the same constituents as we had done in the foods.

I have always had, and still have, a great interest in the similarities and differences between species, and the second approach to body composition, which was really an extension of the first, was to study changes in composition during the development of other species. We included pigs, cats, guinea pigs, rabbits, rats and mice in the investigations (36). As a result of all this work, we were able to establish some general principles, and also some important species differences, which were linked with the state of maturity the young of each species reaches when it is born. The human infant is exceptional in having 16% of fat in its body at birth, whereas most species have only 1-2% (37). The guinea pig, however, has about 10%, and one newborn grey seal, which we found recently dead on a beach on the Isle of Oronsay, Scotland, and brought to Cambridge in the boot of my car, had 9%. Fat was the great variable in the newborn as well as the adult, and it was essential to express the amounts of the other constituents per unit weight of fat-free body tissue to get a true picture of chemical development before and after birth.

In the early 1950s John Dickerson and David Southgate joined us and they stayed with us for many happy years. David's first job was to help with the preparation of the third edition of *The composition of foods* (74). We were very pleased, later, to entrust the fourth edition entirely to him and to Alison Paul. The fifth edition, published in 1991, has involved a larger team.

John Dickerson extended the earlier work on the composition of the body to the separate organs and tissues, but soon after he arrived he came with us on our adventure at Sandhurst. Dr Otto Edholm came to see us one day and told us that the General who had recently inspected the cadets, aged $18\frac{1}{2}$ to 20, was convinced that they were not gaining weight as they should, and this was because they were not getting enough 'good red meat'. We agreed to collaborate with Dr Edholm in an investigation of the food intakes and energy expenditures of the cadets.

We made two visits to Sandhurst, each lasting for a week or so. We found that the cadets got a large ration of meat, which they ate. The total energy from the food supplied amounted to 3714 Cal/d, but the cadets ate only 68% of this, and most of the missing 32% was accounted for by uneaten bread. They preferred to go to the canteen and buy cakes and pastries providing almost the same amount of energy as would have been supplied by the bread they did not eat. More interesting perhaps were the discoveries about their energy expenditure. We had been led to believe that they lived lives of ceaseless strenuous activity. In fact we found that they spent $8\frac{1}{2}$ hours out of the 24 in bed, $9\frac{1}{4}$ hours sitting, some of it at lectures, and these two together accounted for 50% of their total energy expenditure. Dressing, cleaning uniforms and getting about the grounds accounted for another 28% and drill, sport and parades, which were regarded as so important in their training, took up only 7% of the time and 12% of the energy (52,53).

Another person who joined us during the 1950s was Gordon Kennedy and it was he who introduced us to the idea of rearing rats in large and small groups. If two litters of rats born on the same day are mixed and three returned to one mother and the remainder, 16-20 to the second, those suckled in the small group get more milk per rat and grow faster than those in the large group, so that by weaning at three weeks they are two to three times as heavy. We confirmed Kennedy's observation that, even though all the rats had access to unlimited food from weaning onwards, those that were small at weaning remained small, and showed no sign of the catch-up growth so characteristic of rehabilitation after undernutrition at older ages (71,72,77). We ourselves used these large and small litter rats for a variety of studies, and since that time they have been used by investigators all round the world.

Our studies on severely undernourished pigs arose out of our work in Germany, and were possible because Professor McCance had facilities at his home in Bartlow for keeping pigs, and these pigs became an important part of our lives for about 15 years. We found we could undernourish them so severely from ten days of age that by one year they weighed only 3% as much as their well-nourished littermates (70). This is, I believe, the most severe growth retardation that has ever been produced and was only possible because the difference between the weight of a newborn pig and an adult is so large. We made many studies on these animals, anatomical, physiological, chemical and psychological.

In 1966, Professor McCance went to Uganda for two years and I became more adventurous. I continued the undernutrition for two and three years before I rehabilitated the pigs (91). They had to be allowed to gain weight very slowly all the time, for if they lost weight they died. When the animals were rehabilitated after one, two or three years, they ate a great deal of food and gained weight rapidly for a time, but the longer they had been undernourished the sooner they stopped growing, and the final weight of those rehabilitated after three years, the age at which the normal pig stops growing, was only half that of pigs well-nourished throughout. In spite of this they matured sexually, and when rehabilitated males and females were mated, the females produced good litters with normal sized piglets which they suckled satisfactorily, and these piglets bore no mark of the nutritional adventures their parents had undergone.

We had always been interested in trace elements, and in the 1950s we measured the absorption and excretion of iron, copper and zinc by young babies. We found that, unlike adults, breast-fed babies one week old excreted far more iron and zinc in their faeces than they received in their food, so that they were losing more than 1% of the body's total iron and zinc each day (80). This could obviously not go on indefinitely, and we thought the iron might have come from unabsorbed bile and the zinc from pancreatic secretions, but unfortunately we had no way of getting any further with this at that time. We also became interested in the ability of young babies to absorb calcium and fat from various kinds of milk. We found that there is a fairly well defined limit to the amount of fat that infants can absorb. This varies from baby to baby, and the level depends on the nature of the fat and the age of the baby. Breast milk fat is absorbed in the greatest quantity, cows' milk fat in the least, and a milk with vegetable and animal fat came in between.

Rex Dean, who had been with us in Germany for the three years we were there, and was my partner and supporter in the experiments with bread and the growth of undernourished children, was asked by Sir Harold Himsworth, then Secretary of the Medical Research Council, to go to Uganda to look into the malnutrition among young children that had been reported there. This was in the early 1950s, and the Infantile Malnutrition Research Unit was subsequently set up in Kampala. Rex Dean was in charge of it until he died in 1964. He had often invited me to visit him and I eventually went early in 1964, but by this time he was not at all well, and I wished I had gone before. Roger Whitehead, who looked after the biochemical work, was really running the Unit. He took me on a wonderful trip to the Queen Elizabeth Game Park. I went to Uganda twice more, once shortly after Rex Dean died, and Roger was Acting Director, and again during the period when Professor McCance was there and Roger was working with me in Cambridge. Those three visits to Uganda made a lasting impression on me, not only the colour and beauty of the African scene, but the other side of the picture, the severe malnutrition among the young children, and the way they recovered in response to treatment with the right kind of food.

In 1968 I moved to the Dunn Nutrition Laboratory, as Head of the Infant Nutrition Research Division. Then in 1973, I retired for the first time. I moved to the Department of Investigative Medicine at Addenbrooke's Hospital. This was the successor to Professor McCance's Department of Experimental Medicine, for the hospital had always disliked the word 'experimental'. The authorities there had never heard of Claude Bernard! For a time I had laboratory accommodation and some PhD students, and even when laboratory space was no longer available, I still had an office which Professor Ivor Mills allowed me to keep until he retired in 1988. I then retired for the second time.

When the British Nutrition Foundation's Research Conference in Cambridge on Nutritional Problems in a Changing World was being organised in 1973, I became involved in the planning of the session on Infant Feeding. It was this that inspired us to analyse infant milks on sale in different European countries, and in the course of this we discovered that the Dutch formula Almiron, which was used for nearly all babies in Holland who were not breast fed, had all the cows' milk fat replaced with maize oil. This has 60% of its total fatty acids as linoleic acid compared with 1% in cows' milk fat, or even 8% in the fat of breast milk. This made us wonder what was happening to the fatty acid composition of the fat of babies living on it.

We investigated this and found that it was indeed having a remarkable effect. In three months the linoleic acid in the body fat of the Dutch infants had risen to 46% of the total, whereas in the artificially fed British infants who were having cows' milk fat, it remained at about 1% (92). In breast-fed infants linoleic acid contributed 3-4% to the total. These results are expressed as a percentage of the total fatty acids, but to appreciate the magnitude of the difference between the composition of the bodies of Dutch and British babies brought about by the kind of fat in the milk they receive we must remember that by 3 or 4 months 25% of the baby's weight may consist of fat. If this fat has 40% of linoleic acid in it, then 10% of the weight of the baby fed on the Dutch infant food will consist of this one polyunsaturated fatty acid. The corresponding figure for breast-fed babies was less than 1%. So the body composition of babies had been altered on a national scale in a remarkable way. The question is, does this matter? Are the Dutch people any the better or worse off for having had such a highly unsaturated body fat in infancy? This question is relevant to UK too, for the fatty acids in the fat of our babies must have become more unsaturated with the newer type of infant foods that are now being used. The composition of the depot fat may not matter very much, but what about the other lipids of the body? We had to go to animal experiments to look into this further. We used guinea pigs because the guinea pig is one of the few small mammals that deposits fat in its adipose tissues before birth (37).

We fed a group of pregnant guinea pigs on a diet containing maize oil and therefore much linoleic acid, and another group on the same basic diet with beef dripping, which has very little linoleic acid in it. At birth the body fat of the young of the maize oil mothers was similar in fatty acid composition to that of the Dutch infants, while the fat in the young of the beef dripping mothers was like that of British infants. We then looked at the fatty acid composition of the phospholipid fractions of red cells, muscle and liver and found that they were also very different (95). Not only so but the myelin in all parts of the brain was affected by the nature of the dietary fat consumed by the mother during pregnancy (97). The lipids of the brain are not immutable but can be altered quite readily at the time when myelination is proceeding rapidly. Although much of the myelination of the human brain has occurred before birth, it continues for some time afterwards, and if I was able to have another adventure in nutrition, I should use this ready made experiment to look further at the implications of feeding such very different fats in infancy.

I still had pigs available in the late 1960s and early 1970s and I turned my attention to two other aspects of nutrition and early development, for both of which the pig was a particularly suitable experimental animal. The first was the effect of slow growth before birth and a small size at full term on subsequent growth and development (91). When a sow has a large litter there is sometimes one, the runt, which weighs only a third as much as its littermates because it was undernourished before birth. We investigated the physiological and chemical development at birth compared with that of the larger littermates and followed growth to maturity. The pig born small never caught up in weight.

The second study (86) concerned the effects on the digestive tract of the newborn pig of its first experience of food by mouth. Some members of a litter were removed from the sow before they had suckled and they received only water by stomach tube for 24 hours. Others in the litter were allowed to suckle. The digestive tract of those having colostrum grew very rapidly both in weight and length, far more rapidly than any other part of the body (93,94). I suggested that this was related to the absorption of gamma globulins just after birth and this has since been shown to be true.

In 1986 I went to Washington DC for a few weeks to work in the Nutrition laboratory at the Zoo. It came about in this way. In 1975 I was invited to Cornell to lecture. My plane to New York was delayed, I missed the connection to Ithaca, and I finally arrived there at midnight one snowy winter's night. I was afraid there would be no one to meet me, and I did not know where I was staying. But there stood a solitary figure, a young man, who greeted me by telling me I was the only person in the world who would appreciate what he was doing for his PhD. This was Olav Oftedal. He was collecting together information about the composition of the milk of all the species whose milk had been analysed, and he was filling in the gaps by analysis where possible. We have remained friends ever since. Olav later became nutritionist at Washington Zoo.

In 1984, he and two colleagues mounted an expedition to the pack ice off Labrador to measure the milk intake and milk composition of two species of seals born and suckled on the pack ice. One of the species, the hooded seal, doubles its birth weight of 20kg in four days on a milk containing 60% fat, of which it takes 10kg a day. The mother then leaves it and goes back to the sea. Olav had brought to Washington 20 frozen bodies of newborn and suckled seals, killed according to the Canadian Sealing Regulations. These bodies remained in the cold store at the Zoo for two years, along with the bodies of newborn and suckled black bears, born and suckled while their mothers were 'hibernating' and taking no food or drink for four months. I visited Olav several times during those two years. Each time he took me to the cold store to view the frozen bodies, and I realised that nothing was going to be done with them unless I lent a hand. So I offered to go and help.

I got a grant from the Smithsonian Institution, the laboratory was cleared of all other work, and we had a hectic few weeks dissecting the animals, weighing and measuring the various parts of the body and preparing the material for analysis. This was rather a complicated job, wrapping up and labelling the various parts of the body from so many animals. I thoroughly enjoyed being associated with it all, and getting my hands, or rather rubber gloves, dirty again. A paper describing this study has now been published (99) and another, on the nutrition and growth of suckling black bears will appear in the British Journal of Nutrition. This work has given me many new problems to think about in comparative nutrition.

January 1993
Sharing in the preparation of this book and reading the frank comments of some of the people who have worked with us in our somewhat unconventional Department has been an enjoyable, if enlightening, experience.

We should like to thank all the contributors who have spent time and trouble recording their recollections of life with McCance and Widdowson. There are many others who have been with us for various lengths of time; some of them coming from other parts of the world. European colleagues who have been authors or co-authors of papers describing investigations they made with us include Per Lous from Copenhagen, Joseph Lat and O Koldovsky from Prague, Ernst Zweymuller from Vienna, Peter Schmidt from Budapest, Vera Cabak from Sarajevo, Cleo Economou-Mavrou and 'Poppy' Artavanis from Athens and N Hatemi from Istanbul. Others came from farther afield; from USA and Canada, Ed Ferguson, Jack Crawford, John Boylan, Bob Bradfield, John Forrest, Elinor Glauser, Bernice Hines, Inge Radde, Pat Cavell, Rae Schemmel, Frances Zeman and Helen Chan; from South Africa Ian Holman and Jack Booyens, and from New Zealand Patricia Harris. We have kept in touch with many of them and we are sorry that the limitations on the size of this book did not allow us to include their impressions of the Department of Experimental Medicine. They probably found it even less like what they had expected than those whose recollections have been recorded.

We should also like to pay tribute in this book to members of our Department in one or other of its locations who have since died. They include Alec Haynes, Margery Masters (Peggy Cutting), Winifred Young, Rex Dean, Eric Glaser, Dick Berridge, Ian Holman, John Boylan, Paul Fourman, Gordon Kennedy, Hilda Bruce, Laurie Lawn, Kate Rintoul and Wayne Shaw. We remember them all with affection.

Selected publications of McCance and Widdowson

When I decided to include a list of McCance and Widdowson publications in this book, it soon became clear that if all references were given, it would contain nearly 600 items, covering nearly 50 pages. Professor McCance and Dr Widdowson were therefore asked to select 100 for special mention

Those listed were chosen partly to cover their range of interests, partly because they were milestones in their many years of research together, and partly because, for some reason, they were particularly memorable—either because of the interest they aroused, the unusual circumstances in which they were written, for example, on board a liner on the Atlantic in a Force Nine gale, or because they led to long-lasting friendships.

MA

1 *McCance RA, Lawrence RD.* **The carbohydrate content of foods.** London. Medical Research Council Special Report Series No. 135. London: HMSO, 1929.

2 *Widdowson EM.* **A method for the determination of small quantities of mixed reducing sugars and its application to the estimation of the products of hydrolysis of starch by taka-diastase.** Biochem J 1931; **25:** 863-879.

3 *Widdowson EM.* **Chemical studies in the physiology of apples. XIII, The starch and hemicellulose content of developing apples.** Ann Bot 1932; **46:** 597-631.

4 *McCance RA, Shipp HL.* **The chemistry of flesh foods and their losses on cooking.** London. Medical Research Council Special Report Series No. 187. London: HMSO, 1933.

5 *Widdowson EM.* **A comparative investigation of urine- and serum-proteins in nephritis.** Biochem J 1933; **27:** 1321-1331.

6 *Widdowson EM, McCance RA.* **The available carbohydrate of fruits. Determination of glucose, fructose, sucrose and starch.** Biochem J 1935; **29:** 151-156.

SELECTED PUBLICATIONS

7   *McCance RA, Lawrence RD*. **The secretion of urine in diabetic coma.** Q J Med 1935; **4:** 53-79.

8   *Widdowson EM*. **A study of English diets by the individual method. Part I. Men.** J Hyg Camb 1936; **36:** 269-292.

9   *Widdowson EM, McCance RA*. **A study of English diets by the individual method. Part II. Women.** J Hyg Camb 1936; **36:** 293-309.

10   *McCance RA*. **Experimental sodium chloride deficiency in man.** Proc Roy Soc B 1936; **119:** 245-268.

11   *McCance RA, Widdowson EM, Shackleton LRB*. **The nutritive value of fruits, vegetables and nuts.** Medical Research Council Special Report Series No. 213. London: HMSO, 1936.

12   *McCance RA, Widdowson EM*. **The fate of the elements removed from the blood-stream during the treatment of polycythaemia by acetylphenylhydrazine.** Q J Med 1937; **6:** 277-286.

13   *Widdowson EM, McCance RA*. **The absorption and excretion of iron before, during and after a period of very high intake.** Biochem J 1937; **31:** 2029-2034.

14   *McCance RA, Widdowson EM*. **Absorption and excretion of iron.** Lancet 1937; **ii:** 680-684.

15   *McCance RA, Widdowson EM*. **The secretion of urine in man during experimental salt deficiency.** J Physiol 1937; **91:** 222-231.

16   *McCance RA, Luff MC, Widdowson EE*. **Physical and emotional periodicity in women.** J Hyg Camb 1937; **37:** 571-611.

17   *Richards AI, Widdowson EM*. **A dietary study in north-eastern Rhodesia.** Africa 1937; **9:** 166-196.

18   *McCance RA, Widdowson EM*. **The absorption and excretion of iron following oral and intravenous administration.** J Physiol 1938; **94:** 148-154.

19   *McCance RA, Widdowson EM*. **The fate of calcium and magnesium after intravenous administration to normal persons.** Biochem J 1939; **33:** 523-529.

20   *McCance RA, Widdowson EM*. **The fate of strontium after intravenous administration to normal persons.** Biochem J 1939; **33:** 1822-1825.

21   *McCance RA, Widdowson EM*. **Chemical composition of foods.** Medical Research Council Special Report Series No. 235. London: HMSO, 1940.

22   *McCance RA, Young WF*. **The secretion of urine by newborn infants.** J Physiol 1941; **99:** 265-282.

23 *Young WF, Hallum JL, McCance RA.* **The secretion of urine by premature infants.** Arch Dis Childh 1941; **16:** 243-252.

24 *McCance RA, Widdowson EM.* **Mineral metabolism of healthy adults on white and brown bread dietaries.** J Physiol 1942; **101:** 44-85.

25 *McCance RA, Widdowson EM.* **The absorption and excretion of zinc.** Biochem J 1942; **36:** 692-696.

26 *Wilson DC, Widdowson EM.* **A comparative nutritional survey of various Indian communities.** Indian Med Res Mem No. 34. Kampur, India, 1942.

27 *McCance RA, Widdowson EM.* **Seasonal and annual changes in the calcium metabolism of man.** J Physiol 1943; **102:** 42-49.

28 *McCance RA.* **The excretion of urea, salts and water during periods of hydropenia in man.** J Physiol 1945; **104:** 196-209.

29 *McCance RA, Widdowson EM.* **An experimental study of rationing.** Medical Research Council Special Report Series. No. 254. London: HMSO, 1946.

30 *Widdowson EM.* **A study of individual children's diets.** Medical Research Council Special Report Series No. 257. London: HMSO, 1947.

31 *McCance RA, Widdowson EM.* **The digestibility of English and Canadian wheats with special reference to the digestibility of wheat protein by man.** J Hyg Camb 1947; **45:** 59-64.

32 *McCance RA.* **Osteomalacia with Looser's Nodes (Milkman's Syndrome) due to a raised resistance to vitamin D acquired about the age of 15 years.** Q J Med N S 1947; **16:** 33-46.

33 *Venn JAJ, McCance RA, Widdowson EM.* **Iron metabolism in piglet anaemia.** J Comp Path Ther 1947; **57:** 314-325.

34 *Widdowson EM, McCance RA.* **Sexual differences in the storage and metabolism of iron.** Biochem J 1948; **42:** 577-581.

35 *Dean RFA, McCance RA.* **Inulin, diodone, creatinine and urea clearances in newborn infants.** J Physiol 1947; **106:** 431-439.

36 *Spray CM, Widdowson EM.* **The effect of growth and development on the composition of mammals.** Br J Nutr 1950; **4:** 332-353.

37 *Widdowson EM.* **Chemical composition of newly born mammals.** Nature 1950; **166:** 626-628.

38 *Widdowson EM, Spray CM.* **Chemical development *in utero*.** Arch Dis Childh 1951; **26:** 205-214.

SELECTED PUBLICATIONS

39   *Widdowson EM, McCance RA, Spray CM.* **The chemical composition of the human body.** Clin Sci 1951; **10:** 113-125.

40   *McCance RA, Widdowson EM.* **The metabolism of iron during suckling.** J Physiol 1951; **112:** 450-458.

41   *McCance RA.* **The history, significance and aetiology of hunger oedema. Studies of undernutrition, Wuppertal, 1946-9.** Medical Research Council Special Report Series No. 275. London: HMSO, 1951; 21-82.

42   *Widdowson EM.* **The response to unlimited food. Studies of undernutrition, Wuppertal 1946-49.** Medical Research Council Special Report Series. No. 275. London: HMSO, 1951: 313-345.

43   *McCance RA, Widdowson EM.* **Famine.** Postgrad Med J 1951; **27:** 268-277.

44   *Widdowson EM.* **Mental contentment and physical growth.** Lancet 1951; **i:** 1316-1318.

45   *McCance RA.* **Practice of Experimental Medicine.** Proc Roy Soc Med 1951; **44:** 189-194.

46   *McCance RA, Widdowson EM.* **A method of breaking down the body weights of living persons into terms of extracellular fluid, cell mass and fat, and some applications of it to physiology and medicine.** Proc Roy Soc B 1951; **138:** 115-136.

47   *McCance RA, Widdowson EM.* **Renal function before birth.** Proc Roy Soc B 1953; **141:** 488-497.

48   *McCance RA, Widdowson EM.* **Normal renal function in the first two days of life.** Arch Dis Childh 1954; **29:** 488-494.

49   *McCance RA, Widdowson EM.* **The influence of events during the last few days *in utero* on tissue destruction and renal function in the first two days of independent life.** Arch Dis Childh 1954; **29:** 495-501.

50   *McCance RA, Naylor NJB, Widdowson EM.* **The response of infants to a large dose of water.** Arch Dis Childh 1954; **29:** 104-109.

51   *Widdowson EM, McCance RA.* **Studies on the nutritive value of bread and on the effect of variations in the extraction rate of flour on the growth of undernourished children.** Medical Research Council Special Report Series No. 287. London: HMSO, 1954.

52   *Widdowson EM, Edholm OG, McCance RA.* **The food intake and energy expenditure of cadets in training.** Br J Nutr 1954; **8:** 147-155.

53   *Edholm OG, Fletcher JG, Widdowson EM, McCance RA.* **The energy expenditure and food intake of individual men.** Br J Nutr 1955; **9:** 286-300.

54 Widdowson EM. **Assessment of the energy value of human foods.** Proc Nutr Soc 1955; **14:** 142-154.

55 Widdowson EM, McCance RA. **Physiological undernutrition in the newborn guinea-pig.** Br J Nutr 1955; **9:** 316-321.

56 McCance RA, Widdowson EM. **Protein catabolism and renal function in the first two days of life in premature infants and multiple births.** Arch Dis Childh 1955; **30:** 405-409.

57 McCance RA, Widdowson EM. **The response of puppies to a large dose of water.** J Physiol 1955; **129:** 628-635.

58 McCance RA, Widdowson EM. **Metabolism, growth and renal function of piglets in the first days of life.** J Physiol 1956; **133:** 373-384.

59 McCance RA, Widdowson EM. **Breads white and brown. Their place in thought and social history.** London: Pitman Medical Publishing Co Ltd, 1956.

60 Widdowson EM, McCance RA. **The effects of chronic undernutrition and of total starvation on growing and adult rats.** Br J Nutr 1956; **10:** 361-373.

61 McCance RA, Ungley GC, Crosfill JWL, Widdowson EM. **The hazards to men in ships lost at sea, 1940-44.** Medical Research Council Special Report Series No. 291. London: HMSO, 1956.

62 Masterton JP, Lewis HE, Widdowson EM. **Food intakes, energy expenditures and faecal excretions of men on a polar expedition.** Br J Nutr 1957; **11:** 346-358.

63 McCance RA, Widdowson EM. **Hypertonic expansion of the extracellular fluids.** Acta Paediatr Stockh 1957; **46:** 337-353.

64 McCance RA, Widdowson EM. **The response of the new-born puppy to water, salt and food.** J Physiol 1958; **141:** 81-87.

65 Widdowson EM and McCance RA. **The effect of food and growth on the metabolism of phosphorus in the newly born.** Acta Paediatr Stockh 1959; **48:** 383-387.

66 McCance RA, Widdowson EM. **The effect of colostrum on the composition and volume of the plasma of new-born piglets.** J Physiol 1959; **145:** 547-550.

67 McCance RA, Widdowson EM. **The effect of lowering the ambient temperature on the metabolism of the new-born pig.** J Physiol 1959; **147:** 124-134.

68 Dickerson JWT, Widdowson EM. **Chemical changes in skeletal muscle during development.** Biochem J 1960; **74:** 247-57.

SELECTED PUBLICATIONS

69   Widdowson EM, Dickerson JWT. **The effect of growth and function on the chemical composition of soft tissues.** Biochem J 1960; **77:** 30-43.

70   McCance RA. **Severe undernutrition in growing and adult animals. 1. Production and general effects.** Br J Nutr 1960; **14:** 59-73.

71   Widdowson EM, McCance RA. **Some effects of accelerating growth. I. General somatic development.** Proc Roy Soc B 1960; **152:** 188-206.

72   Dickerson JWT, Widdowson EM. **Some effects of accelerating growth. II. Skeletal development.** Proc Roy Soc B 1960; **152:** 207-217.

73   McCance RA, Widdowson EM. **Renal aspects of acid base control in the newly born. I. Natural development.** Acta Paediatr Stockh 1960; **49:** 409-414.

74   McCance RA, Widdowson EM. **The composition of foods. 3rd edition.** Medical Research Council Special Report Series No. 297. London: HMSO, 1960.

75   Widdowson EM. **Nutritional individuality.** Proc Nutr Soc 1962; **21:** 121-128.

76   McCance RA. **Food, growth and time.** Lancet 1962; **ii:** 621-626; 671-676.

77   Widdowson EM, Kennedy GC. **Rate of growth, mature weight and life-span.** Proc Roy Soc B 1962; **156:** 96-108.

78   Widdowson EM, McCance RA. **The effect of finite periods of undernutrition at different ages on the composition and subsequent development of the rat.** Proc Roy Soc B 1963; **158:** 329-342.

79   McCance RA, Widdowson EM. **The effect of administering sodium chloride, sodium bicarbonate and potassium bicarbonate to newly born piglets.** J Physiol 1963; **165:** 569-574.

80   Cavell PA, Widdowson EM. **Intakes and excretions of iron, copper and zinc in the neonatal period.** Arch Dis Childh 1964; **39:** 496-501.

81   Davies JS, Widdowson EM, McCance RA. **The intake of milk and the retention of its constituents while the newborn rabbit doubles its weight.** Br J Nutr 1964; **18:** 385-392.

82   Widdowson EM and Dickerson JWT. **Chemical composition of the body.** In: Comar CL and Bronner F, eds. Mineral Metabolism. New York: Academic Press. 1964; **IIA:** 1-247.

83   Schmidt P, Widdowson EM. **The effect of a low-protein diet and a cold environment on calorie intake and body composition in the rat.** Br J Nutr 1967; **21:** 457-465.

84 Widdowson EM. **Harmony of growth.** Lancet 1970; **i:** 901-905.

85 McCance RA, Hamad El Neil, Nasr El Din et al. **The response of normal men and women to changes in their environmental temperatures and ways of life.** Phil Trans R Soc 1971; **259:** 533-561.

86 Widdowson EM. **Intra-uterine growth retardation in the pig. I. Organ size and cellular development at birth and after growth to maturity.** Biol Neonate 1971; **19:** 329-340.

87 Bilby L, Widdowson EM. **Chemical composition of growth in nestling blackbirds and thrushes.** Br J Nutr 1971; **25:** 127-134.

88 Widdowson EM, Chan H, Harrison GE, Milner RDG. **Accumulation of Cu, Zn, Cr and Co in the human liver before birth.** Biol Neonate 1972; **20:** 360-367.

89 Widdowson EM, Crabb DE, Milner RDG. **Cellular development of some human organs before birth.** Arch Dis Childh 1972; **47:** 652-655.

90 Widdowson EM, Shaw WT. **Full and empty fat cells.** Lancet. 1973; **ii:** 905.

91 Widdowson EM. **Changes in pigs due to undernutrition before birth and for one, two and three years afterwards and the effects of rehabilitation.** Adv in Exp Med and Biol 1974; **49:** 165-181.

92 Widdowson EM, Dauncey MJ, Gairdner DMT, Jonxis JHP, Pelikan-Filipkova M. **Body fat of British and Dutch infants.** Br Med J 1975; **1:** 653-655.

93 Widdowson EM, Crabb DE. **Changes in the organs of pigs in response to feeding in the first 24 hours after birth. I. The internal organs and muscles.** Biol Neonate 1976; **28:** 261-271.

94 Widdowson EM, Colombo VE, Artavanis CA. **Changes in the organs of pigs in response to feeding for the first 24 hours after birth. II. The digestive tract.** Biol Neonate 1976; **28:** 272-281.

95 Pavey DE, Widdowson EM, Robinson MP. **Body lipids of guinea pigs exposed to different dietary fats from mid-gestation to 3 months of age. II. The fatty acid composition of the lipids of liver, plasma, adipose tissue, muscle and red cell membranes at birth.** Nutr Metabol 1976; **20:** 351-363.

96 McCance RA. **Perinatal physiology.** In: Hodgkin et al, ed. The Pursuit of Nature. Cambridge, Cambridge University Press, 1977: 133-168.

97 Pavey DE, Widdowson EM. **Body lipids of guinea pigs exposed to different dietary fats from mid-gestation to 3 months of age. V. The fatty acid composition of brain lipids at birth.** Nutr Metab 1981; **24:** 357-366.

SELECTED PUBLICATIONS

98 *Widdowson EM.* **Animals in the service of human nutrition.** Nutr Revs 1986; **44:** 221-227.

99 *Oftedal OT, Bowen OD, Widdowson EM, Boness DS.* **Effects of suckling and the post-suckling fast on weight of the body and internal organs of harp and hooded seal pups.** Biol Neonate 1989; **56:** 283-300.

100 *McCance RA, Widdowson EM.* **The birth and early development of infant physiology.** Annales Nestlé. 1992; **50:** 1-12.

Citation facts about McCance and Widdowson publications

Some of the McCance and Widdowson papers have, at various times, been classified as 'Citation Classics', so I thought it would be interesting to generate some statistics about the annual citation rate of all their joint papers.

With the advance of information technology and the supposed ease of computerised literature searches, I expected this to be a relatively straightforward operation. But, as Professor McCance and Dr Widdowson have commented in their *Advice to a Young Scientist*, on pages 63 to 66, computerised records only go back a certain number of years. In the end, the most practical option was to use the printed version of the *Science Citation Index* which, even then, only went back as far as 1945.

This citation analysis has therefore been restricted to the 45-year period 1945 to 1989. A further limitation, when using the *Science Citation Index* to generate facts about a joint scientific partnership, is that the recorded citations refer only to first authors of papers. 'McCance' citations are therefore those where McCance is first author of any paper and 'Widdowson' citations are those where Widdowson is first author.

For each of the currently available cumulative indexes (ten-year periods between 1945 and 1964, and five-year periods between 1965 and 1989), two exercises were undertaken: first an average annual citation rate was derived separately for McCance citations and for Widdowson citations. The results are shown in the Figure on page 54. Over the whole 45-year period, McCance papers were cited 7892 times and Widdowson papers 5148 times, giving an overall average annual citation rate, over 45 years, of 175 and 114 respectively.

Between 1945 and the second half of the 1960s, the McCance citations greatly outnumbered those by Widdowson. The peak period for McCance citations was the latter half of the 1960s. Between 1975 and 1979, the Widdowson papers were cited at much the same frequency as those of McCance. After 1980, the Widdowson citations took the lead and peaked in the first half of the 1980s. Thus we observe two overlapping distribution curves, so characteristic of any master/disciple relationship.

Citations of McCance and Widdowson publications

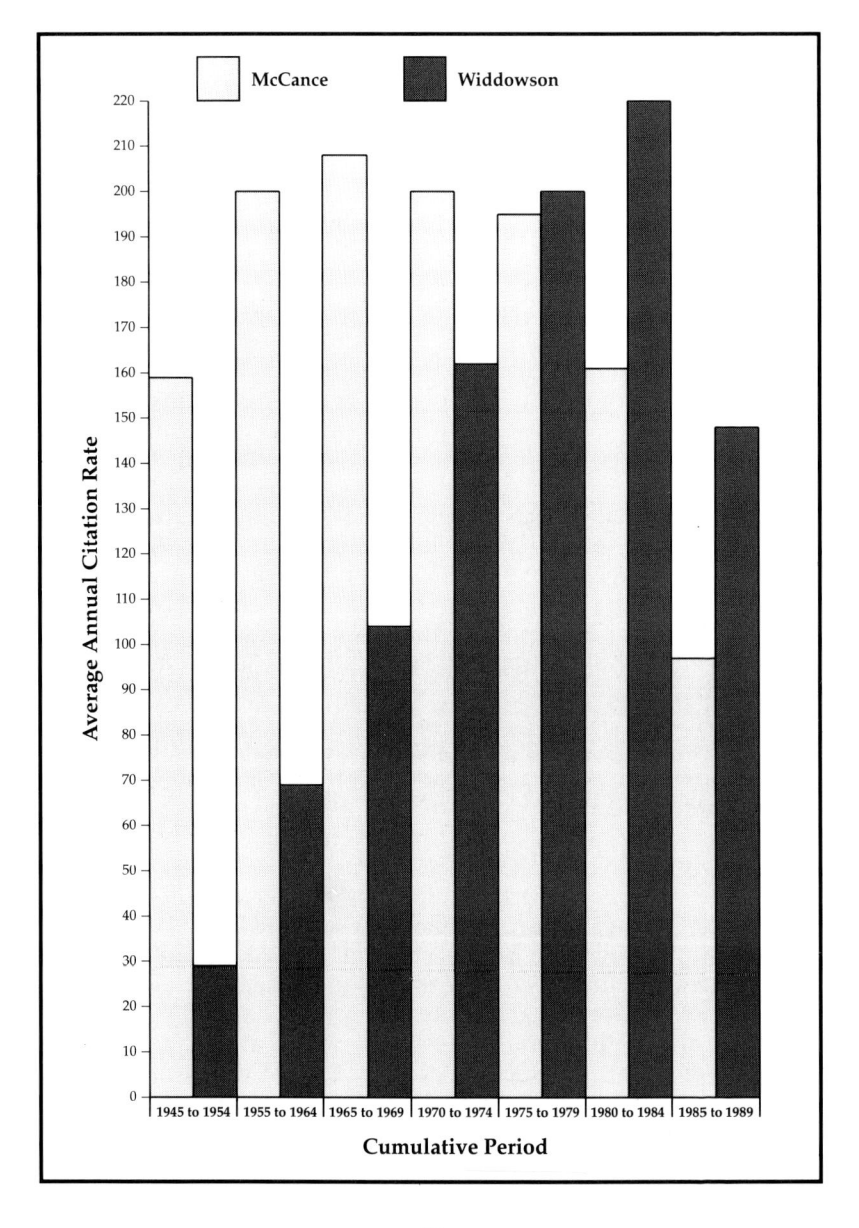

CITATION FACTS

CUMULATIVE PERIOD	MOST CITED PAPER WITH McCANCE AS FIRST AUTHOR	MOST CITED PAPER WITH WIDDOWSON AS FIRST AUTHOR
1945-1954	McCance RA, Young WF. (1941) The secretion of urine by newborn infants. [22]	Widdowson EM, McCance RA, Spray CM. (1951) The chemical composition of the human body. [39]
1955-1964	McCance RA, Widdowson EM. (1951) A method of breaking down the body weights of living persons into terms of extracellular fluid, cell mass and fat, and some applications of it to physiology and medicine. Proc Roy Soc B, 1951; 138: 115-130.	Widdowson EM, McCance RA, Spray CM. (1951) The chemical composition of the human body. [39]
1965-1969	McCance RA. Severe undernutrition in growing and adult animals. I Production and general effects. Br J Nutr. 1960; 14: 59-73.	Widdowson EM, McCance RA. (1960) Some effects of accelerating growth. I General somatic development. [71]
1970-1974	McCance RA, Widdowson EM. (1960) The Composition of Foods. Third edition. Medical Research Council Special Report Series No. 297. 1960. London: HMSO.	Widdowson EM, McCance RA. (1960) Some effects of accelerating growth. I General somatic development. [71]
1975-1979	McCance RA, Widdowson EM. (1962) Nutrition and Growth. Proc Roy Soc B. 1962; 156: 326-337.	Widdowson EM, McCance RA. (1960) Some effects of accelerating growth. I General somatic development. [71]
1980-1984	McCance RA, Widdowson EM. (1942) Mineral metabolism of healthy adults on white and brown bread dietaries. [24]	Widdowson EM, McCance RA. (1960) Some effects of accelerating growth. I General somatic development. [71]
1985-1989	McCance RA, Widdowson EM. (1942) Mineral metabolism of healthy adults on white and brown bread dietaries. [24]	Widdowson EM, McCance RA. (1960) Some effects of accelerating growth. I General Somatic development. [71]

The numbers in square brackets refer to the reference number in the Selected Publications (see pages 45 to 52)

The second exercise was to see which of the papers, with either McCance or Widdowson as first author, was cited most frequently. So, for each cumulative index period, the most commonly cited McCance or Widdowson paper was identified (see Table on page 55).

In Professor McCance's list, it is surprising that *The Composition of Foods* only qualified as the most cited paper in one period (1970 to 1974), although the third edition, in particular, has received frequent citation on a very regular basis. As McCance citations have waned throughout the 1980s, it has been his 1942 'bread' paper that has been most frequently cited.

Dr Widdowson's list shows a remarkable consistency. *The Chemical Composition of the Human Body*, published in 1951, was her most cited paper until the mid-1960s, but then it was overtaken by the first of several publications describing the effects of accelerating growth, usually known as the 'small and large rat litter' paper published in 1960. The continuing popularity attached to this paper and the technique it describes is evident by its frequent citation, even in the latter half of the 1980s.

Perhaps the most impressive fact to emerge from this analysis is that, with two exceptions, the most frequently cited papers of either McCance or Widdowson have been their joint papers: either McCance and Widdowson, or Widdowson and McCance. Is there any better illustration of the enduring strength of such a successful partnership?

MA

Twenty questions and their answers from McCance & Widdowson

'What questions would you put to Professor McCance and Dr Widdowson if you had the chance?'

During the past couple of years, I have asked this of the book's contributors and many others—some from the world of science, some from outside. Having identified 20 questions which seemed to cover the full range of interest, I asked Professor McCance and Dr Widdowson for their responses. They are joint replies except where indicated :

Q   Which of your scientific achievements gave you most satisfaction?

A   No particular scientific achievement, but discovering how something we have said, written or done has helped somebody in his or her scientific career gives us a great deal of satisfaction.

Q   What has been the greatest honour ever bestowed upon you?

A   Being elected to the Fellowship of The Royal Society.

Q   How would you describe the working relationship between McCance and Widdowson?

A   (EW) Professor McCance had the adventurous spirit and the ideas for unusual scientific activities, for instance, to make an experimental study of rationing; to go to Germany; to go to Khartoum as part of a study of responses to high and low temperatures. I readily fell in with the ideas, we worked out the plan of action together, and then I looked after the day-to-day running of the enterprise.

Q   What were the elements of the chemistry between McCance and Widdowson that led to such a successful working partnership?

A (EW) Professor McCance was the acid, and I was the neutralising base.

Q Who were your own mentors?

A (EW) My first mentor was Helen Archbold, later Helen Porter FRS, in the Department of Plant Physiology at Imperial College. She taught me the principles and practice of research, and how to write a scientific paper. To a lesser extent, I also regard Professor VH Mottram and Margery Abrahams as my mentors, for they got me interested in nutrition.

A (RM) I would regard Sir Joseph Barcroft as my greatest mentor.

Q Which of your ex-colleagues/pupils are you most proud of?

A We would not differentiate between them. We are proud of almost all of them.

Q Did you ever make any mistakes during your research career?

A A very small mistake in the first edition of the *Food Tables* caused considerable annoyance. There was a printer's error in the nitrogen value for blackcurrants (a decimal point had slipped) so that it appeared that they contained ten times as much as they really did. Certain people never let us forget that one!

(EW) On a more serious note, I am quite prepared to admit that I got it wrong when I said in the *Lancet* that vitamin D sulphate was higher in human than in cows' milk. We later realised that the analyses had been at fault.

Q If you could start your career all over again, would you choose nutrition? If not, what would you choose?

A (EW) I did not choose nutrition. Nutrition as a subject did not exist when I started. I have been a chemist, biochemist, plant physiologist, medical researcher, neonatologist, physiologist, but not a nutritionist; except as part of all these other disciplines.

A (RM) I was a biochemist, physiologist, physician, registered medical practitioner, neonatologist, but not a nutritionist.

Q Many of your studies were based on self-experimentation. Would more such studies improve the present quality of nutrition science?

A   We did not believe that we should use human subjects in experiments that involved any pain, hardship or danger, unless we had made the same experiment on ourselves. This has always been our policy. Yes, more self-experimentation might improve the quality of nutrition science.

Q   Your papers were characterised by an attention to scientific detail and were written in a very relaxed and personal style. What do you think of today's editorial policy which demands a more terse, impersonal style and much more statistical detail?

A   If you look at the scientific literature in the early part of the 20th century, you will find much more detail about individual experimental subjects, both human and animal, than we gave, and a very chatty style. We were a sort of halfway house between that and the present style which is unreadable except to the experts. It probably is the editorial policy of the journals that is to blame for the change.

Q   You were always very interested in inter-individual variation in your scientific data. Do you feel that this variation tends to be disregarded now?

A   It was the study of individual diets of men, women and children in the 1930s that got us interested in individual differences. We called it 'nutritional individuality'. Yes, we do think it is neglected nowadays. Papers tend not to be accepted today if the experiment has not been made on a large number of human/animal subjects, so that the results can be analysed statistically. You only need a small number of subjects when the differences are large and then you may need no statistics at all. We were interested in the extremes as well as the means of the range. Nowadays it is only the means or median values that seem important.

Q   You were always very interested in inter-species variation in response. Why?

A   Our interest in inter-species differences arose when we realised that different species are born at different stages of development. We are fond of a quotation from Claude Bernard (The Father of Experimental Medicine):

'The whole success or failure of an experiment may depend on the choice of the right experimental animal.'

TWENTY QUESTIONS

Q   You always stressed age and sex differences in response to any factor. Do these get overlooked these days?

A   Age and sex are important—this is self-evident. When we were doing experimental work, sex, or gender, was very much neglected and so many experiments were made only on men and male animals. Many of our experiments demonstrated differences due to age and sex.

Q   Do you agree that treating macronutrients as single chemical entities has handicapped the development of our understanding of nutrition and its relationship to degenerative disease?

A   Yes. The study of osteoporosis provides a good illustration. Loss of calcium from the bones is emphasised again and again, and no mention is made of the loss of nitrogen, phosphorus and potassium that is going on in parallel in the body at the same time.

Q   You have visited scientists in many countries. If you had chosen to work abroad permanently, which country would you choose and why?

A   (EW) I have never wanted to work in any other country. I enjoyed working in Germany, but we were not working with Germans at a scientific level. If I had to choose somewhere, I suppose I would choose the USA because of my friendship with scientists there.

A   (RM) I have never wanted to work anywhere else, not even the USA.

Q   What do you consider the most important unanswered question in nutrition?

A   The importance of genetic influences.

Q   Do you believe that individual nutrition scientists can still make a worthwhile contribution to the science, or must we inevitably move towards multidisciplinary teams?

A   This all depends on the scientists themselves. So long as they have a broad outlook and range of skills, and know where to get help when they need it, there is no reason why they should not make a worthwhile contribution to the science of nutrition—if the organisation that supports them will let them.

Q What do you think about the people who make fortunes out of pseudo-nutrition?

A Less than nothing, and we fear the Register of Accredited Nutritionists and similar schemes won't stop them.

Q What role can the food industry play in promoting nutrition education and research?

A It can play a vital role in supporting education and research and in the dissemination of sound information, for example, through the Nutrition Foundations.

Q Do you attribute your own longevity to your dietary knowledge and interest in nutrition?

A (EW) No. I eat butter, eggs and white bread, which some people think are bad for you but I do not. However, I do eat plenty of fruit and vegetables and drink lots of water. I think my longevity is largely due to my genes (Father died aged 96 and Mother 107). Perhaps having been breast-fed has helped!

Advice to a young scientist

When I first asked McCance and Widdowson to give some advice, their first reaction was to say, 'No'. How could *they*, who started their research careers in human nutrition 60 years ago, have any advice to offer young scientists who are starting in the 1990s? A laboratory today is a very different place from when they began. Their tools were Bunsen burners, burettes, pipettes, beakers, measuring cylinders and visual colorimeters. Scientists today have the use of sophisticated equipment such as they never dreamed of.

When they began, there was no learned Society, and no specialist journal dealing with nutrition. They were physiologists, biochemists, physicians and agriculturalists interested in some aspects of nutrition of man or animals as part of their particular subject. There has been an enormous advance in knowledge and proliferation of literature in the past 60 years, which in one way makes things more difficult, but on the other hand, the ease with which literature searches can be made makes it less likely that important papers will be missed. But a word of warning must be issued. These literature searches only go back a certain number of years, and all the papers published before that time are not indexed. This is why people are busy nowadays rediscovering what McCance and Widdowson knew more than half a century ago.

To come back to where I started, that McCance and Widdowson should offer some advice. When they thought further about it, they came to the conclusion that the changes over the years have really all been matters of technical improvements and sophistication in methods of measuring, analysing, recording, calculating and being able to make studies on living people. But the principles of research have not changed, nor has there been any fundamental alteration in the physiology and biochemistry of people and animals being investigated. The components of the plants and animals that form the basis of the food they eat have not changed either, except in matters of detail, for example the amount of fat in meat.

So in the end, McCance and Widdowson decided to set out a few principles of research which they believe are as important today as they always were.

MA

Advice to a young scientist from McCance & Widdowson

Treasure your exceptions

You must realise that there are two main types of research, observational and experimental. We have dabbled in both. Dietary surveys and food analysis are observational. You may compare food intakes in two areas or two countries, but this is still observational unless you have deliberately changed the conditions in one of the groups to be compared. If you get a result that does not fit in with all the others, or your results show wide variations, think about the extremes. Don't just regard them as a nuisance because they increase your standard error. They may be the most interesting part of your study.

Vary your conditions

This is the experimental type of research. Conditions are varied in some way, and two or more groups of animals or people, or their products, eg blood or urine, are compared. Each group may be studied on more than one occasion, so that each serves as its own control. Generally speaking, in making such studies it is better to have only one variable at a time, otherwise the results may be difficult to interpret. However, two variables sometimes give results that neither would give alone. For example, we found many years ago that young rats fed on a diet low in energy and low in protein did not grow but they survived, whereas those having a diet low in energy and high in protein died. What is the explanation?

Do not be afraid of owning up to a mistake, even if your results have already been published

We all make mistakes from time to time. We once quoted *'The man who makes no mistakes does not usually make anything'*. It is far better for you to publish a correction yourself than to give someone else the pleasure of doing so.

If you are using an animal as a model for human adults or children, be careful to choose an appropriate species of the right age for your experiments

The classical example of choosing the right species was in 1907, when Holst and Frölich wanted to repeat Eijkman's work on beri-beri. Eijkman had used pigeons but, for convenience, Holst and Frölich used guinea pigs. They fed them on a refined cereal diet, but what the guinea pigs developed was not beri-beri but scurvy. If they had chosen almost any other experimental animal the problem of the cause of human scurvy would have remained unsolved.

Just as important as the right species is the right age, particularly if you are making experiments on very young animals. Animals are born at different stages of development. A newborn rat corresponds in many ways to a human fetus, and a newborn guinea pig to an infant several months old.

If your results don't make physiological sense, think! You may have made a mistake or you may have made a discovery

Check everything, repeating your experiment if you can. If you are sure you have not made an error, think hard about the explanation! For many years we were busy measuring various aspects of renal function in newborn infants and animals, and comparing them with those of adults of the same species. Whatever test and method of comparison was used, for example, body weight or surface area, the newborn always appeared to have very inefficient kidneys. Its ability to excrete nitrogen, electrolytes and phosphorus was low in all the species we studied.

This in itself was a discovery at the time, but we were always worried that this didn't make physiological sense, because the animals and infants were healthy. They grew, and the composition of their body fluids remained normal. It took us a long time to realise what by hindsight is so obvious, that the newborn does not need to have kidneys as efficient at excreting nitrogen and mineral salts as an adult, because so much of the intake of those substances is used for growth, that they do not reach the kidney for excretion.

In animals that grow very rapidly like the rabbit, almost the whole of the nitrogen in the protein of the milk is used for protein synthesis and growth. It is only when you feed newborn infants and animals with milks containing higher concentrations of nitrogen, electrolytes or phosphorus than their mothers' milk contains, that you get into trouble.

If your results seem impossible, think and think again

While we were in Germany after the war, we made nutritional studies in several orphanages. Food was severely rationed and the children somewhat undernourished but not exceptionally so. We weighed and measured the children regularly in two orphanages for six months while they lived on their German rations. We planned at the end of this time to provide unlimited bread, with some margarine and jam to spread on it, to the children in one Home, while nothing extra was to be given to the children in the other. At the end of six months, the second Home would get extra food.

We found that during the first six months, when no extra food was supplied, the children in one Home (A) were growing faster in height and weight than those in the other (B). It so happened that we had chosen Home A to receive the extra food, and we had to go on with our plan. To our astonishment the children in Home A, who had originally grown faster and now received the extra food, immediately began to grow more slowly, while those in Home B began to grow rapidly in weight and height, although they had nothing but their German rations.

What could the explanation be? Did extra food actually hinder growth? This seemed to be too absurd to consider. Did the children in Home A eat the extra food? They did. A dietitian supervised their meals all the time. Did the children eat the same amounts of their German rations in the two homes? They did. Was there some noxious agent that somehow moved from one Home to the other just when we began to give the extra food? There was.

It so happened that the housemother who presided over Home B during the first six months was moved by the authorities to Home A just when we began to give the extra food to Home A. Thanks to the smartness of our research nurse, we discovered that the housemother was a most unpleasant woman and very unkind to the children. Her unkindness and the unhappiness of the children was sufficient to delay their growth in spite of the extra food.

Tender loving care of children and careful handling of animals may make all the difference to the successful outcome of a carefully planned experiment.

The scientific achievements of McCance and Widdowson

How do you condense 60 years of scientific achievements of two prolific researchers into one section of a commemorative volume such as this?

As ever, McCance and Widdowson helped me with the solution to this editorial problem. They were prepared to classify their joint achievements into six broad categories and then to nominate six of their former colleagues to review their main achievements in each.

I was delighted when all six nominees, Professor David Southgate, Sir Douglas Black, Professor John Dickerson, Dr Brian Wharton, Dr David Lister and Dr Roger Whitehead responded with enthusiasm, not only by providing a paper for this book, but also by agreeing to present their paper at the British Nutrition Foundation's Conference, held in London on 29th June 1993, to pay tribute to The Scientific Achievements of McCance and Widdowson.

MA

About the authors

David Southgate graduated from the University of London in Biological Sciences and Chemistry in 1954. He joined Professor McCance and Dr Widdowson in 1955 and was initially concerned with the analytical work required for the third edition of the Food Tables which was followed by studies of the energy value of foods. He moved with the Department of Experimental Medicine to the Dunn Nutritional Laboratory in 1968 and initiated the programme for the preparation of the fourth edition of the Food Tables which was completed in 1978. He then started up the Nutrition Division at the Agricultural and Food Research Council's Food Research Institute in Norwich, from where he retired in 1992.

Douglas Black spent six months in the Department of Medicine in Cambridge in 1942. Subsequently he joined the Department of Medicine in Manchester, where he spent 26 years, ending up as Professor. During that time, he also practised general medicine, with a special interest in kidney disease. From 1977 to 1983, he was President of the Royal College of Physicians and he became a Knight Bachelor in 1973.

John Dickerson joined the Department of Experimental Medicine at the end of August 1952. He gained his PhD in 1959 for his work on aspects of body composition during normal development, and as a result of undernutrition. He left the Department in 1965, just before Professor McCance retired, and went to work with John Dobbing in Professor Tanner's Department at the Institute of Child Health in London. In 1967, he became a Reader in Human Nutrition in the Department of Biochemistry at the newly formed University of Surrey, and in 1973 he became Professor. He retired in 1988 and was later appointed Emeritus Professor.

Brian Wharton graduated in medicine at Birmingham in 1960. This was followed by two years at the MRC Infantile Malnutrition Research Unit in Uganda studying kwashiorkor, the subject of his MD thesis. After returning to the UK, he worked at the University of Bristol, the Institute of Child Health in London and the Sorrento Maternity Hospital at Birmingham. Most recently, he held the position of Rank Professor of Human Nutrition in Glasgow. He is a member of various national and international committees advising on child nutrition.

David Lister was Professor McCance's PhD student and then a post-doctoral worker in the Department of Experimental Medicine in Cambridge from 1961 to 1966. After holding a fellowship at the University of Wisconsin, he returned to Cambridge between 1966 and 1984 to work at the Low Temperature Research Station which was subsequently moved to Bristol as part of the Meat Research Institute. From 1985 to 1989, he was Assistant Director and Head of Shinfield Station at the Agricultural and Food Research Council's Institute of Grassland and Animal Production. He is currently Head of the Animal Production and Human Nutrition Division at CAB International in Oxfordshire.

Roger Whitehead was a member of the Medical Research Council's (MRC) staff in the Infantile Malnutrition Research Unit in Uganda from 1958 to 1973 and was Director of the Unit from 1968 to 1973. He returned to the UK in 1973 to take up the Directorship of the MRC Dunn Nutrition Unit which is located within the University of Cambridge. He holds important advisory roles to the UK Government and became a Commander of the Order of the British Empire (CBE) in 1992.

The composition of foods
by David Southgate

INTRODUCTION

The names McCance and Widdowson for virtually all nutritionists in the United Kingdom, and throughout the world, are synonymous with tables of food composition. Since the first edition was published in 1940[1], these tables have become the dietitians' 'bible' and an essential source of information for the development of quantitative studies of human nutrition.

The contribution to nutrition science made by the compilations of the nutritional composition of foods, originally as printed tables and more recently as nutritional databases, is a tribute to McCance and Widdowson's original ideas and to the inspiration that they have given to those who have followed in their footsteps. The task of the compiler of nutritional data on the composition of foods is one that never ceases, thanks to the innovative skills of the food industry, the evolution of dietary patterns and the changing interests of nutritionists themselves.

In my own experience, as one of those fortunate to have worked in this field, one often meets with some surprise that a nutrition research scientist should have an interest in, let alone embark on, studies of the composition of foods. This reflects a surprising ignorance of the fact that a knowledge of the composition of foods 'is the first essential in the dietary treatment of disease or in any quantitative study of human nutrition'[1].

In this paper, I should like first to pay tribute to the research partnership of McCance and Widdowson and secondly, to show how their interest in the composition of foods provided the basis for many of their other contributions to the nutritional and physiological sciences which others will discuss in other parts of this book.

A WORKING TOOL FOR NUTRITIONAL RESEARCH

I think that it is important to recognise that McCance and Widdowson were not interested in the composition of foods as an end in itself, but as a means to an end, usually some other research end. In this, they shared their motivation with one of the other great compilers of food compositional data, Atwater, who also needed compositional data for his researches on energy balance[2].

One characteristic that distinguished McCance and Widdowson's approach to research was their response to an interesting idea or problem. The immediate reaction was, 'Well, let's get on with the analysis or experiments needed to resolve the problem'. If a piece of work or research needed doing, everyone had to set to and get it done. So, when information on food composition was needed, they started to analyse the foods.

Of course, they were working in those halcyon days when one did not have to spend time writing a research proposal and wait for the 'expert peer-review process' to tell one whether it was worth doing; one could just get on and do it. I leave posterity to judge whether the taxpayer got better value from the researchers then, or under the present system. For certain, the description of any scientific post as a full-time one by the Medical Research Council (MRC) was interpreted literally in the Department of Experimental Medicine and one accepted it as the norm.

CARBOHYDRATES—THE INITIATORS OF A PARTNERSHIP

The story of the beginning of the partnership has been told several times[3] and, since I was only an infant at that time, I cannot add any further detail, only some comments. It is interesting to note that the partnership really started with a shared interest in the carbohydrates in foods, at a time when most nutritionists were chasing after vitamins and protein in what would now be called the 'front end' of nutrition research. For McCance, the interest was a pragmatic clinical one, involving the management of the diabetic patient, for whom the carbohydrate values for foods in the late 1920s were unsatisfactory because they were obtained 'by difference', so that the glucogenic available carbohydrates were not distinguished from the unavailable, indigestible carbohydrates.

McCance and Lawrence[4] prepared a review of the carbohydrates in foods supplemented with McCance's own analyses. The parts of the review which dealt with the unavailable carbohydrate (dietary fibre in modern terms), are quite extraordinarily pertinent today, and should be required reading for present-day workers in the field of dietary fibre[5]. It was the analyses in the report that interested Elsie Widdowson because she had been working on the carbohydrates in the developing apple. In the light of current interests in complex carbohydrates[6], this provides another example of how forward-looking McCance and Widdowson were in their research interests.

FRUITS, VEGETABLES AND NUTS

The partnership properly starts with the work on the composition of fruits, vegetables and nuts[7]. This generated a series of research studies on the analysis of the individual carbohydrate species in these foods[8]. Delicate methods were evolved for measuring glucose, fructose and sucrose, in mixtures, using a range of reducing sugar methods, and for starch using enzymatic hydrolysis followed by measurements of glucose and maltose. To those of us brought up in the chromatographic era, analyses of these mixtures with HPLC have only recently become routine; and incidentally, the results from these new methods substantially confirm those exacting measurements made nearly 60 years ago[9].

The work on food composition had some other interesting methodological innovations, some of which had been carried over from the earlier work on flesh foods[10], eg, the emergent microanalytical techniques that were coming into use in clinical laboratories. The use of these would have seemed perfectly natural to McCance, but in food analysis, this was an important innovation. First, it greatly speeded up the analyses and also enabled McCance and Widdowson to start accumulating data on minerals in foods. Secondly and more importantly, it established a common analytical resource for measuring inorganic constituents in foods, blood, urine, faeces and tissues, that supported all the metabolic work on mineral metabolism and salt and water metabolism, where McCance & Widdowson established themselves as researchers of international repute.

PUTTING THE FIRST EDITION TOGETHER

Once the work on the composition of the fruits, vegetables and nuts had been completed, it was obvious to Dr Widdowson that she and Professor McCance had the foundations for a comprehensive set of Food Composition Tables; all they needed to do was to analyse the other foods, eg, cereals, milk and dairy products. So, true to form, they set to and did it. This was not, as far as one can tell, a decision from on high but because they could see how useful such tables would be in their nutritional research. For example, Dr Widdowson had ideas for a study on the food intakes of children[11] and this could only be done with a full set of data. This interest in the tables as a research tool (just as Atwater had done earlier), is a clear example of doing the work on the research infrastructure because of the benefits that would then accrue.

As users of food composition data, McCance & Widdowson recognised that virtually all existing tables only gave values for the composition of raw foods, which limited their usefulness when studying the food and nutrient intakes of individuals. Clearly, the new tables had to include cooked foods. This was another innovation which marked the first edition of McCance and Widdowson[1] as belonging to a new generation of Food Composition Tables. One can see real practical touches in evidence. Some of the recipes were taken from Dr Widdowson's mother's cookery book and Dr Widdowson realised that the composition of many dishes could be calculated from the composition of the ingredients, the recipe and measured cooking losses. Calculating cooked dishes before the days of computers or calculating machines was a formidable task but it needed to be done, so it was.

The first edition included another new feature which reflected McCance and Widdowson's research interests at that time: values were given for a measure of ionisable iron to provide some estimates of the bioavailability of iron in foods[12]. The interest in bioavailability is further reflected in the inclusion of phytate values, as it was becoming apparent that phytate was an inhibitor of calcium and iron absorption[13].

One of the most important features of the first edition was the inclusion of textual introductions describing the sources of data, the recipes used for calculating the composition of the cooked dishes and above all, a description of the samples of foods analysed.

INCLUSION OF WAR-TIME DISHES IN THE SECOND EDITION
The second edition[14] was a relatively minor revision, which included a number of economy dishes developed in the War years and the format and content were little changed from those of the first edition.

EXPANDING AND DEVELOPING: THE THIRD EDITION
The next phase in the activities in the area of food composition was one in which I was directly involved, so that my personal impressions of working in the Department of Experimental Medicine with Professor McCance and Dr Widdowson on food composition now form part of the account.

The nutrition sciences had evolved considerably over the period since the first edition and not only was it necessary to extend the food tables to include the processed foods, which were increasingly important in the UK diet, but the coverage of nutrients needed to be expanded to include the vitamins where the methods for their measurement were more or less well established. Interest in protein nutrition was also being supported by application of microbiological assays and ion-exchange chromatography for the analysis of amino acids and there was considerable demand for tables giving the amino-acid composition of foods.

Support from the MRC enabled Professor McCance and Dr Widdowson to convert a house in Shaftesbury Road into laboratories to start on the preparation of the third edition. The analytical work for this was led by Dr Ian Holman, who had been the biochemist for the studies of undernutrition in Germany after the war[15]. Ian Holman was a specialist in vitamin analysis, and I joined him in the autumn of 1955 to start on the analyses for the third edition.

Our first task was to set up and test all the methods to be used for the major constituents and minerals. We decided that the volume of literature on the vitamins in foods was such that it would not be practicable or prudent to embark on the analysis of all the vitamins in foods. We therefore decided that we would depart from the McCance and Widdowson principle of only using their own analytical data in The Composition of Foods and rely on literature data for the vitamins. So method development and testing was limited to proximates and minerals. This required setting up a range of new colorimetric and flame-photometric methods and evaluating the results on a range of foods, initially in order to ensure that the new data we generated were compatible with the existing data. This was necessary because we proposed to carry forward values from the first and second editions into the third edition, where we had evidence that the values were reliable and applicable to the foods available at that time.

We decided that methods for the carbohydrates would be a special area for study because the developments in colorimetric and chromatographic methods for carbohydrates[9] would permit more specific analyses. It was this work that led me into the dietary fibre field in due course. Once the analytical resource was set up, I began to see at first hand how it could contribute to the research of the Department; methods for foods transfer very well to tissues and are essential in metabolic studies. One quickly became integrated into some of the other research in progress in the laboratory[16].

When Ian Holman left to go to South Africa, I had to look after the analyses; I was joined by Irene Barrett who began compiling the vitamin data, using, as a base, the literature collection on punched cards that Ian had left behind.

It is very difficult to convey the atmosphere in the Department of Experimental Medicine in those days. A succession of visitors and research students trooped through, each bringing new ideas and skills; many of them needing advice or training in the analytical techniques being used for the food-table work. At the same time, I quickly became involved with those people using the food composition tables so that my appreciation of the requirements of the users became sharper, and I hope more useful, as we entered the compilation stage.

This was where I saw one of Dr Widdowson's skills come into play in the evaluation of data as we went through the compilation process. It was as if any suspect figures were ringed in ink that was only visible to her eyes. Each query involved going back to the original analytical data, rechecking calculations and in many cases, going back to resample and analyse the food. Dr Widdowson also had the facility to relate values and to challenge them if there were inconsistencies. These characteristics are the major reason why much of the data generated in the 1930s remains valid today. They are essential skills for a compiler of food tables or nutritional databases[17,18].

The third edition was published in 1960[19] and it included vitamins and amino acids and many of the values from the earlier editions.

A PARTNERSHIP WITH THE MINISTRY: THE FOURTH EDITION

Although the third edition was very well received, the diet of the UK population was continually evolving and the food industry was constantly searching for, and developing, new or improved products. Nutrition science was also developing continuously and by the second half of the 1960s, it became clear to me that a new edition was needed. Dr Widdowson received my initial ideas with interest, and together we produced a proposal for the preparation of a fourth edition. In this we decided to involve the specialist Institutes and Research Associations concerned with foods, in the review of the existing data, and to assist in generating proposals for analysis, where the composition of the foods had changed.

This proposal was put by Dr Widdowson to the Ministry of Agriculture, Fisheries and Food (MAFF) Committee on Food Composition. I must say that the MRC was not too keen on carrying the work of revision on its own but MAFF was very enthusiastic and agreed to second a nutritionist to the Dunn Nutrition Laboratory where I was working in Dr Widdowson's Infant Nutrition Research Division.

Alison Paul was selected to come to Cambridge and a Steering Panel of Users was set up, that included a representative of the Laboratory of the Government Chemist (who was going to undertake the analytical work). Dr Widdowson was an active member of that panel; contributing guidance and advice and making sure that the stylistic standards of the text met the exacting standards of McCance and herself, and of course, scrutinising the data with continued rigour. At this stage, Dr Widdowson said that she felt that she had handed the food-composition table baton on to me but she still continued her interest, making sure that the standards and traditions of the past were retained.

When we had the draft fourth edition completed, both McCance and Widdowson contributed stylistic additions to the text to round it off. We decided that the title of the fourth edition should include their names. We expect that this will be retained in future, in recognition of their special contribution to the development of nutrition compositional data[20,21].

One of the developments included in the proposals for the fourth edition was computerisation and, in this, we had great assistance from MAFF. Dr Widdowson, clearly remembering her hours of toil with slide rule and log tables, was very keen on this idea and a computer-readable tape was available at the same time as the printed book was published. This tape is the source material for most of the nutritional databases in use in the UK and elsewhere.

Another aspect of Dr Widdowson's involvement in the food composition tables was an international one. She had a good rapport with Bernice Watt, one of the compilers of the original US Department of Agriculture Handbook No 8, although Dr Widdowson was always proud of the fact that the UK could produce food composition tables of the same international standing, but with rather fewer resources than the Americans.

In Europe, as a member of the Group of European Nutritionists, she was co-chairman of a working party on the Principles for Preparing National Tables of Food Composition. True to her character, she insisted that I should come to the meeting, 'as I was doing the work',[22]. This has led, in due course, to developments in Europe[23], the EC FLAIR Eurofoods-Enfant Concerted Action on developing nutritional databases in Europe and to the world-wide INFOODS initiative for coordinating nutritional databases across the world[17].

In all these activities—using up-to-date methods, including the foods in the form that they are eaten, insisting that the carbohydrates in foods are measured directly and, above all, maintaining high standards of documentation to support the analysis and the compilation itself—the principles evolved by McCance and Widdowson, in making tables of the nutritional composition of foods into tools to serve nutrition research, are central to the principles being followed, wherever nutrition compositional compilations are being made.

References

1   *McCance RA, Widdowson EM.* **The chemical composition of foods**. Medical Research Council Special Report Series No. 235. London: HMSO, 1940.

2   *Atwater WO, Bryant AP.* **The chemical composition of American food materials**. Bulletin US Official Experimental Station No. 28. Storrs Conn USA, 1905.

3   *Widdowson EM.* **Adventures in nutrition over half a century.** Proc Nutr Soc 1980; **39:** 293-306.

4   *McCance RA, Lawrence RD.* **The carbohydrate content of foods**. Medical Research Council Special Report Series No. 213. London: HMSO, 1929.

5   *Southgate DAT.* **The dietary fibre hypothesis; a historical perspective**. In: Schweizer TF, Edwards CA eds. Dietary fibre: a component of food. London: Springer-Verlag, 1992: 3-20.

6   *British Nutrition Foundation.* **Task Force Report. Complex carbohydrates in foods**. London: Chapman & Hall, 1991.

7   McCance RA, Widdowson EM, Shackleton LRB. **The nutritive value of fruits, vegetables and nuts**. Medical Research Council Special Report Series No. 213. London: HMSO, 1936.

8   Widdowson EM, McCance RA. **The available carbohydrates of fruits. Determination of glucose, fructose, sucrose and starch.** Biochem J 1935; **29:** 151-156.

9   Southgate DAT. **Determination of food carbohydrates.** 2nd ed. London: Elsevier Applied Science Publishers, 1991.

10 McCance RA, Shipp HL. **The chemistry of flesh foods and their losses on cooking.** Medical Research Council Special Report Series No. 187. London: HMSO, 1933.

11 Widdowson EM. **A study of individual children's diets.** Medical Research Council Special Report Series No. 257. London: HMSO, 1947.

12 McCance RA. **The ionisable and available iron in foods.** Chem & Ind 1939; **58:** 528.

13 McCance RA, Widdowson EM. **Mineral metabolism of healthy adults on white and brown bread dietaries.** J Physiol 1942; **101:** 44.

14 McCance RA, Widdowson EM. **The chemical composition of foods.** Medical Research Council Special Report Series No. 235. 2nd ed. London: HMSO, 1946.

15 Widdowson EM, McCance RA. **Studies on the nutritive value of bread and the effects of variations in the extraction rate of flour on the growth of undernourished children.** Medical Research Council Special Report Series No. 287. London: HMSO, 1954.

16 Widdowson EM, Southgate DAT. **Haemorrhage and tissue electrolytes.** Biochem J 1959; **72:** 200-204.

17 Southgate DAT, Greenfield H. **Principles for the preparation of nutritional data bases and food composition tables.** In: International Food Data Bases and Information Exchange. Simopoulos AP, Butrum RR eds. World Review of Nutrition. Vol 68. Basel: Karger, 1992: 27-48.

18 Greenfield H, Southgate DAT. **Production and management of food composition data.** London: Elsevier Applied Science Publishers, 1992.

19 McCance RA, Widdowson EM. **The composition of foods.** 3rd edition. Medical Research Council Special Report Series No. 297. London: HMSO, 1960.

20 *Paul AA, Southgate DAT.* McCance and Widdowson's **The Composition of Foods.** 4th edition. London: HMSO, 1978.

21 *Holland B, Welch AA, Unwin ID, Buss DH, Paul AA, Southgate DAT.* McCance and Widdowson's **The Composition of Foods**. 5th ed. Cambridge: Royal Society of Chemistry, 1991.

22 *Southgate DAT.* **Guidelines for the preparation of tables of food composition**. Basel: Karger, 1974.

23 *West CE* ed. **Eurofoods: towards compatibility of nutrient data banks in Europe**. Annals of Nutrition & Metabolism 1985; **29:** Supplement 1.

Mineral metabolism
by Douglas Black

INTRODUCTION

It is a privilege to be associated with the celebration of what must be, through its combination of duration and productivity, a unique scientific partnership. It has lasted for upwards of half a century, and has made major discoveries in several fields of nutritional science and physiology. This chapter is limited—if that be the right word—to the contribution of RA McCance and EM Widdowson to knowledge of mineral metabolism. Even so, the diversity of their contribution suggests that it should be reviewed selectively rather than comprehensively. Further, although what is sometimes called the 'lead role' may have varied from one study to another, there was in all the studies the closest intellectual and practical collaboration between Mac and Elsie; visiting workers orbited irregularly around that binary star of the first magnitude.

THE BACKGROUND

Some parts of what was known of mineral metabolism by the early 1930s had been laid down in the previous century. As early as 1873, Bunge had written on the significance of sodium chloride, and its occurrence in the human body; he had even observed in balance experiments a reciprocal relationship between sodium and potassium. Sidney Ringer had demonstrated the sensitivity of heart muscle to changes in the electrolyte composition of the surrounding medium. It had been discovered, forgotten, and rediscovered that the replacement of the fluid lost by the vomiting and diarrhoea of cholera required salt as well as water.

More important, perhaps, than those isolated observations, was the imaginative generalisation of Claude Bernard, that constancy of the internal environment is a precondition of the proper functioning of cells, and thus of life itself (*'La fixité du milieu interne est la condition de la vie libre'*). In the earlier decades of the present century, some of the clinical syndromes arising from disturbances of body fluid were beginning to be recognised—the circulatory collapse of body fluid depletion, the iatrogenic alkalosis of peptic ulcer therapy, water intoxication after administration of pituitary antidiuretic hormone as a provocative test for epilepsy.

Retroscopic analysis (that dangerous tool) may allow us to distinguish several reasons why, around 1930, the time had become ripe for highly significant advances in the knowledge of mineral metabolism, and in the application of that knowledge in clinical medicine and surgery. At the most general level, the discovery of insulin had shown that major therapeutic advance could come directly from a basis of biochemical knowledge, in contrast to previous major discoveries like that of digitalis, which had stemmed from serendipitous clinical observation.

From a completely different discipline, Moynihan had ventured the claim, 'We have made surgery safe for the patient, we must now make the patient safe for surgery'—an enterprise which called for informed pre-operative and post-operative fluid replacement. And the development of paediatrics, and especially of 'neonatology' as a discipline, revealed the vulnerability of infants and children to fluid loss—it is not an accident that so much of the pioneer work on mineral metabolism came from paediatricians such as Gamble, Darrow and Kerpel-Fronius. Of course age-related changes in mineral metabolism and renal function have been an abiding interest, reviewed with typical breadth of vision by McCance himself[1].

These prior incentives to take an interest in mineral metabolism were reinforced by improved analytical methods. The most important advance in these, the use of flame photometry, still lay in the future; but reliable methods of estimating sodium and potassium were supplementing the estimation of chloride and bicarbonate, and making possible what was to prove a more significant means for unravelling the skein which Gamble called 'the companionship of water and electrolytes'.

It would be both inappropriate and unfair to regard the studies of Mac and Elsie on mineral metabolism simply as manifestations of the *Zeitgeist*, even though that may have made some contribution to their inception, technical possibility, and timely acceptance. Fortunately, the studies themselves are innovative enough to dispel any such notions. Not only did they introduce a valuable technique of investigation, that of self-conducted balance studies on experimental diets; but also their first major foray into the field of mineral metabolism led to the clear separation of salt and of water depletion, previously lumped together under the term 'dehydration'.

EXPERIMENTAL SALT DEPLETION

In 1635 a bequest from Dr Theodore Goulston to the Royal College of Physicians provided for an annual series of lectures, to be given by one of the four youngest Fellows of the College, and 300 years later, the Goulstonian lectures[2] were given by RA McCance; in them he described a group of observations which have arguably had greater influence than any other comparable studies on our knowledge of the metabolism of body fluid, and on the practical application of that knowledge.

There are many clinical situations in which salt deficiency is one component of the biochemical disturbance—for example, diabetic coma, miner's cramp, heat exhaustion, Addison's disease, infantile gastro-enteritis, and cholera. Much had already been written about them, and McCance's second lecture reviews what can be gleaned from the literature and from clinical observation. But it is at the beginning of the third lecture that he sets out the rationale for the experimental study of salt depletion in man.

Many patients with clinical salt depletion are too ill to be studied in adequate detail. The clinical picture is complicated, and possibly distorted by the features of the disease, which is responsible for the loss of salt; and there are liable, in a clinical situation, to be disturbances of body fluid other than salt depletion, such as acidosis or alkalosis, depletion of water and of electrolytes other than salt. Then comes the forecast, simply and clearly expressed: 'It occurred to me that if I could produce a simple sodium-chloride deficiency in a normal animal or person, uncomplicated by forced dehydration, change of reaction, or any other concurrent morbid process, I might be able to throw some light on the pathology of this group of diseases.'

The studies which followed were not only important in themselves, they also foreshadowed future studies on other aspects of body fluid, using an experimental design whose marks were the production of an uncomplicated deficiency; the use of a previously *normal* subject; and a preference for the *human* model: 'Man is the best experimental *animal* to employ in this type of research, and I decided to use him.'

The method chosen for inducing salt depletion was profuse thermal sweating in a radiant heat bath, combined with a diet very low in salt. The losses of salt and of water in the sweat were measured, only the loss of water being replaced. Even with this exacting regime of mineral intake and induced massive losses of salt, an unequivocal state of sodium deficiency took over a week to achieve, by which time biochemical changes and associated symptoms had appeared. The ultimate sodium deficit was of the order of 800 milliequivalents, representing about a sixth of all the sodium in the body, but about a quarter of that which is not sequestrated in the bones, and as much as a half of what is normally present in extracellular fluid.

As might be expected from the predominance of sodium among the cations of plasma and extracellular fluid, there was not only a decrease in sodium concentration in plasma, which may be related to the muscle cramps experienced by the subjects; but also evidence of the decreased volume of plasma and extracellular tissue fluid. This was hinted at by breathlessness on exertion, but perhaps more directly indicated by a threefold rise in blood urea, indicative of substantial decrease in blood flow to the kidneys.

Subjective symptoms are difficult to assess in the subjects of self-experiment; but there is an internal consistency in the reported experiences which may give them objective validity, especially as similar symptoms are encountered in clinical states of sodium depletion. The symptoms included taste disturbance, loss of appetite, and frank nausea with abdominal discomfort; breathlessness and tiredness, especially on what might be quite minimal exertion; muscle cramps and tiredness, again especially on exertion—one subject found that his arm became tired with shaving, and his jaw with eating. Further validation of these subjective elements came from their rapid disappearance when sodium balance was restored.

This clear delineation of the effects of sodium depletion, attended by only minimal depletion of water, was a milestone in the understanding of the separate effects of sodium and water depletion. But the significance of these experiments and their interpretation goes beyond theoretical understanding into practical application, and this has indeed been characteristic of much of the work done by Mac and Elsie. To give just one example, in the context of heat stress which was soon to become a practical hazard in desert warfare, it enabled the syndrome of 'heat exhaustion' to be identified with moderate salt depletion, and appropriate measures to be undertaken[3].

EXPERIMENTAL WATER DEPLETION

As we have just seen, the studies on experimental salt depletion arose mainly from the wish to understand more fully what was happening in various clinical situations, but were followed later by practical application. In partial contrast, the studies on water depletion themselves arose at least in part as direct responses to two problems in 1942: namely, those of soldiers isolated in the desert and of shipwrecked mariners in lifeboats. But rational practical measures presuppose some science-based analysis, and the search for practical steps may then contribute to scientific knowledge.

In this group of experiments, two normal subjects were studied by the techniques of metabolic balance[4], and a further ten were observed with particular reference to renal function[5]. In the metabolic studies, a self-selected, somewhat dry, diet was kept constant throughout a preliminary period when fluids were drunk as desired, a dehydration period when no fluid was given, and a rehydration period of controlled intake of water. There is, of course, no such thing as a completely 'dry' diet, for almost all foods contain some water, and water is also generated in the metabolism of the major nutrients. However, water derived in these ways averaged only 183ml/day (from food) and 399ml/day (from metabolism).

That the dehydrating regime was nevertheless effective is shown by a negative water balance of 3530ml in both subjects after three to four days of dehydration. In striking contrast to the situation in salt depletion, this considerable loss of water was not associated with net loss of electrolyte, there being a small retention of sodium and chloride, and a still smaller negative balance of potassium. In further contrast to salt depletion, plasma volume was well maintained. Loss of water with no corresponding loss of those electrolytes which determine the osmolality of body fluids must lead to an increase in their osmolality, and this was indeed indicated by a rise in plasma sodium of the order of 10% in both subjects. As might be expected from the amount of water lost, both subjects lost weight (3.8kg) during the dehydration period. Subjectively, there was of course some thirst, but this was less troublesome than the difficulty of masticating and swallowing dry foods. The days of dehydration passed slowly, but there was no very definite feeling of illness.

It is of course difficult to infer from the findings after a short, but rigorous, period of water depletion what might be the cause of death after prolonged water deprivation; but the inexorable increase in the osmolality of body fluid was put forward as a likely mechanism, consistent with earlier work in animals suggesting that 'the rise in the total osmotic pressure of the body and not the accumulation of any specific substance was the cause of death'. Used as a working hypothesis, this view naturally directs attention to the kidneys, one aspect of whose function is the maintenance of the osmolality of the body fluids. Under the particular stress of water deprivation, the requirement is to excrete in the urine the maximum quantity of osmotically active substances (mainly urea and electrolytes) in the least possible amount of water—in other and possibly plainer words, to excrete a maximally concentrated urine.

The studies on the performance of the kidneys[5] showed that under conditions of dehydration renal blood flow and glomerular filtration rate were well maintained, and the urine reached osmolalities (calculated from urea, sodium and potassium) of the order of 1000 milliosmoles/l. Not unexpectedly, the loss of water in the urine was greater on a diet high in salt than on one low in salt; and a high protein intake would also increase the osmotic load requiring excretion.

These observations on the effects of water depletion on the composition of body fluid and on renal function, carried practical implications. Men lost in the desert without water had been known to drink their own urine, but 'a dehydrated man can do himself no good by drinking his own urine. By so doing, he is merely asking his kidneys to repeat work which they have already done, and cannot be expected to do better'[5]. Animals such as the gerbil can of course survive in the desert without water, other than that derived from their diet, but they do so by being able to produce urine several times more concentrated than maximally concentrated human urine.

There was a conflict in the advice given to lifeboat crews early in the War—whether to take small amounts of sea water, to add some sea water to the fresh-water ration carried in limited amount, or to abstain entirely from sea water. Since sea water has an osmolality much greater than that of maximally concentrated human urine, it would seem likely that any temporary relief would be outweighed by greater long-term damage arising from the addition of osmotically active salts, which cannot be fully disposed of, to the body.

CALCIUM ABSORPTION

A notable feature of the scientific collaboration which we are celebrating has been the ability to pursue effectively and simultaneously more than one major theme. The results of the salt-depletion experiments were published in the same year (1940) as the first edition of Food tables. And at the same time as the studies on water deprivation, work was in full progress on the factors determining calcium absorption in the Wartime diet.

Before the outbreak of the Second World War in 1939, much of Britain's bread had been made from imported grain, and much of it was white, ie, made with flour of about 70% extraction, the discarded elements of the grain, including 'unavailable carbohydrate' being diverted to animal feeding—'the husks that the swine did eat', to their nutritional benefit. When shipping space was diverted to Wartime needs, and further restricted by submarine warfare, economy in grain imports was achieved in part by the introduction of the 'National loaf', made from 85% flour. At the same time, there were restrictions on the supply of dairy products, the major source of dietary calcium; and the question arose whether an increase in the extraction percentage of flour, together with diminished intake of calcium from other sources, might impair an optimal balance of calcium.

It takes a measure of boldness to claim that any biological question has been answered, for one problem tends to lead to another; but such a claim might be justified, at least at the practical level, on behalf of the studies carried out in Cambridge[6], on the effects of bread of different extractions on mineral absorption. Balance experiments were carried out on five men and five women over a period of nine months, on diets in which 40-50% of the calorie intake came from flour of 69% or 92% extraction.

The effect of fortifying each type of flour with calcium carbonate was studied; of adding sodium phytate (known to form complexes with calcium) to 69% extraction flour; and of taking calciferol made up in arachis oil on a crust of bread made from 92% extraction flour (calciferol as it turned out had little effect on calcium absorption from the diets made up with the 92% flour). But it was clearly shown that less calcium was absorbed when the flour was of the higher extraction; that the addition of sodium phytate depressed the absorption of calcium; and that fortification of flour with calcium salts was an effective way of increasing calcium absorption.

Clear-cut results can justify clear-cut recommendations. These were set out thus:

> 'It has been recommended that flours for national use during the present emergency should have calcium carbonate added to them in the following proportions: white flour, 65mg of calcium per 100g; National 85% wheatmeal, 120mg of calcium per 100g; 92% wheatmeal, 200mg of calcium per 100g.'

The triumph of common sense is seldom rapid. Some critics, the forerunners of the opponents of fluoridation, invoked the propriety of adding 'chemicals' to something consumed by all. Others had worries superficially more specific, like a possible increased risk of heart disease. But in the end, Wartime fortification of bread with calcium salts was accepted and implemented.

Before leaving this theme, I cannot resist quoting in full a paragraph which sets out the distinction between the 'medicine of individuals' and the 'medicine of populations', in terms which should be a constant guide to those who advise on dietary matters:

> 'In making these recommendations, it seems wise at the same time to sound a note of warning. The Ministry of Food thinks—and must think—in terms of national requirements. If the nation is short of calcium because its milk supplies have been curtailed, the simplest way of putting this right (from the Government's point of view) is to add calcium to bread—because everyone eats bread. But people will not change their dietary habits to please the Ministry of Food. The large milk consumer may—or may not—become the big bread eater when his favourite beverage is restricted. Hence, many who were well supplied with calcium may go short, and, vice versa, many who were taking very little may suddenly find themselves with more than they had before. It is clear, therefore, that although the addition of calcium to bread may maintain the nation's calcium intake at its previous level, there will be a great deal of watchful care needed on the part of those responsible for the well-being of individuals'[6].

CONCLUSION

I am well aware that three vignettes of particular studies, however important, cannot do full justice to the breadth and depth of the contribution which Mac and Elsie have made to our knowledge of mineral metabolism. Some further aspects of their contribution are the proper province of the chapters on the composition of food and of the body. A leading article in the *Lancet* of 1936, commenting on the

Goulstonian Lectures, predicted that, 'Dr McCance's lectures should stimulate others to pay more attention to fluid metabolism'. This seems to have happened; and the technique of detailed studies of 'pure' distortions of body fluid in normal human subjects, pioneered by them, has been exploited by others, including some who derived it from the fountainhead[7,8].

References

1. *McCance RA.* **Age and renal function**. In: Black DAK, ed. *Renal Disease*, 1st ed. Oxford: Blackwell Scientific Publications, 1962: 157-170.

2. *McCance RA.* **Medical problems in mineral metabolism**. Lancet 1936; **i:** 643- 650, 704-710, 765-768, 823-830.

3. *Ladell WSS, Waterlow JC Hudson MF.* **Desert climate. Physiological and clinical observations**. Lancet 1944; **ii:** 491-497, 527-531.

4. *Black DAK, McCance RA, Young WF.* **A study of dehydration by means of balance experiments**. J Physiol 1942; **102:** 406-414.

5. *McCance RA, Young WF.* **The secretion of urine during dehydration and rehydration**. J Physiol 1944; **102:** 415-428.

6. *McCance RA, Widdowson EM.* **Mineral metabolism of healthy adults on white and brown bread dietaries**. J Physiol 1942; **101:** 44-85.

7. *Black DAK, Milne MD.* **Experimental potassium depletion in man**. Clin Sci 1952; **11:** 397-417.

8. *Fourman P.* **Depletion of potassium induced in man with an exchange resin**. Clin Sci 1954; **13:** 93-110.

Body composition
by John Dickerson

INTRODUCTION

It is a pleasure to be able to contribute to this very special book in honour of two colleagues and friends, Professor McCance (Mac) and Dr Elsie Widdowson, who have made a unique and unsurpassed contribution to nutrition science. Their lively professional interest in body composition was already well developed when I joined the Department of Experimental Medicine in Cambridge in 1952. Well known for their work on the composition of food, perhaps it was not surprising that they should have turned their attention to the composition of the body.

A paper on the *Composition of the body*, published in an issue of the *British Medical Bulletin* in 1951[1], contained references to eight of their own papers. My first introduction to the subject, if I may thus describe it, was seeing tanks containing thick brown sludge, on and under the laboratory bench, labelled 'Pig 1, 2 or 3', etc. There were also Winchester bottles containing similar 'brews' which periodically became exhibits at one of Elsie's Part 2 physiological lectures. Solutions of urea and sodium thiocyanate were also made up for practicals associated with these lectures and used by the students to measure their total body water and extracellular fluid.

Two or three years later, I was given the opportunity to start work on aspects of body composition with them. Opportunities like this often mould careers and this one has made a generous contribution to mine. It was characteristic of Mac and Elsie that they drew others into the various aspects of their work and in so doing shared their enthusiasm and vision. In retrospect, it is clear that it is in no small part this ability to stimulate others that has enabled them to make such a lasting contribution to nutrition science. Those we honour have not only won our respect as scientists, they have our affection as friends.

In trying to put their work on body composition in perspective, I shall give what amounts to no more than a thumbnail sketch of some of our work. In doing so, I am conscious of the limitations of mere words. It is somewhat like trying to present the beauty of a sunset in a black and white photograph. For me, revisiting this work brings back memories of a personal kind—regular visits and discussions, keen interest, Mac's 'cycling thoughts', the many tables, as each set of analytical results was added to the picture. All these are peculiarly mine. They are part of the 'colour' which cannot be conveyed on the printed page.

WHOLE BODY

In our review on the *Chemical composition of the body*[2], Elsie and I compared the composition of the body as revealed by chemical analysis to 'a snapshot of a busy street full of pedestrians and automobiles...essentially the static reproduction of a dynamic scene, full of individual and collective activity'. Determination of the composition of adult man by chemical analysis presents considerable difficulties; particularly if one wants a picture of a healthy body, for healthy persons do not die, except as a result of accident or suicide. Having identified and obtained a suitable body, with permission from its custodians for its disposal in this way, one is still left with the problem of its quantitative analysis.

Up to 1945, our knowledge of the chemical composition of the adult human body was limited to that published by Moleshott in Germany in 1859. Then, in 1945 values appeared for the composition of a man who had died of a heart attack. In 1953-1956, values were published, also from the US, for the composition of three more men[2]. In the meantime, Mac and Elsie had published their results for the bodies of two men and a woman. The technique used to handle quantitatively the 62kg, 72kg and 45kg respectively of material was to macerate it in hydrochloric acid and then to analyse the mixture for fat, total nitrogen (N), calcium (Ca), magnesium (Mg), phosphorus (P), sodium (Na), potassium (K), iron (Fe), zinc (Zn) and copper (Cu), by standard chemical procedures. Water was obtained by difference.

When we put together the results for the analyses of these bodies and those from the US, we came to the conclusion that the sum total of the information available for the composition of adult man in the best degree of health was limited to that for four men and one woman[2]. These included two of those analysed in Cambridge. Thus, 40% of the worldwide information came from the Cambridge laboratory.

Human fetuses and stillborn babies are of a more manageable size and a number of them were analysed in Europe around 1900. For the results of such analyses to be used as a basis for the calculation of nutrition requirements for fetal growth by the factorial method, it is essential that they are obtained in a systematic fashion over the period of gestation. The Cambridge laboratory undertook such a study and the results for 24 fetuses, varying in weight from 0.75g to 4373g have been published[2].

This work included determinations of water, total N and fat in each fetus, of K, Ca, P and Mg in most, and of Fe, Cu and Zn in about two-thirds. The results showed a fall in the proportion of water from 924g to 585g per kg body tissue between the youngest and the oldest fetus. Fat began to be deposited at a body weight of about 670g, reaching about 150g per kg at about 3000g, with the heaviest fetus containing 283g per kg. Much of the fat in man at all ages is subcutaneous and hence acts as a layer of insulation. Babies of low birth weight, and especially those of very low birth weight, contain very thin layers of fat, which has an important influence on their care.

Systematic determinations of the changes in body composition during fetal growth make possible the calculation of the probable accretion rates of different body constituents. These are then a basis for the elaboration, for instance, of nutrient solutions for the intravenous feeding of very low-birth-weight babies in which it seems desirable to try to reproduce outside the uterus, the growth rate which would have been likely, had the baby remained in the uterus for the proper time[3].

Man is one of the few species which at birth contains large amounts of fat; others include the guinea pig. The bodies of newborn rats, rabbits, cats and pigs contain only about 10g per kg of tissue. Considerable amounts of fat are then laid down during suckling. Information about comparative aspects of body composition and physiology are an essential prerequisite if such species are to be used in experiments with relevance to man. At the same physiological milestone, birth, mammals differ widely in their degree of development and this is reflected in the composition of their organs and tissues.

About a quarter of a century before Mac and Elsie's systematic studies on chemical development, Moulton[4] had put forward the concept of 'chemical maturity'. This was defined as the stage in development at which the water, N and salts reached a constant proportion of the fat-free body tissue. The work done at Cambridge showed that the inorganic constituents do not all reach a constant proportion at the same time, and that although the idea of 'chemical maturity' has been useful, it requires elaboration and further definition, if it is to be used for detail. It is doubtful if the age of chemical maturity of man can ever be determined due to the extent of individual variation[1].

The challenge in the assessment of body composition, 'the central problem', as it was described with the prophetic insight[1], 'has always been the determination of the composition of living men, women and children at different stages of health and development'. Often the impetus for the development of techniques in physiology and nutrition has been the need for information about disease processes. Around 1945, FD Moore was starting his work on body composition in surgical patients using 'dilution methods'. This work did much to popularise in clinical work the appreciation of the value of measuring body compartments and was summarised in the equation:

$$\text{MAN} = \underbrace{\text{Body Cell Mass} + \text{Extracellular Mass}}_{\text{Lean Body Mass}} + \text{Fat}$$

At the same time, Sir David Cuthbertson was continuing his work on the metabolic response to injury, following his original paper in 1930[5] in which he described the considerable increase in urinary N excretion which follows bone injury. From the ratios of N:S in the urine, Cuthbertson concluded that the bulk of the N excreted came from the breakdown of muscle protein.

The importance of these changes in body composition, to recovery after injury or operation, has been one factor contributing to the continued search for techniques that can be used to measure the constituents of the living human body. A recent review from the Dunn Nutrition Laboratory in Cambridge[6], concluded that *in vivo* neutron activation[7] is probably the most useful of the techniques available. Instead of depending on the measurement of the volume of distribution of radioisotopes and other substances, as Moore, and indeed our colleagues, had done, this technique makes use of the fact that when the body is irradiated with fast neutrons, gamma rays are emitted as products of interactions between neutrons and the nuclei of elements in the body. It may be that the solution to the 'central problem' is within sight.

SKELETAL MUSCLE

The structure and chemical composition of the adult mammalian organism is reached by a process of differential growth. Skeletal muscle accounts for about 20% of the body weight of a newborn baby, whereas in the adult the proportion has increased to about 40%. Muscle proteins represent a reserve of amino acids that can be drawn upon in periods of nutritional deprivation, or as a result of metabolic stress, such as that after injury. It seemed logical that this tissue should receive our attention. Others had analysed muscle in various nutritional and medical conditions, but ours was, and I think still is, the only systematic detailed study of the effects of growth and development on this tissue. Histological examination alone indicated that growth is associated with an increase in cell mass. In the human sartorius muscle the adult number of fibres is acquired by the end of gestation and subsequent increase in size is due to increase in size of existing fibres.

The challenge presented to us was to find if there is a change in the composition of the muscle cell during growth, recognising that it is practically impossible to separate these cells for analysis. Constituents had to be partitioned between the cellular and extracellular components of the tissue. We were interested particularly in the ratio of fluid to solid, ie, the degree of hydration of the cells. Earlier, Marion

Harrison (later Marion Robinson) had studied the composition of the liver cell[8] and the effects of starvation upon it[9], using DNA as a base of reference for other cellular constituents, on the assumption that the amount of DNA in a diploid nucleus is species specific and constant. Since the major 'solid' component of the cells is protein, it seemed reasonable to use intracellular protein N as a base of reference in our studies[10].

The amount of water per kg of fat-free quadriceps muscle falls steadily during development, due to an increase in the deposition of protein. The large increase in cell mass which this represents causes a decrease in the volume of extracellular fluid as shown by a fall in the amount of chloride (Cl). These changes agree with the changes in histological structure, as also do the changes in the amount of extracellular protein; this increases during fetal life as the number of fibres increases and falls during postnatal life when growth is by increase in size of existing fibres. The amount of protein relative to water in the cells increases within the progress of development.

Following their studies of the effects of undernutrition in Germany after the Second World War, Mac and Elsie initiated in-depth studies in experimental animals. Interest in the effects of undernutrition on growth was not new. Jackson in 1925[11] had produced a book on the subject. However, it is probable that the studies done by our colleagues were on a scale not previously attempted and not likely to be repeated. Pigs, rats and chickens were used, each with advantages for the particular study in which they were involved. As a reminder of the words of Claude Bernard in his *Introduction to the study of experimental medicine* (1865), Elsie quoted in her EV McCollum International lecture[12], 'The solution of a physiological or pathological problem often depends solely on the appropriate choice of the animal for the experiment'.

The studies on pigs, in particular, became internationally well known. Some of the undernourished animals weighed only about 4-5kg at one year of age; their well-nourished litter mates weighed about 170kg at the same age. Among the many investigations carried out on these animals[13], we analysed the quadriceps muscle. The composition resembled in some ways that of muscle from a 90-day-old fetus with a large amount of extracellular fluid (measured as the 'Cl space'), increased concentrations of Na and decreased concentrations of K. The muscle cells had evidently shrunk as a result of the undernutrition, for the amount of cellular protein was greatly reduced and the cells were over-hydrated. In contrast, the amount of extracellular protein was greatly increased, possibly due to the 'metabolic inertia' of collagen in some parts of the body[14].

In the 1950s, it was still considered that kwashiorkor was due to a diet that contained too little protein relative to energy. In an experiment in which young rats were given a restricted amount of a high-protein diet in order to keep their body weight at a similar level to those of animals receiving a low-protein diet, some of the animals receiving the high-protein diet died. In another experiment of a similar sort[15], a number of animals receiving limited amounts of a high-protein diet again died. The muscles of these animals contained much higher concentrations of Na (136 mmoles/kg) and lower concentrations of K (47 mmoles/kg) than those of the animals that survived (92.3 and 71 mmoles/kg respectively). It seemed that the muscle cells of the animals that died had lost the ability to extrude Na and retain K; that the low-energy, high-protein diet had interfered with the energy-dependent sodium pump mechanism.

There is no doubt that using a variety of species increases the flexibility of experimental design. In our studies, the larger the animal, the greater the degree of growth retardation that could be achieved by undernutrition. Pigs were perhaps ideal, but expensive. The fowl is a compromise species. By feeding a small amount of a good diet to chicks from two to three weeks of age, their growth can be restricted to 100g in six months. Controls that were fed the diet *ad lib* grew to 3500g in the same time.

The muscular system is composed of a number of different muscles which grow at different rates, a fact exploited in the production of domestic meat animals[16]. We found that the pectoral muscles which grow later than the sartorius, were affected much more by undernutrition, and showed similar changes in composition to those we had found in the pigs[17].

Dr Robert Montgomery had been studying the effect of protein-energy malnutrition (PEM) on the structure of human sartorius muscles in Jamaica, and when he joined us the opportunity was taken to compare the chemical and histological changes in the sartorius muscles of the undernourished chickens[18]. There was a good degree of agreement between the results of the two approaches. Chemically, the changes induced by underfeeding were not very different from those induced in human infants by PEM but differences in histology convinced us that the chemical approach had severe limitations and should always be supported by morphological study. Childhood malnutrition has a complex aetiology[19] and it is therefore not surprising that its effects are not reproduced by simple dietary deficiency. Be this as it may, in many hospital patients the effects of dietary deficiency are superimposed on the metabolic consequences of disease[20]. Our work has emphasised the vulnerability of skeletal muscle and helps us to understand why, after a severe illness, the ability to do a full day's work often takes a long time to return to normal.

SKIN

'The skin is an organ that all can see'[21] but its contribution to the composition of the body has often been overlooked. The effects of malnutrition on its structure and integrity may be an important cause of life-threatening disease in children in poor countries. Skin may also lose its integrity as a secondary consequence of disease in countries like our own. In adult man, the skin may account for about 7% of the fat-free weight and about 10% of the body protein. Subcutaneous fat, besides being an energy reserve, and playing an important role in temperature control, acts as a protective 'cushion' for underlying organs and tissues.

From an analytical view, the skin presents unique problems because of its form and structure. The composition, expressed per unit fat-free weight, gives only part of the picture. During growth there is the usual fall in the proportion of water and increase in the amount of protein, with increasing age between a fetal age of 13-14 weeks to a postnatal age of three to five months[22].

In contrast to skeletal muscle, there are difficulties in calculating the distribution of water due to the fact that some of the Cl, and possibly Na, is inside the cells and that the principal protein of the dermis, collagen, binds the Cl ion. The concentration of this protein increases rapidly during the second half of gestation and during the first few months of postnatal life. At all ages, over 66% of the water in human skin is outside the cells, though its distribution changes as more collagen is laid down. The proportion of water associated with the cells increases to a maximum in the newborn baby and falls to a lower level in the adult. This change roughly parallels the cellular constituents.

When we reviewed the literature on the composition of skin[2] we noted a large discrepancy in the values reported for potassium by different workers. Workers who had analysed the entire skin of either man or the rat reported values for K which were about twice those in which pieces had been analysed. Our study of shaved rat skin[23] showed that the composition varied from different sites of the same animal and from the same site in the two sexes. It is affected by the thickness of the epidermis relative to the dermis, by the density of hair follicles and glands and by the presence of other structures such as muscle fibres.

In man, variations in skin composition and structure may account for the proneness of certain areas of skin to certain diseases. Furthermore, variations in structure might help us to understand why, in a generalised disease, such as kwashiorkor, some areas of skin are affected more than others.

We have seen that the extracellular protein of skeletal muscle, predominantly collagen, is resistant to metabolic breakdown in even severely undernourished animals. However, the collagen of the dermis of the skin does not show the same 'metabolic inertia'. It is, in fact, quite rapidly broken down. The susceptibility of skin collagen to nutritional deprivation, together with the effect of such deprivation on cell multiplication in the epidermis, and loss of subcutaneous fat, is an important factor in the aetiology of pressure sores in malnourished and elderly patients.

THE SKELETON
Mac and Elsie have had a long-standing interest in calcium metabolism. Some 99% of the body's content of this mineral is in the skeleton. The fact that development is associated with growth and age-related mineralisation of secondary centres of ossification in the long bones is used to assess physiological age in children. The development of cortical bone tissue is associated with an increase in the degree of calcification, as shown by a rise in the Ca:N ratio[24]. However, none of these studies included fetal and postnatal bones and in no study that we could find was the development of a long bone and its cortex addressed.

With Mac and Elsie's encouragement, I undertook what is, I believe, the only study of its kind of the chemical development of the human femur[25], which included femora from 62 subjects varying in age from 12 weeks gestation to 35 years. At all ages, cortical bone, and up to 12 years of age, epiphyses were analysed. The remainder of each bone was also analysed so that the composition of the whole bone could be obtained. Perhaps the most interesting finding from these analyses was that the Ca:N ratio in the cortex, after increasing during gestation, did not rise significantly during the first nine months of postnatal life. This was reminiscent of the fall in the percentage of calcium which had been reported previously in the cortex of kitten bones during early postnatal life.

The cancellous bone of the metaphysis is more susceptible to calcium deficiency than cortical bone. When this was included in our bone samples, the Ca:N ratio of the non-epiphysial parts of the bone fell significantly during early postnatal life. This suggested that the dietary mineral supply during the first few months after birth is insufficient to keep pace with the growth of the bone. Kitten bones show this fall in mineralisation after birth to a greater degree than human bones, and an experiment in newborn kittens[26] showed that it could be partially prevented by giving a supplement of calcium phosphate. We have now concluded that competition for dietary phosphate, induced by the rapid growth of soft tissues, is the probable cause of the fall in bone calcification in the kitten and possibly also in human babies.

Malnutrition reduces bone growth and delays skeletal development. Conversely, overnutrition accelerates these processes[27]. When bone age, as indicated by radiological evidence, is compared with chronological age, the assumption is made that the latter is what should determine bone development. This is true up to a point, but forcing or restricting nutrition may so alter the rate at which bone develops that it masks the usual effect of chronological age, that is that it disturbs the 'harmony of growth'[28].

For obvious reasons, little information is available about the capacity of the human skeleton to recover from a period of retarded growth. In the rat, the capacity for recovery varies in different bones of the skeleton, according to the timing of retardation with respect to the age at which the peak rate velocity of growth of the individual bones occurs[29]. The growth and development of the pelvis seems to be particularly vulnerable to nutritional deprivation early in life; a fact which I believe is recognised in countries in which childhood PEM is endemic.

THE BRAIN

The brain is unique among the organs of the body in that it contains practically no neutral fat and that its high-lipid content is due to complex lipids present in its membranes. We had only a passing interest in the chemical composition of the brain until John Dobbing showed in the rat that undernutrition early in life retarded brain growth and reduced myelination[30]. At that time Davison and Dobbing were formulating their ideas about myelination as a vulnerable period in brain development[31] and we were able to show that this applied also to our undernourished pigs[32].

This introduction to a particular aspect of the chemical composition of the brain led to a series of studies on the effects of development and of PEM on the chemical composition of the human brain. In this we have had the generous collaboration and interest of a number of people, including Professor John Waterlow and Dr Edmond Hey. Dobbing and others had used cholesterol as a marker for assessing the degree of myelination. We continued to do this but we have also been interested in assessing the degree of synaptic development, for which we have used a disialoganglioside as marker.

Our work[33] has shown that the development of dendritic arborisation is specifically retarded in malnourished children, and it is tempting to suggest that this deficit in neuronal connections may contribute to the behavioural defects found in these children. However, the apparent relationship between malnutrition and the development of specific structures, as reflected by chemical composition, is not a simple one, for synaptic development (and possibly other aspects of brain development) are retarded by sensory deprivation, a common feature of the environment in which malnourished children are reared.

CONCLUSION

Body composition is a crucial subject in the science of nutrition, for, 'We are what we eat'. Mac and Elsie have made their own distinctive contributions to it, arising from their interests in infant nutrition and growth. There is a harmony in growth[28] which is manifested by changes in the composition of organs and tissues with time as they acquire their mature structure and function. Undernutrition distorts this harmony by retarding, or even reversing to varying degrees, aspects of the developmental process.

What our colleagues started, others have been able to continue. They lit a torch which they passed on. For me, with John Dobbing's help, it has led to an interest in brain growth, development and function[34]. But beyond this, as I have already hinted, it has led me into clinical nutrition[35]; some of the effects of PEM that we studied are not limited to children in poorer countries but have real relevance for the seriously ill in our own.

As one of those privileged to work with Mac and Elsie, I owe much to their teaching, encouragement and example. Both individually and together, they have been a source of continuing inspiration, help and support.

References

1 *McCance RA, Widdowson EM.* **Composition of the body**. Br Med Bull 1951; **7:** 297-306.

2 *Widdowson EM, Dickerson JWT.* **Chemical composition of the body**. In: Comar C, Bonner F, eds. Mineral Metabolism. London: Academic Press, 1964; **IIA:** 1-247.

3 *Morgan JB, Kovar IZ.* **The low birth weight infant and parenteral nutrition**. Nutr Res Revs 1992; 5; 115-229.

4 *Moulton CR.* **Age and chemical development in mammals**. J Biol Chem 1923; **57:** 79.

5 *Cuthbertson DP.* **The disturbance of metabolism produced by bony and non-bony injury, with notes on certain abnormal conditions of bone**. Biochem J 1930; **24:** 1244-1263.

6 *Coward WA, Parkinson SA, Murgatroyd PR.* **Body composition measurements for nutrition research**. Nutr Res Revs 1988; **1:** 115-124.

7 *Burkinshaw L.* **Measurement of human body composition** *in vivo*. Prog in Med Rad and Phys 1985; **2:** 113-137.

8 *Harrison MF.* **Composition of the liver cell**. Proc Roy Soc B 1953; **141:** 203-216.

9 *Harrison MF.* **Effect of starvation on the composition of the liver cell**. Biochem J 1953; **55:** 204-211.

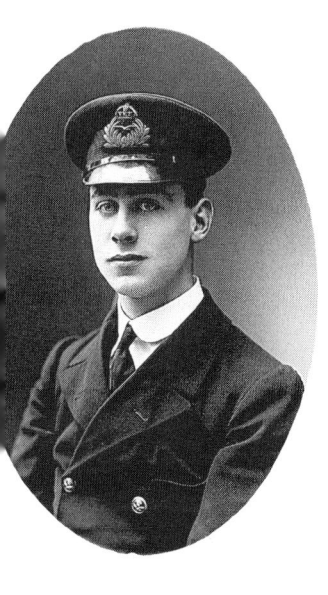

Left
Professor McCance in the uniform of the Royal Naval Air Service, 1917.

Right
Dr Widdowson in London's Hyde Park after the presentation of her Bachelor's degree (BSc) in the Albert Hall, 1928.

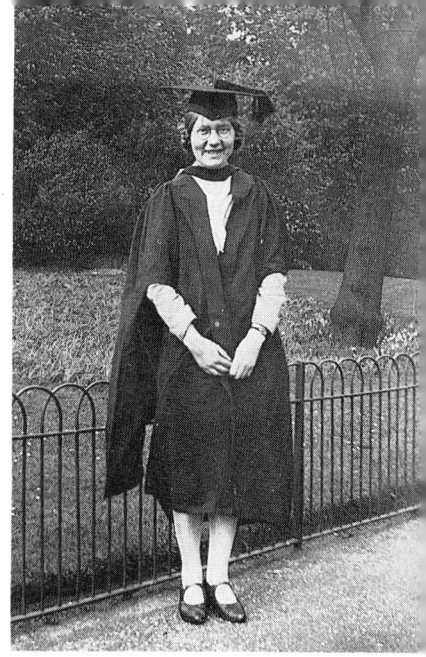

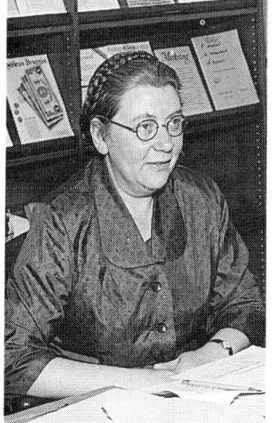

Far left Professor McCance at the Liga dos Combatentes da Grande Guerra, Oporto, Portugal, 1943.

Left Dr Widdowson in Columbus, Ohio, 1959.

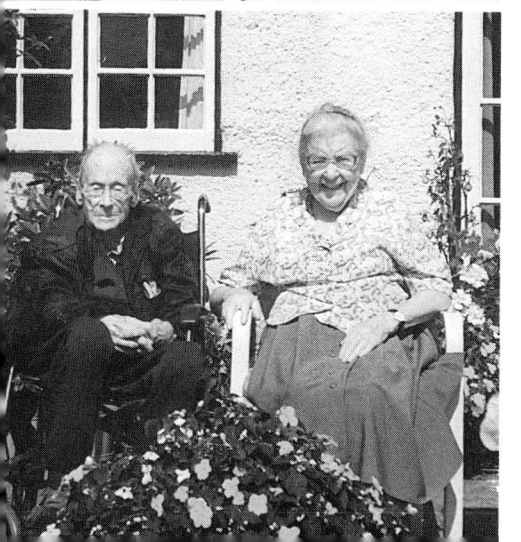

Professor McCance and Dr Widdowson in Dr Widdowson's garden in Barrington, Cambridgeshire, 1991.

I

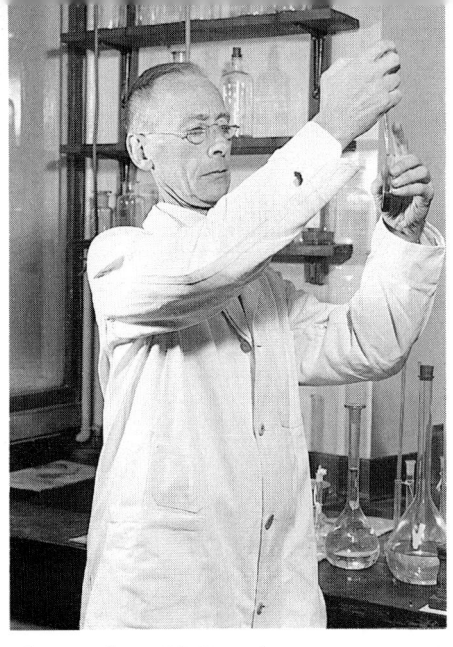

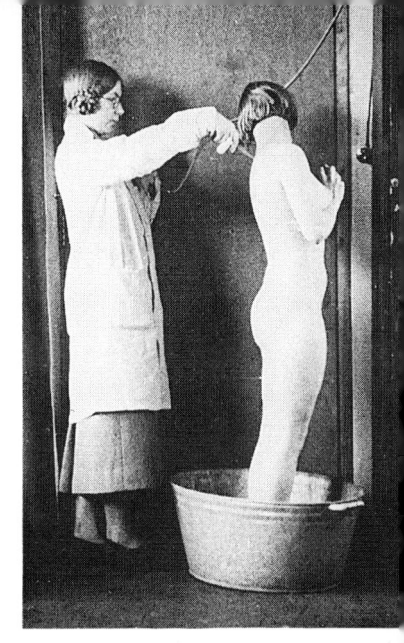

Above Professor McCance in the laboratory at King's College Hospital, 1935.

Above right Dr Widdowson 'washing down' one of the subjects in the salt deficiency experiments, 1934.

An experimental meal in the laboratory at King's College Hospital, 1935.
Left to Right:
Monica Verdon-Roe, AN Other, Dr Widdowson, Margery Masters.

Dr Widdowson injecting herself with solutions of calcium, magnesium and iron, 1934.

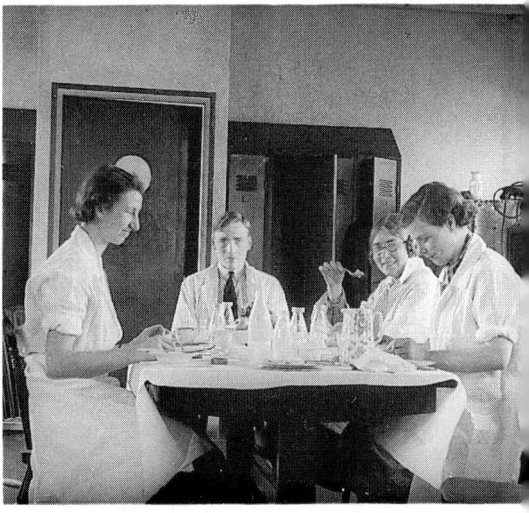

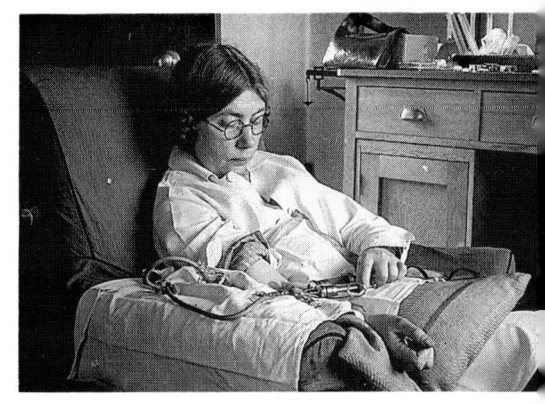

Andrew Huxley resting and calculating his diet after walking in the Lake District. Professor McCance's son, Colin, watches with interest, January 1940.

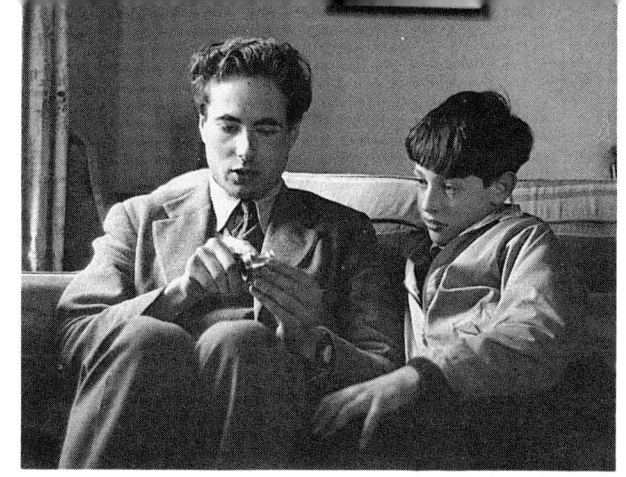

Professor McCance, Dr Widdowson and Andrew Huxley in the Lake District during the Experimental Study of Rationing, January 1940.

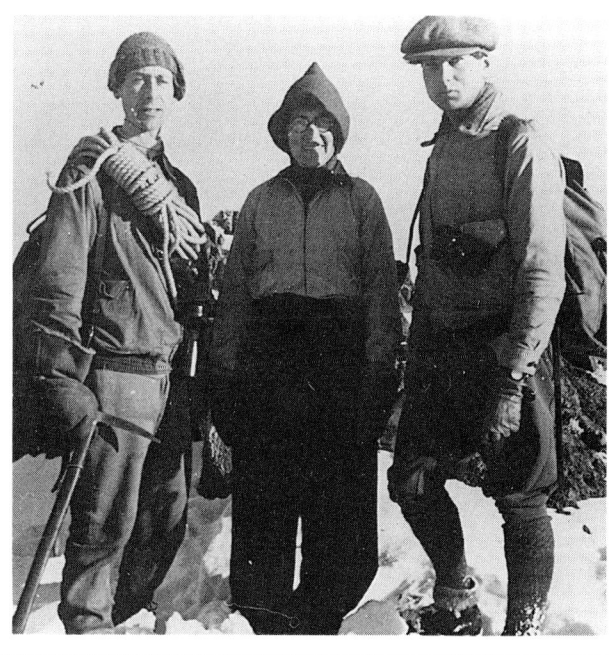

Below Andrew Huxley, Widdowson and Colin McCance on the way home from one of their expeditions in the Lake District, January 1940.

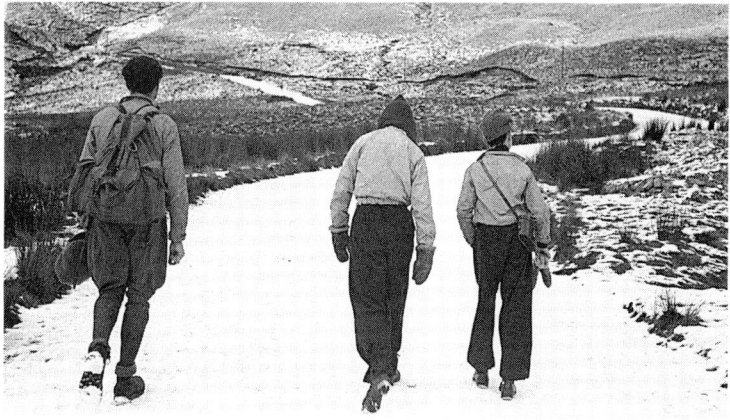

Some of the experimental subjects involved in determining mineral metabolism of healthy adults on white and brown bread dietaries, 1940.
Left to right:
E Bassadone, Norman Kent, Rosamund Wilson, Professor McCance, Dr Widdowson, Barbara Alington, P Steiner, Amicia Melland.

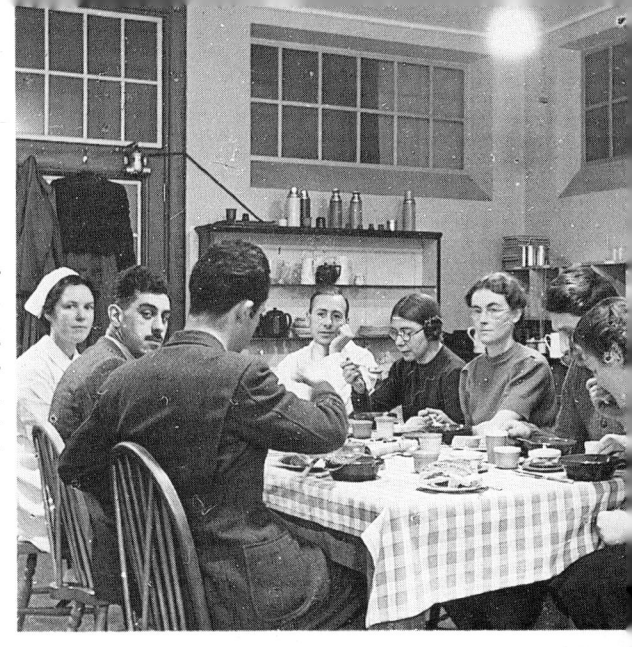

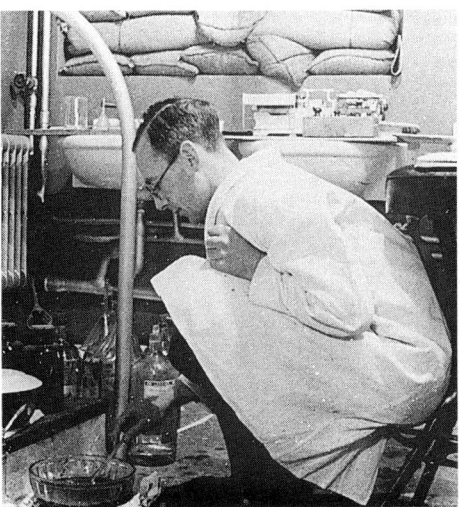

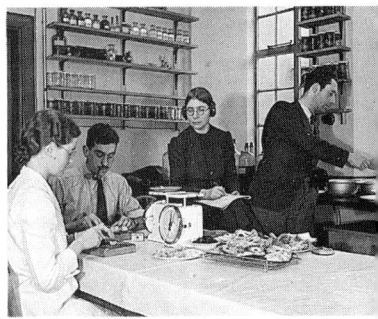

Left Professor McCance in the gentlemen's toilet 'mashing up' faeces of the subjects in the bread experiment, 1940.

Above Preparing the duplicates for the analytical part of the bread experiment.
Left to right: Barbara Alington, Norman Kent, Dr Widdowson, E Bassadone

Left Professor McCance and Dr Widdowson with Mr de Valera (the Taoiseach of Ireland) after giving a lecture on the effect of wholemeal bread on the absorption of calcium, Dublin, 1943.

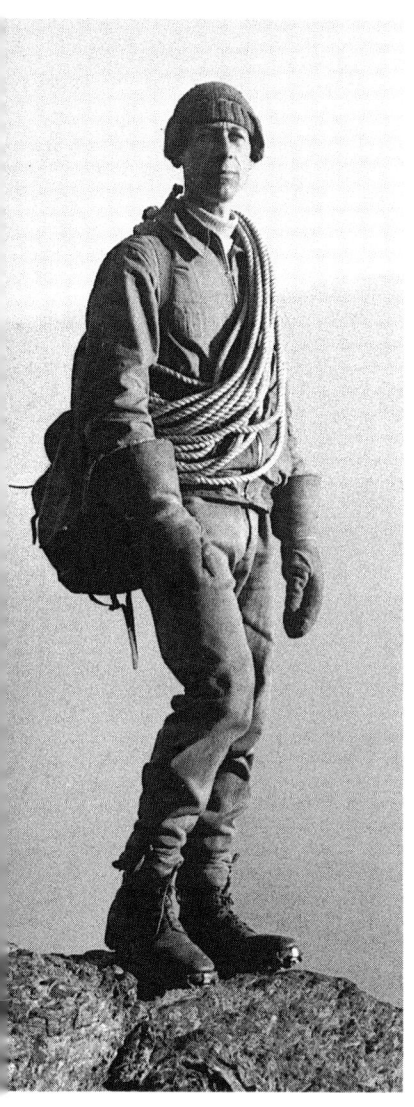

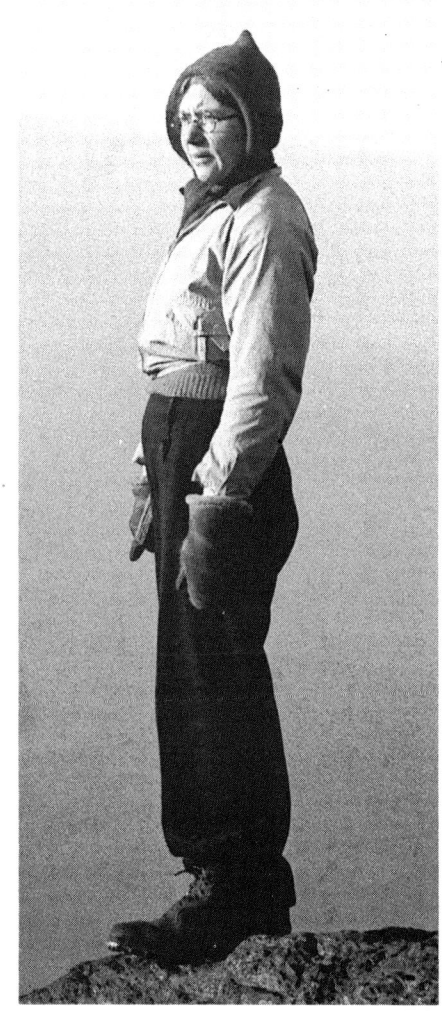

Professor McCance and Dr Widdowson testing their physical fitness in the English Lake District as part of the Experimental Study of Rationing, January 1940.

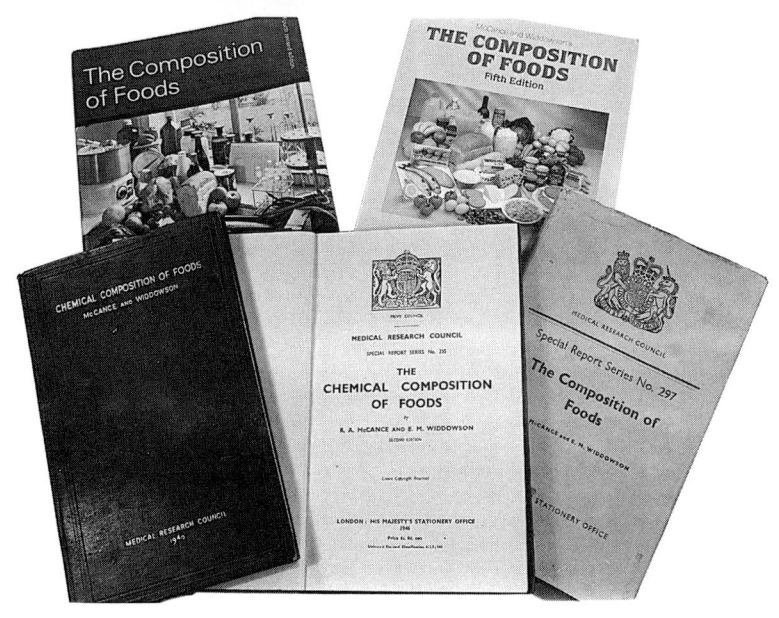

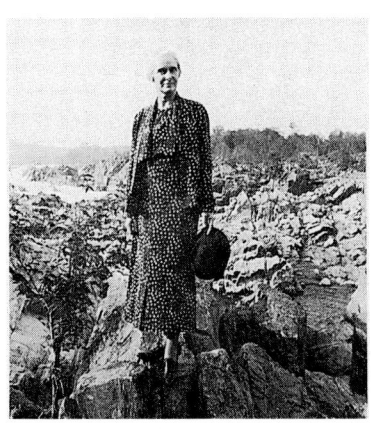

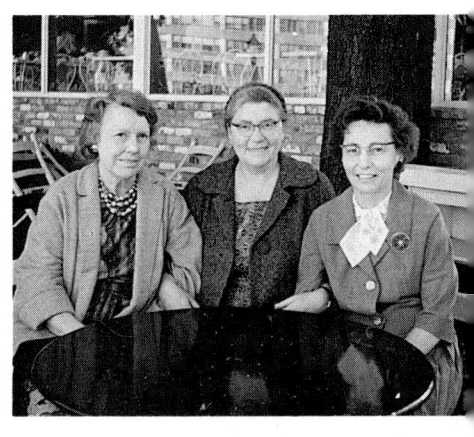

```
12          CHEMICAL COMPOSITION OF FOODS
                                     3 eggs
407. LEMON CURD                      Juice of 3 lemons (4¼ oz.)
     8 oz. sugar
     2½ oz. butter
Place the butter, sugar and lemon juice in a double pan and stir till melted.
Add the eggs one by one and cook slowly, stirring all the time until the mixture
coats the back of a wooden spoon.

                                     5 oz. golden syrup
413. TOFFEE                          1 tablespoon water
     8 oz. sugar
     1 oz. butter
     1 teaspoon vinegar
Place all the ingredients in a saucepan and heat gently till melted.  Boil
rapidly for 10 minutes or until a small portion, dropped into cold water,
becomes brittle.  Pour into buttered tins and mark into squares while still
warm.
```

Top **The five British editions of** *The Composition of Foods*, **1940, 1946, 1960, 1978, 1991.**

Above left **Miss Charlotte Chatfield, one of the first compilers of the American Food Tables, Washington DC, 1936.**

Above right **Dr Widdowson with Bernice Watt (right) and Annabel Merrill (left), compilers of Hand Book Number 8—the American Food Tables Washington DC, 1962.**

Left **Two of the recipes in the first edition of** *The Chemical Composition of Foods* **which were taken from Dr Widdowson's mother's recipe book**

A page from the first edition of *The Chemical Composition of Foods*, 1940. Note the names of foods still familiar today (eg Kellogg's All-Bran and Hovis).

Middle The equivalent page from the third edition of *The Composition of Foods*, 1960. Some new brand names have been added (eg Bemax, Allinson's and Procea).

Bottom The equivalent page from the Japanese edition of *The Composition of Foods* which is based on the third British edition, 1960. All-Bran, Allinson's and Bemax appear in the tables, even though they were unlikely to be on Japanese meal tables.

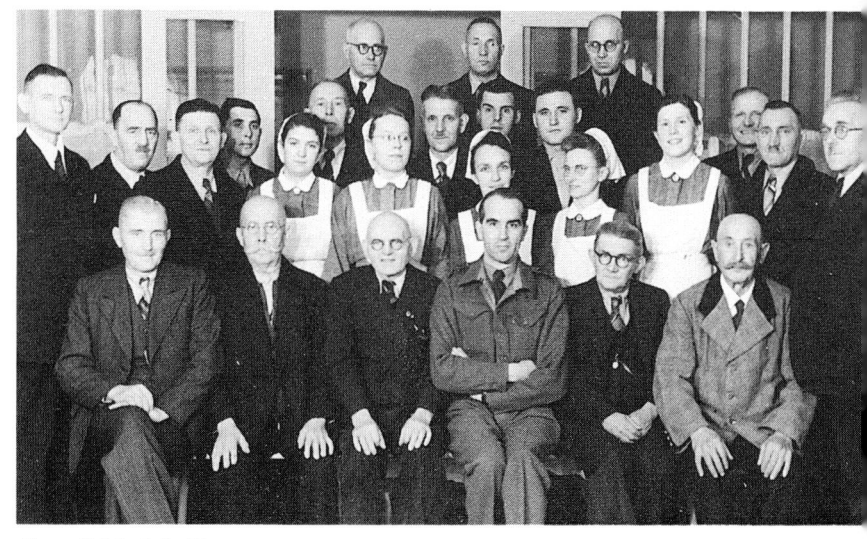

Above Subjects in Dr Widdowson's study of the effects of unlimited food on undernourished men, 1946. Rex Dean is in uniform in the centre of the group.

Right A leisure trip along the Rhine, 1947. *Left to right:* AN Other, Rex Dean, Dr Widdowson, Lois Thrussell.

Below Sir Edward Mellanby, Secretary of the Medical Research Council and his wife visiting Professor McCance and Dr Widdowson in Wuppertal, 1947.

Professor McCance's photograph of Dr Dorothy Rosenbaum, returning home from a 'hamstering' trip, Summer 1947.

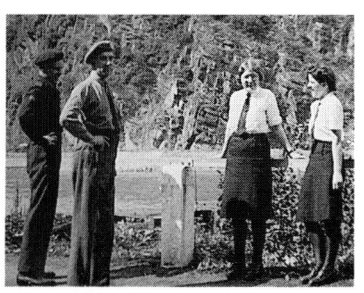

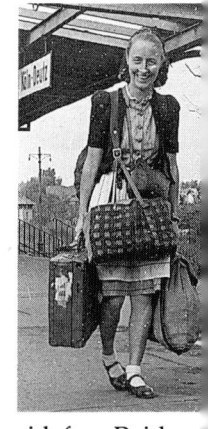

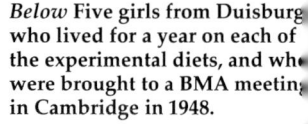

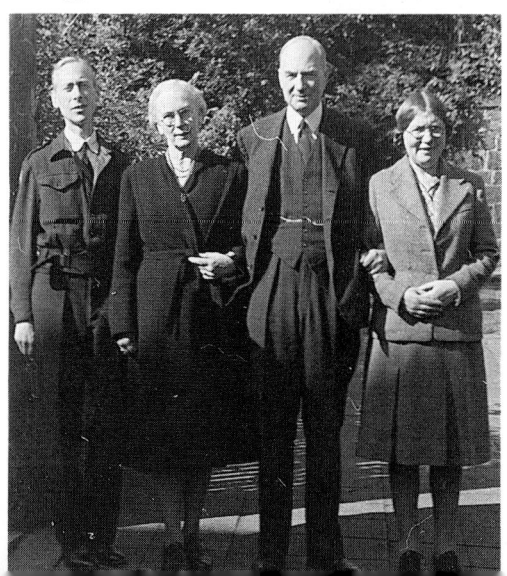

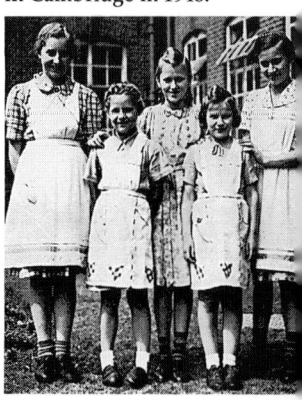

Below Five girls from Duisburg who lived for a year on each of the experimental diets, and who were brought to a BMA meeting in Cambridge in 1948.

10 Dickerson JWT, Widdowson EM. **Chemical changes in skeletal muscle with development.** Biochem J 1960; **74:** 247-257.

11 Jackson CM. **The effects of inanition and malnutrition upon growth and structure.** London: Churchill, 1925.

12 Widdowson EM. **Animals in the service of human nutrition.** Nutr Revs 1986; **44:** 221-227.

13 Widdowson EM, Dickerson JWT, McCance RA. **Severe undernutrition in growing and adult animals 4. The impact of severe undernutrition on the chemical composition of the soft tissues of the pig.** Br J Nutr 1960; **14:** 457-471.

14 Neuberger A, Perrone JC, Slack HGB. **The relative metabolic inertia of tendon collagen in the rat.** Biochem J 1951; **49:** 199-204.

15 Cabak V, Dickerson JWT, Widdowson RA. **Response of young rats to deprivation of protein or of calories.** Br J Nutr 1963; **17:** 601-616.

16 Hammond J. **Growth and the development of mutton qualities in the sheep.** Edinburgh: Oliver and Boyd, 1932.

17 Dickerson JWT, McCance RA. **Severe undernutrition in growing and adult animals. 3. Avian skeletal muscle.** Br J Nutr 1960; **14:** 331-338.

18 Montgomery RD, Dickerson JWT, McCance RA. **Severe undernutrition in growing and adult animals 13. The morphology and chemistry of development and undernutrition in the sartorius muscle of the fowl.** Br J Nutr 1964; **18:** 587-593.

19 Golden MHN. **Free radicals in the pathogenesis of kwashiorkor.** Proc Nutr Soc 1987; **46:** 53-6.

20 Dickerson JWT. **Hospital induced malnutrition: a cause for concern. Professional Nurse 1986;** August: 293-296.

21 McCance RA, Barrett AM. III. **The effects of undernutrition on the skin.** In: Studies of Undernutrition, Wuppertal 1946-9. Medical Research Council Special Report Series No. 275. London: HMSO, 1951: 83-96.

22 Widdowson EM, Dickerson JWT. **The effect of growth and function on the chemical composition of soft tissues.** Biochem J 1960; **77:** 30-43.

23 Dickerson JWT, John PMV. **The effect of sex and site on the composition of skin in the rat and mouse.** Biochem J 1964; **92:** 364-368.

24 Rogers HJ, Weidman SM, Parkinson A. **Studies on the skeletal tissues 2. The collagen content of bones from rabbits, oxen and humans.** Biochem J 1952; **50:** 537-542.

25 Dickerson JWT. **Changes in the composition of the human femur during growth.** Biochem J 1962; **82:** 56-61.

26 Slater JF, Widdowson EM. **Skeletal development of suckling kittens with and without supplementary calcium phosphate.** Br J Nutr 1962; **16:** 39-48.

27 Dickerson JWT, Widdowson EM. **Some effects of accelerating growth. II. Skeletal development.** Proc Roy Soc B 1960; **152:** 207-217.

28 Widdowson EM. **Harmony of growth.** Lancet 1970; **1:** 901-905.

29 Dickerson JWT, Hughes PCR. **Growth of the rat skeleton after severe nutritional intrauterine and post-natal retardation.** Resuscitation 1972; **1:** 163-170.

30 Dobbing J. **The influence of early nutrition on the development and myelination of the brain.** Proc Roy Soc B 1964; **159:** 503-309.

31 Davison AN, Dobbing J. **Myelination as a vulnerable period in brain development.** Br Med Bull 1966; **22:** 40-44.

32 Dickerson JWT, Dobbing J, McCance RA. **The effects of undernutrition on the development of the brain and cord in pigs.** Proc Roy Soc B 1967; **166:** 396-407.

33 Dickerson JWT, Merat A, Yusuf HKM. **Effects of malnutrition on brain growth and development.** In: Dickerson JWT, McGurk H, eds. **Brain and Behavioral Development.** London: Surrey University Press (Blackie), 1982: 73-108.

34 Dickerson JWT, McGurk H eds. **Brain and Behavioral Development.** London: Surrey University Press (Blackie), 1982.

35 Dickerson JWT, Lee HA eds. **Nutrition in the clinical management of disease.** 2nd ed. London: Arnold, 1988.

The physiology of the newborn
by Brian Wharton

INTRODUCTION

I first *saw* Mac at a meeting of the Neonatal Society which he was chairing in 1965. A colleague of mine was presenting a paper on hypoglycaemia and strayed over time; you can guess the consequences! I first *met* him at another meeting of the Neonatal Society in Bristol later that year. He was planning his move to Uganda and wanted a young paediatrician (those were the days!) to go with him.

I met Elsie in Cambridge before going to Uganda, but did not get to know her well until we sat on various government committees together, trying to decide what babies should eat and drink.

Neonatal medicine and physiology were my entrée, therefore, to the distinguished world of McCance and Widdowson. It has been a great privilege and pleasure to review their distinctive contribution to neonatal physiology, which will follow the pathway of the nutrients in the newborn. First I shall discuss the food they eat and its digestion and absorption. Having reached the *'milieu interieur'*, I shall ask how and where the products of digestion are used for growth and development? Finally, how are they excreted?

I have not attempted to refer to all the papers in this area and clearly there is an element of personal choice. Where possible, I have tried to draw out the contribution that McCance and Widdowson have made to the concepts we hold and the explanations we seek today.

FOOD

Elsie has often described how her previous experience in analysing the fructose content of apples allowed her to correct Mac's approach to this, when his interests in diabetes and carbohydrate metabolism were developing at King's[1]. This was the kernel that grew into *The composition of foods*. But what of the newborn's food, that is: breast milk, cows' milk and infant formulae?

Breast milk

The composition of food can be determined by the usual analytical methods, but as these have become more refined, more nutrients and individual parts of the nutrient (eg, amino acids or fatty acids) can be included. Breast milk has a composition which varies according to the stage of the feed (fore or hind milk), the time of day, and the time since birth; but details of sample collection are often not given in published papers on the composition of breast milk.

This limitation and the advent of new analytical methods led a team convened by the Department of Health to establish a modern standard[2]. Elsie was a member of that team. A complete breastful of milk was collected from mothers during a morning of their second month of lactation. Unfortunately, some of the analytical detail did not appear in the report, but it eventually appeared in the fourth edition of *The composition of foods*. A very attractive publication of Elsie's was *Feeding the newborn mammal*[3]. It contains a most comprehensive table, comparing the composition of milks of over 40 species.

I remember in 1967 having to 'mind the shop' in Kampala while Mac and Glan Howells accompanied an elephant cull in the north of the country, around the Nile, ostensibly to collect milk and urine for comparative studies (*c'est la vie!*). The elephant's milk was brought to Cambridge for analysis and a paper was written about it[4]. I presume that is the source for one line in the table.

Infant formulae

Another reason for determining the composition of human milk was to use it as a template for the design of modern infant-feeding formulae. Elsie was a leading contributor to the Department of Health's Panel on *Artificial feeds for the young infant*[5]. The Panel's report was widely influential in Britain, and internationally, in determining the composition of the diet of the newborn bottle-fed baby. It included recommendations on alpha linolenic acid and mentioned the relative contributions of linoleic acid and alpha linolenic acid—and this was 13 years ago!

Quantity

The amount of milk consumed by infants is more difficult to determine. McCance and Widdowson studied this in young rabbits, who took a quarter of their own weight of milk over a few minutes in just one feed[6]. In subsequent balance studies, they frequently measured the intakes of human babies (who take only 2% of their body weight on six to eight occasions each day)—and of many other animals.

They were intrigued to compare the nutrient intakes with rates of growth in different species, eg, the baby rabbit, which doubles birth weight at about one week and the human baby who takes 20 weeks or more. Over this period, the rabbit consumes about 4kcal per gram of weight gain, whereas the human consumes nearly ten times that amount because of the higher proportion of intake required for maintenance. Not even suckling seals have escaped Elsie's interest and attention[7].

Intestinal Events

Numerous balance studies in various species were performed by McCance and Widdowson, often not primarily for intestinal reasons, but the results allowed the calculation of net apparent absorption (intake—faeces) for many nutrients, including protein, fat and minerals.

Protein and Fat

Mac and Elsie, like many others, showed that the absorption of nitrogen and fat from breast milk was always more than 90%. In subsequent years they showed that absorption of fat from relatively modern infant formulae was often much less[8].

There was an early, but subsequently undeveloped, interest in dietary immunoglobulins. In pigs the amount of gamma-globulin absorbed from colostrum was sufficient to raise the serum globulin from 0.9g to 3.6g per 100ml—a substantial transfer of immunological information[9].

In 1959, the significance of dietary transfer of immunoglobulin as secretory IgA in the human, had not yet been appreciated. Indeed the structure, and thence the classification of the immunoglobulins, while imminent, was undeclared.

Minerals

The absorption of minerals attracted a lot of attention from McCance and Widdowson. At the time, when I myself was still a newborn, they had already suggested that variation in the intestinal absorption of iron was the main factor regulating total body iron in adults[10].

But what about iron absorption in the newborn? Some years later, Cavell and Widdowson[11] showed that normal breast-fed infants at one week of age excreted more iron in their faeces than they took in, ie, there was a negative net iron absorption (about 1mg per day) and it was thought this was due to its excretion in bile in a non-absorbed form. A similar mechanism was thought to account for the negative net absorption of manganese, copper and zinc at this age. Cadmium, despite its 'proximity' to zinc in the Periodic Table, showed a net absorption of about 50%[12].

A sad commentary on our modern times was the spur to study strontium absorption in the newborn in the 1960s. Levels of radioactive strontium were increasing in the environment and a detailed study of strontium handling was desirable. Of course, Mac and Elsie had injected strontium into each other three decades previously and found that most of it was excreted by the kidneys[13].

Working with people from Harwell in the 1960s, they showed that the breast-fed baby had a negative net absorption of strontium at the age of one week and was in overall negative balance. By six weeks of age, about half of the strontium was absorbed, leading to a net retention. Even at one week of age, the bottle-fed baby was receiving much more strontium than the breast-fed baby, and since it absorbed a quarter of it, its retention was much higher (14,15).

Following nuclear accidents, therefore, it would seem to be a theoretical advantage for babies to be breast-fed. However, following the Chernobyl disaster in 1986, the problem was circumvented by using formulae manufactured from cows' milk produced before the accident.

Gut growth and adaptation

Some of Elsie's more unusual interests were the changes in the intestinal tract of the newborn piglet that occurred following feeding. The piglet showed substantial increases in the weight of the intestine, particularly in the mucosa of the jejunum, and this occurred to a greater extent than with any other organ. The high protein concentration in colostrum was suggested as the cause[16,17]. Interpretations nowadays would focus on the possible role of biologically active peptides and growth factors in the maternal milk, or the stimulation of trophic gut hormones by the milk; ie, similar observations would lead to different interpretations.

The importance of intraluminal nutrition to the welfare of the enterocyte and intestine generally, has only been appreciated in recent years when it has been possible to keep babies alive on parenteral nutrition without any enteral feeds. Even when all nutrient requirements are being supplied parenterally, current management would include, if at all possible, small amounts of maternal milk enterally, to prevent gut atrophy.

In the 1960s, Mac enjoyed an interesting cooperation with Andrew Wilkinson, Professor of Surgery at the Institute of Child Health in London, studying the progress of newborn piglets following an early intestinal resection—jejunum[18], ileum[19] and colon[20]. Growth in length of the remaining intestine was no more than normal, but there was an increase in its girth and weight, probably representing mucosal hypertrophy. It was thought that this depended largely on the extra functional demand made on it—a further argument for feeding the short or damaged gut, if possible.

INTERMEDIARY METABOLISM

Phosphate

McCance and Widdowson had noted the high plasma phosphorus of babies receiving cows' milk compared with breast-fed babies, and commented that the intake had more than saturated the capacity of the baby to incorporate phosphorus into its growing tissues[21]. Plasma calcium concentration was not determined at that time and so they did not note the accompanying hypocalcaemia, an object of great interest and clinical significance in subsequent years. They argued that since some of the babies getting breast milk excreted only traces of phosphorus on the seventh day, it was possible that their capacity to incorporate phosphorus into growing tissue was not completely saturated.

This observation has early hints of what is now known as the phosphate deficiency syndrome. It occurs in rapidly growing preterm babies usually receiving breast milk. Bone growth quickly outstrips the supply of phosphorus; rickets and osteopaenia occur. The available calcium cannot be used for growth and so hypercalciuria, even with nephrocalcinosis, or renal stone formation, occurs.

When attention was drawn to the clinical problem of neonatal hypocalcaemia (causing convulsions) in later years, McCance and Widdowson looked at the absorption of calcium and the factors interfering with it, such as fat (8). Unfortunately, dietary calcium in the newborn has little effect on the plasma calcium. Nevertheless, intriguing relationships between calcium and phosphorus continued to occupy them. Modest increases in the dietary phosphorus of babies receiving breast milk did not affect absorption of calcium, but its retention was increased—presumably because the extra phosphorus had enabled increased mineralisation of the bone[22].

Sodium

Another interest of clinical importance was hypertonicity of extracellular fluids. McCance and Widdowson showed that the addition of too much sodium chloride to the diet of newborn babies and piglets caused increased tonicity of the extracellular fluid leading to its expansion, and eventually leading to oedema[23]. These observations have some relevance to the problems of hypernatraemia, caused if salt, instead of sugar, is added accidentally to cows' milk. They are also related to the hypernatraemia seen in babies with diarrhoea receiving high solute milks, such as cows' milk. However, in these babies, fluid loss from the bowel results in dehydration with weight loss so that the pathophysiology is different from the effects of adding both sodium and water to the diet.

An intriguing further observation, and one that McCance had seen previously in adults[24], was that piglets given both salt and water, break down less of their tissue proteins than those given water alone; the animals given both salt and milk have lower urinary nitrogen levels than those receiving milk alone[25]. Babies who develop hypernatraemic dehydration when they have gastroenteritis, are often the ones with satisfactory growth curves and some are even overweight. It has been suggested that the increased thirst induced by high solute feeds causes babies to drink more milk, and so they put on more weight. Is this the explanation for the results in piglets, or did the higher salt intake of the babies reduce their protein breakdown?

GROWTH AND BODY COMPOSITION

Growth

The McCance and Widdowson method for producing cohorts of well-nourished and under-nourished suckling animals, by rearing 'small' and 'large' litters, has become a classic technique. They are sometimes referred to affectionately as 'Elsie and Mac' rats, and the method has been repeated in legions of nutritional experiments, since it was introduced in 1960.

Methods such as this were the seedcorn for so much subsequent work but, in particular, the study of the relationships between the timing of nutritional stress, the stage of development of the individual, and the subsequent effects of that stress. Very broadly, rats undernourished throughout the suckling period had more respiratory infection, and a higher mortality rate, and the survivors did not catch up in weight, even though they had unlimited access to food thereafter.

Undernutrition at a later stage did not have this permanent effect and catch-up occurred if the opportunity for rehabilitation was given. That statement is a simplification, and I must beware of over-interpreting, and extrapolating from the original data and conclusions of McCance and Widdowson, as so many others have done.

Nevertheless, with the exception of organogenesis as a critical period, their concepts were some of the earliest, and for so long the only ones relating developmental physiology to nutritional outcome[26-32]. They have been followed by a distinguished group of contributors to this concept—Cheek, Winick, Dobbing, Hirsch, Lucas and Barker. The concepts are encapsulated in Mac's essay on Food, growth and time[33].

Body composition

McCance and Widdowson studied 'real' body composition. By 'real' I mean analyses of actual bodies and tissues, not a mere collection of anthropometric and/or electrical data which are then referred to majestically as body composition! From the neonatal perspective, the most important work was the determination of fetal body composition.

The groundwork was published in 1951 and 1964[34,35]. An extensive series of dissections was made, in association with Edmund Hey in the 1970s, but so far, these have been published only in part[36,37]. The accumulation of trace elements in the fetal liver and cellular development in various organs (as estimated from total protein and DNA measurements) were also determined[38,39].

Generally the analyses showed that fat is mainly deposited during the third trimester of pregnancy; the fetus becomes a fatter, less watery and more solid (in terms of protein and minerals) animal. Extracellular fluid decreases and intracellular increases. At term, the extracellular and intracellular compartments are about equal, and by the age of two to three years, the intracellular volume is double the extracellular volume. This relationship holds into the adult years. What then was the significance of this study for modern neonatal care?

Jonathan Shaw was the first person to use these data, together with studies of fetal growth velocity, to derive daily accumulation rates for different fetal ages, once the age of viability had been reached. This provided one factor in the factorial method for estimating the nutrient requirement of very preterm and very low birth-weight babies once they were outside the uterus. This method showed, in particular, that rates of calcium accretion *in utero* could not be matched by the then available foods. Nor can they be easily matched now, and this is one factor in the metabolic bone disease (osteopaenia, rickets) of preterm babies.

The use of *in utero* accumulation rates to determine nutrient requirement begs the question of which criteria of excellence should the preterm baby be aiming for? Should he mimic the watery fetus or quickly deposit fat like a normal newborn baby? Perhaps the extra fat would help thermal homeostasis—another interest of Mac and Elsie's[40]. One can imagine a McCance and Widdowson essay on this topic, *The preterm infant: extrauterine fetus or an immature baby trying to be normal*.

EXCRETION

Sodium

Mac has already described his own first venture into neonatal physiology, which occurred when Winifred Young went from King's College Hospital, London, to the Children's Hospital in Birmingham, under Sir Leonard Parsons, and alerted him to the absence of chloride in the newborn infant's urine[41]. The series of papers[42-44] on newborn infants was followed by investigations of renal function in newborn rats; this showed that neither loads of sodium nor of water were excreted very well (when compared with the adult), and this was later confirmed in newborn infants[45].

The renal function of premature infants was determined at Sorrento Maternity Hospital in Birmingham. That hospital was to be the place where I did much of my own neonatal investigation 40 years later. By then, Dr Hallum, who had worked with Winifred Young and Mac on the study in 1941, was an obstetrician there. Perhaps the 1940s spirit of enquiry had permeated the fabric affecting all who worked there subsequently? Moreover Rex Dean, who did the work on glomerular filtration rate and sodium loading was later to set up the MRC Unit in Uganda where Roger Whitehead, Mac and I worked.

To square the circle, Winifred Young moved to the Queen Elizabeth Children's Hospital in London, and shortly after her death I moved there and continued her work on gastroenteritis and coeliac disease. It has been a pleasure following the interlocking footsteps of great people.

Metabolic relationships

McCance and Widdowson also studied the effects of excessive dietary intakes of potassium in piglets[46]. This was less of a problem than sodium. In terms of intermediary metabolism, this was correct. Nevertheless, the excess potassium had to be excreted, adding to the total 'renal solute load' which had to be excreted by the baby, and in times of water deprivation this presents a problem. In practice, an unnecessarily high protein intake is even more of a problem in dehydrated children.

Protein, in excess of that required for maintenance and growth, results in a substantial production of urea which has to be largely excreted by the kidney. If the child is dehydrated (say from diarrhoea), the volume of urine available in which to excrete this urea is small. The concentrating power of the kidney would be exceeded and so extra urine would be secreted, even though the dehydrated child could ill afford to lose the water.

Many of McCance and Widdowson's studies of intermediary metabolism were related to the role of the kidney in maintaining the constancy of the internal environment, eg, in control of acid-base balance and the compensatory response of the kidney to acidosis[42]. This could just as easily have been mentioned in the section on intermediary metabolism as here in the kidney section—a sign of their integrative approach.

ENVOI

Most of us enjoy a life of only ephemeral contribution to the scientific literature; for the rare few, their message lives on. This review should have brought out the diversity of approach of our famous couple. This diversity is one of the pleasures of both neonatal paediatrics and nutrition.

What is a nutritionist? When HRH The Princess Royal was opening the Rank Department of Human Nutrition in Glasgow, a number of local and national dignitaries were present. Elsie was my personal guest, also representing Mac. A local dignitary sitting next to Elsie enquired, 'Are you a nutritionist?' Elsie's reply was, 'Well, sort of'.

Mac's approach to his own nutrition was at times unusual. I

sometimes wondered whether, for years, he was performing the experiment to see whether, in man, mild undernutrition led to longevity, as in the rat. I accompanied him on one of the first non-stop flights from Entebbe to Gatwick. The morning snack was refused, as were lunch and tea. This was his normal pattern of eating, but how could he manage on the puny airline dinner he would get, instead of the early evening feast he normally enjoyed?

The airline meal arrived and from his knapsack he produced a 2lb loaf and a carving knife. Everything was eaten, much to the consternation of the nearby passengers; Mac was never ordinary and never disturbed by an unusual environment! As his guest at Sidney Sussex College in subsequent years, similar events unrolled. But they knew him there and gave him lots of vegetables; he had no need to take his own loaf.

McCance and Widdowson are nutritionists in the fullest sense—not limited to a single nutrient, to a single technique, or a single organ. Nor are they blinkered by species or age. They have made an indelible mark on both comparative and developmental physiology. Who else could have discussed food, growth and renal function in man, the pig and the rabbit?

Two of my favourite papers are based on prestigious lectures by McCance and Widdowson, and are reproduced in this book: Mac's *Food, growth, and time*[33] and Elsie's *Harmony of growth*[48]. Both lectures were based on observation. They were developmental and comparative—the changes and comparisons. Above all, they developed concepts.

References

1   *Widdowson EM.* **Adventures in nutrition over half a century**. Proc Nutr Soc 1980; **39:** 293-306.

2   *Christie AA, Darke SJ, Paul AA, Wharton BA, Widdowson EM.* **The composition of mature human milk**. Department of Health and Social Security. Report on Health and Social Subjects No. 12. London: HMSO, 1977.

3   *Widdowson EM.* **Feeding the newborn mammal**. Carolina USA: Carolina Biological Supply Co, 1981: 1-31.

4   *McCullagh KG, Widdowson EM.* **The milk of the African elephant**. Br J Nutr 1970; **24:** 109-17.

5   *Oppé TE, Barltrop D, Belton NR et al.* **Artificial feeds for the young infant**. DHSS Report on Health and Social Subjects No. 18. London: HMSO, 1980.

6   Davies JS, Widdowson EM, McCance RA. **The intake of milk and the retention of its constituents while the newborn rabbit doubles its weight.** Br J Nutr 1964; **18:** 385-92.

7   Oftedal OT, Bowen WD, Widdowson EM, Boness DJ. **Effects of suckling and the post- suckling on weights of the body and internal organs of harp and hooded seal pups.** Biol Neonat 1989; **56:** 283-300.

8   Widdowson EM. **Absorption and excretion of fat, nitrogen and minerals from 'filled' milks by babies one week old.** Lancet 1965; **ii:** 1099-1115.

9   McCance RA, Widdowson EM. **The effect of colostrum on the composition and volume of the plasma of newborn piglets.** J Physiol 1959; **148:** 547-59.

10   McCance RA, Widdowson EM. **Absorption and excretion of iron.** Lancet 1937; **ii:** 680-4.

11   Cavell PA, Widdowson EM. **Intakes and excretion of iron, copper and zinc in the neonatal period.** Arch Dis Childh 1964; **39:** 496-501.

12   Widdowson EM. **Absorption, excretion and storage of trace elements: studies over 50 years.** Food Chemistry 1992; **43:** 203-7.

13   McCance RA, Widdowson EM. **The fate of strontium after intravenous administration to normal persons.** Biochem J 1939b; **33:** 1822-5.

14   Widdowson EM, Slater JE, Harrison GE, Sutton A. **Absorption, excretion and retention of strontium by breast-fed and bottle-fed babies.** Lancet 1960; **ii:** 941-4.

15   Harrison GE, Sutton A, Shepherd H, Widdowson EM. **Strontium balance in breast-fed babies.** Br J Nutr 1965; **19:** 111-17.

16   Widdowson EM, Colombo VE, Artavanis CA. **Changes in the organs of pigs in response to feeding for the first 24h after birth.** 2. The digestive tract. Biol Neonate 1976; **28:** 272-81.

17   Widdowson EM, Crabb DE. **Changes in the organs of pigs in respones to feeding for the first 24h after birth. 1. The internal organs and muscles.** Biol Neonate 1976; **28:** 261-7.

18   McCance RA, Stoddart RW, Artavanis C, Wilkinson AW. **Effects of by-passing the jejunum on the mucosal secretion of the pig.** Biochem Soc Trans 1976; **4:** 151-54.

19   McCance RA, Wilkinson AW. **Experimental resection of the intestine in newborn pigs.** Br J Nutr 1967; **21:** 731-40.

20 *Wilkinson AW, McCance RA.* **Clinical and experimental results of removing the large intestine soon after birth.** Arch Dis Childh 1973; **48:** 121-26.

21 *Widdowson EM, McCance RA.* **The effect of food and growth on the metabolism of phosphorus in the newly born.** Acta paediat 1959; **48:** 383-87.

22 *Widdowson EM, McCance RA, Harrison GE, Sutton A.* **Effects of giving phosphate supplements to breast-fed babies on absorption and excretion of calcium, strontium, magnesium and phosphorus.** Lancet 1963; **ii:** 1250-3.

23 *McCance RA, Widdowson EM.* **Hypertonic expansion of the extracellular fluids.** Acta Paed Scand 1957; **46:** 337-53.

24 *McCance RA.* **Medical problems in mineral metabolism. III Experimental human salt deficiency.** Lancet 1936; **i:** 823-7.

25 *McCance RA, Widdowson EM.* **Metabolism, growth and renal function of piglets in the first two days of life.** J Physiol 1956; **133:** 373-8.

26 *Widdowson EM, McCance RA.* **Some effects of accelerating growth. 1. General somatic development.** Proc Roy Soc B 1960; **152:** 188-206.

27 *Dickerson JWT, Widdowson EM.* **Some effects of accelerating growth. 2. Skeletal development.** Proc Roy Soc B 1960; **152:** 207-217.

28 *Widdowson EM, Kennedy GC.* **Rate of growth, mature weight and life span.** Proc Roy Soc B 1962; **156:** 96-108.

29 *Widdowson EM, McCance RA.* **The effect of finite periods of undernutrition at different ages on the composition and subsequent development of the rat.** Proc Roy Soc B 1963; **158:** 329-42.

30 *Widdowson EM, McCance RA.* **A review. New thoughts on growth.** Pediat Res 1975; **9:** 154-56.

31 *Widdowson EM.* **Intrauterine growth retardation in the pig. 1. Organ size and cellular development at birth and after growth to maturity.** Biol Neonat 1971; **19:** 329-40.

32 *Lister D, McCance RA.* **The effects of two diets on the growth, reproduction and ultimate size of guinea-pigs.** Br J Nutr 1965; **19:** 311-19.

33 *McCance RA.* **Food, growth and time.** Lancet 1962; **i:** 671-4.

34 Widdowson EM, Spray CM. **Chemical development in utero.** Arch Dis Child 1951; **26:** 205-14.

35 Widdowson EM, Dickerson JWT. **Chemical composition of the body.** In: Comar CL, Bronner F, eds. Mineral Metabolism. New York: Academic Press 1964; **2A:** 1-247.

36 Widdowson EM, Southgate DAT, Hey EN. **Body composition of the fetus and infant.** In: Visser HKA, ed. **Nutrition and metabolism of the fetus and infant.** The Hague: Martinus Nijhoff, 1979: 169-77.

37 Widdowson EM, Southgate DAT, Hey E. **Fetal growth and body composition.** In: Linblad BS, ed. Perinatal Nutrition. New York: Academic Press, 1988: 3-14.

38 Widdowson EM, Crabb DE, Milner RDG. **Cellular development of some human organs before birth.** Arch Dis Child 1972; **47:** 652-5.

39 Widdowson EM, Chan H, Harrison GE, Milner RDG. **Accumulation of Cu, Zn, Mn, Cr and Co in the human liver before birth.** Biol Neonate 1972; **20:** 360-7.

40 McCance RA, Widdowson EM. **The effect of lowering the ambient temperature on the metabolism of the newborn pig.** J Physiol 1959; **147:** 124-34.

41 McCance RA. **Early physiological work at Sorrento: recollections of the 1930s.** In: *Wharton BA, ed.* **Topics in Perinatal Medicine 2.** London: Pitman Medical, 1982:17-19.

42 McCance RA, Young WF. **The secretion of urine by newborn infants.** J Physiol 1941; **99:** 265-82.

43 Young WF, Hallum JL, McCance RA. **The secretion of urine by premature infants.** Arch Dis Child 1941; **16:** 243-52.

44 Dean RFA, McCance RA. **Inulin, diodone, creatinine and urea clearances in newborn infants.** J Physiol 1947; **106:** 431-9.

45 Dean RFA, McCance RA. **The renal responses of infants and adults to the administration of hypertonic solutions of sodium chloride and urea.** J Physiol 1949; **109:** 81-97.

46 McCance RA, Widdowson EM. **The response of the newborn piglet to an excess of potassium.** J Physiol 1958; **141:** 88-93.

47 McCance RA, Widdowson EM. **Renal aspects of acid base control in the newly born. 1. Natural development.** Acta Paediatr 1960; **49:** 409-12.

48. Widdowson EM. **Harmony of growth.** Lancet 1970; **i:** 901-5.

Normal and retarded growth
by David Lister

INTRODUCTION

Tucked away at the foot of the record card on which Mac had written his notes on the paper *Compensatory growth* by Wilson and Osbourn[1], was the comment, 'I hope mine will be half as good'. 'Mine' referred to his *Food, growth & time,* which he was shortly to deliver as the Lumleian Lecture to the Royal College of Physicians of London. He need not have worried.

That he should have set such store by a review that deals primarily with the practical agricultural implications of retarded and rehabilitated growth, will come as no surprise to those who know McCance and Widdowson. Their capacity for striking gold in their formidable searching of the literature is a rare talent. Apsley Cherry-Garrard's[2] account of the privations endured during *The worst journey in the world*, were to Mac not just an account of the triumph of the human spirit, but a remarkable scientific appraisal of man's response to hunger, the clinical progress of scurvy and the development of ptomaine poisoning.

I remember also his schoolboy excitement on learning about Oppers' analysis of the growth of Dutch military recruits of the early 19th century[3]. 'Wizard' was the usual epithet for these occasions and they were not restricted to the discovery of new scientific reports; the Bible, or the travel writings of Patrick Leigh Fermor, for example, could induce similar reactions.

The search for simple truths by asking the pivotal questions, using rigorous experimentation, long, thoughtful analysis and careful presentation are the hallmarks of the McCance and Widdowson partnership. The 'What about looking at it this way?' element underlies much of their original and innovative approach to science. Miss Widdowson's particular skills emerged in devising and conducting experiments, and as a practical, down-to-earth assessor of experimental findings.

It may seem strange today when first names are the common currency that I refer to her so formally as Miss Widdowson or Dr Widdowson. But such is how I, and many other members of Experimental Medicine, have known her for more than 30 years. It does not detract from the affection she engenders, typified by my own children's view of her as a Beatrix Potter universal granny, complete with fairy-tale cottage, cats and orchard.

The mix of common and complementary skills formed the backbone of the alliance, but collaboration with others was always a crucial element. Experimental Medicine was never a big Department but rarely a day passed, it seemed, without a visit from some internationally renowned scientist or member of the world's great and good, and an interrogation over lunch. Inevitably, collaborative ventures were spawned by such visits; indeed, people are the 'thread' which sutures the McCance and Widdowson story. At every turn of their scientific progress a new name appears and for both of them it is often the recall of an individual person which prefaces remarks about a scientific advance. The work on growth is no exception.

STUDIES ON GROWTH IN GERMANY

It was inevitable that one day Mac and Miss Widdowson would allow their interest in the analysis and metabolism of food to encompass its effects on the growth of the consumer. The first movements in this direction came during their German interlude shortly after the Second World War, when RFA (Rex) Dean first worked with them. Only recently, Mac referred to Dean in a typical conversational aside: 'I was glad that Dean was able to join us. He was an excellent pianist, you know. He played the piano beautifully—well, maybe not beautifully but he could play anything at sight. A remarkable talent.'

Dean, of course, was later to become an authority on kwashiorkor but, at that time, one of his interests and his particular contribution to the Medical Research Council's Study Group, lay in the state of the German men and women returning from captivity and privation in Russia. His studies on the physical and clinical consequences of starvation and rehabilitation were seminal and included investigations on the newborn child. He was clearly party also to the famous research on the effects of feeding children on different kinds of bread.

Their experience in Germany was clearly a turning point in McCance and Widdowson's scientific outlook and was to set the stage for the remarkable and classical experimental programme which was carried out over the next 25 years or so, on the effects of nutrition on growing and adult animals.

ANIMAL EXPERIMENTS

By 1956 some experiments had already been done with rats and guinea pigs[4,5] and, by 1957, some endocrinological associations were spotted[6]. Gordon Kennedy had moved to the Department of Experimental Medicine from the National Institute for Medical Research in Mill Hill, to continue his investigations on hypothalamic function in relation to eating and satiety. He introduced to the Cambridge laboratory the technique of raising rats in large and small litters which AS Parkes (and Castle[7] before him) had used in a small way to look at various aspects of lactation and reproduction. The unusual feature of this exercise which Mac and Miss Widdowson found intriguing was not that the rats raised in large litters were small at weaning, but that they continued to eat less and remained smaller as adults.

Together with an experienced technician, Pat Pledger, Miss Widdowson refined and developed the methodology to produce hundreds of the world-famous large and small rats. It was these studies that provided some of the first information linking chronological, somatic and behavioural development in retarded growth. More precisely it identified critical stages of development at which interference with an animal's growth could have permanent and far-reaching consequences[8].

In the rat the critical stage occurs within the first, second or third week after birth, when any imposed restriction to growth is likely to lead to a smaller adult size. A few weeks later, a short period of controlled feeding can reduce a rat's growth but this is quickly made up when full feeding is restored. A possible explanation for this rests in the development of the appetite control centres of the hypothalamus. These centres do not mature until about ten days after the rat is born and it was argued that it is the feeding experience at this time which may set their functioning level, the rat's subsequent rate of growth and its final size. Scientific support for such a programming role for the hypothalamus then began to emerge elsewhere.

Short[9] found that the exposure of fetal female lambs to androgens could induce anatomical, behavioural and neuroendocrine effects which are indicative of masculinisation. A single dose of testosterone propionate, given within the first five days after birth to female rats, also induced long-term changes in growth rate and efficiency of feed utilisation[10]. It was suggested that this treatment with sex steroids can programme developmental processes in early life, at a time when the animals are reproductively quiescent. All of this began to confirm the proposed role for sex steroids in initiating certain neuronal circuits in the brain, and other developments concerning hypothalamic anatomy and function[11].

The 'experimental medicine' approach in growth studies inevitably combined the anatomical, chemical and functional aspects of growth. Its origin lay in the metabolic investigations of the 1930s and the studies on human body composition in the 1950s. But it soon became routine in the repertoire of techniques for the study of comparative development. The pioneering approaches of acid digestion of tissues and analysis by visual colorimeters are crude by modern standards, and have long been overtaken by automated microanalysis for a multitude of components of blood and tissues. But the difficult, labour-intensive analytical techniques of yesteryear ensured that questions were well formulated before the work was undertaken. McCance and Widdowson always took the trouble to ask the right questions.

All of this work allowed the conclusion to be drawn that inadequate nutrition, however caused, and for surprisingly short periods of time if imposed early in an animal's life, can induce permanent effects on final size and stature. The inevitable question then to ask was, 'Could undernutrition of sufficient severity and duration have similar profound and enduring effects if imposed at other stages of development?'

CATCH-UP GROWTH

The notion of catch-up, or compensatory growth, is part of the dogma of animal production and child rearing. In farm animals it is usually linked to the seasonal availability of food; in children it may be seen as part of the recovery phase following illness. It does not always occur[1] and McCance and Widdowson's significant contribution was to tease out the fundamental principles which determined why this might, or might not happen.

Before this could be properly reasoned, and even before the research on rats had been effectively exploited, steps had been taken to collect some of the necessary information via what became known as 'the undernourished pigs and poultry' studies.

There were 19 papers published in *The British Journal of Nutrition* between 1960 and 1969 on *Severe undernutrition in growing and adult animals*, all documenting this classical and remarkable undertaking. The first paper *Production and general effects*[12], sets out how the work was established and undertaken and describes some of the early results. As the world of nutrition science now knows, the experiments were designed to control the growth of young pigs so that they weighed only 5-10kg when they were a year old and to do the same with chickens so that they weighed about 200g at six months of age.

The published record is a monumental understatement of the difficulties encountered. Finding the appropriate diet, the feeding regimens and housing conditions for the pigs and poultry, which were highly susceptible to cold, infection and parasitic infestation, provided a new aspect to farm-animal husbandry which the animal technicians, Terry Cowen and his father, Stan, developed as they went along.

In time, however, the procedure became sufficiently routine to provide enough material for a variety of studies to be undertaken of the anatomical development and chemical composition of the bodies, tissues and organs. Some of the animals were used to follow the effects of rehabilitation on metabolism and body temperature, and eventually it was possible to look at reproductive function. The external collaborations were drawn from the leading experts of the time, including LE Mount, GA Gresham, CWM Pratt, CH Tonge and JA

Fairfax-Fozzard, whose outstanding radiographic skills brought a new dimension to the research.

In this way a unique body of information on the fundamental effects of undernutrition in pigs and poultry was built up. It is difficult, however, for anyone who was not involved, to imagine the blend of perseverance, cajolery, enthusiasm, heartache, humour and table-thumping that is needed to keep such a difficult enterprise in motion for so long.

Critics who carp about the size of the experimental groups, or the statistical validation of the observations, cannot begin to know what challenges and difficulties the experimenters undertaking this kind of research have to face. A nocturnal power failure might rob the animals of their vital source of heat, and the researchers of months of work. But experimental investigations of this kind were never going to be an easy option. Apart from the overwhelming practical problems of experimentation, there were ethical and philosophical questions to be handled, that are inevitably attached to such work. Even so, the work on undernutrition was completed and the next, relatively easy, phase of rehabilitating the animals could be started.

At first the greatest care was taken to ensure that the digestive systems of the animals were not overwhelmed by giving them too much food in the early stages of rehabilitation. It was soon realised, however, that this was not going to present the anticipated problem, and the pigs and poultry grew as fast as controls of the same initial size, once they were established on full feeding. In next to no time, the appearance of the rehabilitated animals changed remarkably and within a month, the pigs, for example, had lost much of the evidence of their undernutrition—the 'loose', hairy skin, the excessively large head and the characteristic stance. The chickens too, developed a more appropriate plumage and proportioned appearance, little different from those of normally reared birds.

The rehabilitated pigs, however, never quite reached the size of their normally fed litter mates. Although their rate of growth was adequate in the early stages, it persisted only until the age at which normal pigs cease to grow, and thus did not compensate for the 'lost' year.

The undernourished poultry were restricted for six months, during which time a normal bird would have reached its mature size. The rehabilitated birds, unlike the pigs, continued to grow for a further three or four months after the six months of restriction, though they too suffered a reduction in their final size.

This discovery prompted the question of whether pigs were also capable of extending their period of growth, if growth was severely restricted for the whole length of its usual duration. Inevitably the experiments were done[13]. The results showed that indeed the pig can stretch its period of growth; though by only a little, and the longer its growth is restricted, the less recovery it is able to make.

All of this, of course, fits in well with Oppers' view[3] that there is a fixed time for man to achieve final stature. It may be achieved early (in his late teens) or in his early twenties, but all chance of complete recovery from growth setbacks is lost if it has not been made up by about 25 years of age.

The reproductive performance of rehabilitated chickens and pigs seemed to be relatively little affected by their early experience. The chickens laid eggs in size and number which would be no disgrace to the average chicken, and the pigs produced piglets of normal size, though in smaller litters which were reared without handicap. Indeed, it was the normality of the rehabilitated animals which was perhaps the most remarkable feature of the growth-restriction experiments. The condition of both pigs and poultry was such as would have rendered even the most practised eye incapable of assessing the animals' previous histories.

THE PROBLEM OF THE RUNT

The picture of how growth and chronological age are interrelated was now beginning to emerge. There was, however, still one practical matter which required attention and that was concerning the runt animal, whose fetal growth is considerably impaired but whose subsequent development is a contentious matter.

Smallness at birth presents a widely recognised handicap and it is a particular hazard if the environmental conditions are testing, for runts are ill-equipped with energy substrates to cope with such insults[14]. Farm animals of low birth weight may not, in consequence, survive the perinatal period. If they do, their slow growth and poor development usually preclude their retention to maturity, say, for breeding. Information about the final development of runt farm animals is, therefore, sparse and the situation in man is not much better.

Low birth weight can occur from a variety of causes. Apart from genetic reasons, placental blood supply, or the position of the fetus in the uterine horn, or the numbers in the litter are commonly cited and all reflect either the general or local availability of nutrients to the developing young.

Guinea pigs are surprisingly mature at birth and vary quite widely in weight. They can lead an independent existence essentially from shortly after birth, though they grow better if they continue to suckle. In prospect, therefore, this species should provide an excellent model for growth studies. But the stimulus to use them in experiments came quite serendipitously.

There had always been a certain amount of coming and going between the Cambridge University Pathology Department and Experimental Medicine since the Department's earliest days, and some comparisons were inevitable. Mac noticed that the Path Lab's guinea pigs, which were reared on a diet based on sugar-beet pulp, seemed poor specimens compared with those reared on a 'complete' laboratory diet. Here, he persuaded me, was the basis of an experiment. Following the effect of diet throughout life on reproduction and growth, soon became part of my thesis research.

The research showed that if the mother's diet is inadequate in quantity or quality she will have fewer and smaller young, which are rarely able to reach the adult size of contemporaries of heavier birth weight, no matter how well they are fed thereafter[15]. The same picture can be observed for other laboratory species[16].

The nutrition of the mother during pregnancy has also long been known to influence the birth weight of sheep and cattle, though it appears to be only when feed is severely restricted, or restricted over a long period of time, that the birth weight of piglets is affected. The same seems to hold for the size of the newborn human infant which suffers classically through the deprivations caused by wars[17,18].

The development at birth and the future for runt animals became an interest for Miss Widdowson too. Typically, it did not rest with the science, and in the course of her study of the subject she was able to discover the considerable variety of names for these animals and the locations where they are, or have been, used[19]. Runts, she discovered, resemble more closely a heavier newborn animal than an immature fetus of the same weight. Usually the organs and soft tissues are most retarded whereas the growth of the brain is less affected[14]. A small sample of low birth-weight pigs that she was able to keep until they reached their mature size, bore out the general expectation that their smallness at birth would represent a permanent handicap.

EARLY GROWTH RESTRICTION AND ADULT DISEASE IN HUMANS

The 'critical periods' story has been brought up to date and given a novel twist by Professor David Barker's epidemiological studies of the long-term effects of an adverse environment in fetal life, on cardiovascular disease in adult life[20]. Using historical records of birth weight collected in Hertfordshire from 1911 onwards, and conducting follow-up studies on records on those who have died, and on present-day survivors, Barker has been able to construct a hypothesis which declares that retarded growth in fetal life and infancy is strongly related both to mortality from cardiovascular disease and to the adult levels of some of its known risk factors. In particular, he implicates the long-term effects on physiology and metabolism imposed by an adverse environment during critical periods of development. The effects tend to persist, irrespective of the social class in which individuals are born and reared (just as in the guinea pig and rat work cited above).

These recent discoveries bring even greater importance to the critical nature of programming in early life. The results of the laboratory studies with experimental animals now in progress will be keenly awaited.

The 'people' thread that I mentioned in my Introduction is relevant here too. Professors McKeown, Record and Eckstein of the Birmingham University Medical School Departments of Social Medicine and Anatomy, contributed significantly to our understanding of the physiology of growth during the 1950s and 1960s. There was extensive contact between Cambridge and Birmingham on these matters. David Barker was working in Birmingham's Department of Social Medicine during this time and was party to it all. I would like to think that this indirect link with McCance and Widdowson was instrumental to his later thinking.

POSTFACE

It was fortunate for medical science that the coin determining Mac's future career came down in its favour, rather than ordaining a role for him in agriculture and, thence, undoubtedly in animal science. Miss Widdowson might similarly have become a leading figure in food science (if she isn't already, among her many other specialties). As it happens medicine, food and agriculture have benefited in good, if not equal measure, as this volume amply demonstrates.

So it is that McCance and Widdowson's researches on growth and development also form part of the classical literature in animal science, ranking alongside the work of Lawes and Gilbert, Moulton, Brody, Hammond and Blaxter.

Science to McCance and Widdowson is not split between disciplines so much as areas of interest among which they have freely moved. An Australian called Shields, who was a specialist on the marsupial quokka, came to the Department of Experimental Medicine for a sabbatical. He chose to work on coypus which were then starting to become a problem in the drainage systems in the Fens. The coypu was alleged to have an unusual capacity for staying submerged for extended periods and Mac thought it would be interesting, not to say 'wizard', to see why this should be.

On another occasion, Miss Widdowson was diverted (and, from time to time, still is) into examining how it is that infant bears are able to come to terms with the nitrogen balance of their mothers during long periods of hibernation. A young research worker cannot fail to be stimulated by such curiosity.

Curiosity may still be the prime motivator in science but I, for one, regret the passing of the 'wizard' factor.

References

1 *Wilson PN, Osbourn DF.* **Compensatory growth after undernutrition in mammals and birds.** Biol Rev 1960; **35**: 324-363.

2 *Cherry-Garrard A.* **The worst journey in the world.** London: Penguin, 1937.

3 *Oppers VM.* **Analyse van der acceleratie van der menselijke lengtegroei door bepaling van het tijdstip van de groefasen (Thesis)** Amsterdam: University of Amsterdam, 1963.

4 *Widdowson EM, McCance RA.* **Physiological undernutrition in the newborn guinea pig.** Br J Nutr 1955; **9**: 316-321.

5 *Widdowson EM, McCance RA.* **The effects of chronic undernutrition and of total starvation on growing and adult rats.** Br J Nutr 1956; **10**: 363-373.

6 *Kennedy GC, McCance RA.* **Endocrine aspects of overnutrition and undernutrition.** In: *Gardiner-Hill H ed.* **Modern trends in endocrinology.** London: Butterworths, 1957.

7 *Castle WE.* **Genetic studies of rabbits and rats.** Carnegie Pub No. 320. Washington: Carnegie Inst, 1922.

8 *Widdowson EM, McCance RA.* **The effects of finite periods of undernutrition at different ages on the composition and subsequent development of the rat.** Proc Roy Soc B 1963; **158**: 329-342.

9 *Short RE.* **Sexual differentiation of the brain of the sheep.** In: *Forest MG, Bertrand J eds.* **Sexual endocrinology of the perinatal period.** Paris: INSERM, 1974: 121-142.

10 *Perry BN, McCracken A, Furr BJA, MacFie HJ.* **Separate roles of androgen and oestrogen in the manipulation of growth and efficiency of food utilization in female rats.** J Endocr 1979; **81**: 35-48.

11 *Dyer RG, MacLeod NK, Ellendorf F.* **Electrophysiological evidence for sexual dimorphism and synaptic convergence in the preoptic and anterior hypothalamic areas of the rat.** Proc Roy Soc B 1976; **193**: 421-440.

12 *McCance RA.* **Severe undernutrition in growing and adult animals 1. Production and general effects.** Br J Nutr 1960; **14**: 59-74.

13 *Widdowson EM.* **Changes in pigs due to undernutrition before birth and for one, two and three years afterwards and the effects of rehabilitation.** In: *Roche AF, Falkner F eds.* **Nutrition and malnutrition: identification and measurement. Vol 49: Advances in experimental medicine and biology.** New York: Plenum Press, 1974a; **49**: 165-181.

14 Widdowson EM. **Immediate and long term consequences of being large or small at birth: a comparative approach.** In: **Size at Birth.** Ciba Foundation Symposium 27 (NS). Amsterdam: Assoc Scient Publ, 1974b: 65-76.

15 Lister D, McCance RA. **The effect of two diets on the growth, reproduction and ultimate size of guinea pigs.** Br J Nutr 1965; **19:** 311-319.

16 Blackwell NM, Blackwell RQ, Yu TTS, Weng YS, Chow BF. **Further studies on growth and feed utilization in progeny of underfed mother rats.** J Nutr 1968; **97:** 79-84.

17 Antonov AN. **Children born during the siege of Leningrad.** J Pediat 1974; **30:** 250-259.

18 Smith CA. **Effects of maternal undernutrition upon the newborn infant in Holland** (1944-1945). J Pediat 1974; **30:** 229-243.

19 Widdowson EM. **Environmental control of growth: the maternal environment.** In: *Lister D, Rhodes DN, Fowler VR, Fuller MF eds.* **Meat animals, growth and productivity,** New York: Plenum Press, 1976: 273-284.

20 Barker DJP **The effect of nutrition of the fetus and neonate on cardiovascular disease in adult life.** Br J Nutr 1992; **51:** 135-144.

Third world nutrition
by Roger Whitehead

INTRODUCTION
McCance and Widdowson only became involved *directly* in Third World research relatively late in their careers with the Medical Research Council (MRC). In 1966, Professor McCance, on retiring from Cambridge, was appointed Honorary Director of the MRC's Infantile Malnutrition Research Unit in Kampala, Uganda. In reality, however, their work had a profound effect on the health and wellbeing of the underprivileged children of Africa long before that.

THE BEGINNINGS—1946 to 1964

Germany
The beginning was really the series of studies carried out by an MRC team, under the direction of Professor McCance in Germany between 1946 and 1949. One of the members of this team was Dr RFA (Rex) Dean who investigated the value of plant mixtures as additions to the diets of schoolchildren and children living in orphanages. Among those studied were many between six months and two years, an age range in which it is very difficult to feed children adequately without milk. The routine orphanage diets given to such babies at this critical period in German history contained very little animal protein, however, and the plan was to see whether supplements of balanced mixes of cereal and soya proteins could be as effective as milk proteins in the promotion of growth and health.

Although some difficulties were encountered, it was concluded that the excellent growth achieved by most of the children was a good indication that it should be possible to develop a cheap vegetable diet, satisfactory even for children at this vulnerable age. Dean published these findings in a special MRC Report[1].

Plant proteins in the treatment of kwashiorkor
The relevance of this work to the feeding of babies in what we now call the Third World did not escape the attention of the MRC and in 1951, it decided to set up a small research group in Uganda to investigate these possibilities further. This group eventually became a unit which

Dean continued to direct until his premature death in 1964. I myself joined the staff in 1959.

Although Dean developed a scientific style which was in many ways very different from either that of McCance or Widdowson, the debt he felt towards them was always very apparent. While McCance was clearly the 'role model', it was to Elsie Widdowson that he poured out his scientific worries, knowing that he would receive sympathetic advice and encouragement. Dr Widdowson has often related how Dean, when debating whether or not to employ myself, wrote to see if she would be responsible for the interview. Unfortunately, or perhaps fortunately, the letter got lost *en route* and I arrived unvetted by the matriarch!

The main quality that Dean had inherited from his mentors was the ability to define the precise questions which needed to be answered and then to develop the simplest research protocol capable of testing the relevant hypotheses. With Dr Widdowson's advice, he quickly set up a sympathetic dietary study on undernourished Ugandan children between one and three years of age, who had suffered from kwashiorkor[2]. This was at a time when ideas about protein requirements had not yet been placed on a sound scientific basis and a primary aim was to produce diets that contained 'as much protein as possible'. The food had also to be low in fat and the carbohydrate 'should not give rise to any digestive disturbance'. Although Dean found that his diets, fortified with plant protein, could be very beneficial in the treatment of kwashiorkor, he gradually realised that milk-based therapeutic diets were usually more efficient. In retrospect, one can say that the main value of these early studies lay in *prevention*, and providing mothers with practical advice on how they could optimise the health of their growing babies, using only locally available and affordable food stuffs.

In the McCance and Widdowson tradition, these practical studies were operated by Dean in parallel with more fundamental investigations, and ultimately, in which I myself became more and more involved. The basic thrust of this work continued to be reported back to Cambridge and thus when Dean died in 1964, it was not too difficult for his 'teachers' to pick up the mantle of their student.

'GOOD HOUSEKEEPING' IN UGANDA—1964 to 1966
Prior to McCance being asked by the Medical Research Council to take up the directorship of Dean's old unit in Kampala, both he and Dr Widdowson paid separate visits in order to ensure that the initiatives that were already in progress could be brought to a successful conclusion.

Protein and energy status
By this time, Dean and I had become interested in the use of various

biochemical 'markers' as indicators of latent protein deficiency or subclinical kwashiorkor, in contrast to chronic calorie undernutrition or subclinical marasmus. A distortion in the pattern of the free plasma amino acids appeared to be characteristic of the former but not of the latter, thus opening up the possibility of a differential diagnosis at an early stage[3].

Growth stunting had always been a well-recognised feature of both pre-kwashiorkor and marasmus. The fact that the excretion of hydroxyproline-containing peptides, a product of collagen metabolism and hence of bone growth, was reduced in both nutritional disorders[4], offered a biochemical, as opposed to an anthropometric way, of assessing this retarded growth velocity. The working hypothesis was that a combination of plasma-free amino acid and urinary hydroxyproline measurements would enable the public health investigator to determine not only the presence within the community of calorie undernutrition, but also whether this was associated with primary protein undernutrition.

McCance and Widdowson were intrigued with this possibility because they were becoming increasingly concerned by the growing vogue of bundling together protein deficiency and energy undernutrition, under the single descriptive term protein-energy malnutrition or PEM. They were convinced they represented two distinct syndromes. Dr Widdowson set up animal studies in Cambridge and successfully verified the above biochemical differences[5]. Although subsequent work was to cast doubt on the simultaneous measurement of these two parameters as of practical value for public health purposes, the associated human and animal studies did perhaps help to caution the scientific world not to leap too readily into an oversimplified conclusion about kwashiorkor and marasmus having a common nutritional aetiology.

Malnutrition and the immune response

Another ongoing study that McCance found intriguing was one which had been initiated by a young paediatrician, Dr Erasmus Harland. Although it had been assumed for many years in Uganda that malnutrition must cause an impairment of the immune response, this had never been quantified, especially in subclinical malnutrition associated only with growth faltering. Under McCance's guidance, Harland[6] was able to demonstrate that children with subnormal growth had reduced tuberculin reactions after BCG vaccination and that a short period on a diet rich in protein improved the response.

The writing of scientific papers

These are but a few examples of how McCance and Widdowson were able to bring to fruition pieces of work which might otherwise have been lost with Dean's death. In this context, it is well worthwhile recounting another of their fortes that influenced me greatly at this formative stage in my career. This was the great care they always took in the writing up of their work, as well as in the preparation of public lectures. I had expected that two people with such worldwide reputations might have become blasé about such matters, but nothing could have been further from the truth. What was even more important, they made certain that anyone working with them took the same trouble as they did!

One important lesson I had from McCance concerned the writing of scientific papers, particularly those destined for that very demanding journal, the *Lancet*. Two things still stand out in my memory: first, that the introduction should not be a mini-essay but be specific and to the point, leading up to the purpose of the research; secondly, the results and the discussion sections should be kept quite separate in their content. McCance was correcting one of my scripts and pointed out, quite correctly as it turned out, that while the discussion would probably become out-of-date and be in need of modification as knowledge developed, the experimental data were a description of exactly what had happened, and as such should stand the test of time. Now I try to pass on the same advice to others!

With spoken papers, I was amazed by the fact that this famous and experienced pair carefully rehearsed them at least once before they were finally delivered.

Some may feel that these reminiscences are out of place in a chapter which is supposed to be devoted to scientific achievements, but I have included them because they illustrate well the discipline and attention to detail always shown by McCance and Widdowson, even when just called upon to 'housekeep' another MRC establishment.

DIRECTORSHIP IN UGANDA—1966 to 1968

Around the end of 1965, Sir Harold Himsworth, the Secretary of the MRC, decided to ask McCance if he would become the Honorary Director of the Kampala Unit until a more permanent person could be identified. On retiring from the Department of Experimental Medicine in Cambridge in 1966, he spent the following two years resident in Uganda. By way of a swap, I was transferred to Cambridge to work with Dr Widdowson.

This was to be one of the most valuable periods of my career. From the foregoing comments, it might have become apparent that my seven years in Uganda, immediately following a PhD, had left me in danger of being somewhat isolated and too over-specialised. Although I did not wish to leave the field of protein-energy malnutrition, I was badly in need of a period of research in which I would be encouraged to broaden my horizons. There could have been no better person to have worked with than Elsie Widdowson! Not only did she go to endless lengths to find me a house when it was known

I would be leaving Uganda, she also supervised the structural alterations, to make it more suitable for my growing family. When I was ultimately appointed to replace McCance in Uganda, she agreed to take out the appropriate *power of attorney* so she could administer the letting of my property while I was away.

This story is important because it illustrates the total support that Elsie gave to her junior staff. Her great humanism as well as strict scientific guidance has served many a young scientist and enabled them to emulate both her own and McCance's achievements. That she was like this should not really have come as a surprise as Dean had often spoken about his indebtedness to Elsie, but his adulation seemed too good to be true. It was a great experience to find out personally that he had been right all the time.

Although the close relationship between McCance and Widdowson now had to operate across a distance of over 4000 miles, if anything, it became stronger than ever. It is interesting looking back to examine their strategy for this new challenge. After all, it is no mean task at the age of 67 to take on a research unit in the heart of Africa. Essentially, McCance was a *caretaker Director,* but this is certainly not the way that he saw his task. He was clearly keen to make as big an impact in this job as he had with previous challenges. He quickly recruited two bright young medically qualified scientists, Dr Brian Wharton and Dr David Hadden (both now professors) to inject into the unit the modern clinical and paediatric thought that is so clearly needed. Later he introduced a budding medical physiologist, Dr John Ablett. These three clinical scientists, plus a wise and mature physician, Dr Tom Hall, were to form the basis of McCance's research strategy during his stay in Uganda.

Clinical challenges in the therapy of severe protein-energy malnutrition

The therapy of severely malnourished children requires great skill and care. Ingrid Rutishauser provided a font of nutritional knowledge and Dr Wharton's up-to-date experience in the treatment of premature babies, and others needing the specialised services of an intensive baby care unit, was to become an invaluable asset.

Like Dean before him, McCance appreciated that controlling the precise intake of dietary energy, protein and the micronutrients, and spreading the regimen throughout the day, was crucial for the rapid and complete recovery of children with kwashiorkor and marasmus. McCance and Rutishauser were able to demonstrate an essentially linear relationship between energy intake and catch-up growth: at least 150kcal/kg body-weight was deemed necessary for an optimal response[7]. Protein intake was also important, but no additional benefit accrued bove 4g/kg body weight; nevertheless, this was two to three times the need of a normal well-nourished young preschool child.

In the dietary therapy of *protein-energy* malnutrition, there had also been a tendency to ignore the micronutrients, especially vitamins. McCance's team did not make this mistake and recommended generous additional allowances in order to ensure that they did not become further factors limiting catch up.

Dietary problems were just one of the clinical issues that complicated effective treatment. Wharton identified a wide range of pathologies arising from the malnutrition which also needed to be tackled. These included congestive cardiac failure and pulmonary oedema, hypothermia, hypoglycaemia, drowsiness and stupor, diarrhoea, as well as a multiplicity of infections.

Cardiac failure could be a serious problem in the treatment of kwashiorkor in Uganda. Wharton and McCance showed that this became exacerbated in the ward by the use of relatively high sodium-containing regimens (6mEq/kg/d). Extra salt had originally been introduced into the therapeutic diets in order to rectify as quickly as possible deficiencies in sodium that were also known to be present. When low-sodium regimens were introduced (1mEq/kg/d), far fewer children went into cardiac failure[8].

Haemodilution and temporary fluid retention were only partly responsible for the cardiac failure. There was additional evidence of underlying myocardial lesions in kwashiorkor[9]. The cardiothoracic ratio became abnormally high during treatment and there were indications of increased ventricular voltage in the electrocardiogram. Changes in the T-wave pattern and histology were also suggestive of myocardial disease and this was supported by raised levels of the appropriate isoenzyme of serum lactate hydrogenase which fell with nutritional repletion.

The acute encephalopathy of kwashiorkor was also investigated[10]. While apathy and misery were invariably observed in the untreated child, this usually disappeared quickly with successful treatment. A few children, however, became increasingly drowsy during early treatment, often with frank blunting of the conscious level. This was found not to be due to the predictable pathologies of severe brain disruption, infection, drug toxicity, hypoglycaemia, uraemia, or cholaemia. It was, however, associated with a low-serum sodium and it was suggested that a more likely explanation for the drowsiness was abnormal movements of water and electrolytes across the blood-brain barrier.

Hypothermia was also very common during the first three days after admission to the hospital wards of Uganda and in severe cases it was also associated with an increased mortality rate. Practical measures were recommended to deal with the problem of hypothermia, including nursing in beds which provided shelter and warmth. This was not always easy in hospitals designed to take full advantage of any cooling breezes. In 'at risk' cases, those below 70%

weight for age, the frequent taking of rectal temperatures was also found to be informative.

Ultimately, a heated cubicle was prepared in which a cold kwashiorkor patient could be slowly warmed up under carefully controlled conditions, mimicking the then standard procedures used for true cold injury patients. Hypoglycaemia was often associated with this hypothermia and further simple, yet effective, measures were developed to manage this condition as well.

The authorship of the paper describing the hospital treatment of kwashiorkor and marasmus demonstrates McCance's elegant way of avoiding the cumbersome long list of names associated with multi-authorship papers[11].

The abnormal endocrinology of children with severe kwashiorkor

The studies of David Hadden, the second of McCance's young clinical scientists, while tending to be more fundamental in nature, were by no means lacking in potential practical significance. McCance and Hadden investigated a selection of endocrine factors, in the hope that this might shed light on hormonal aids to treatment. Human growth-hormone administration was tried but produced no significant beneficial effect on children with either kwashiorkor or marasmus when given in the second week after admission[12]. Hadden's studies on insulin concentrations in kwashiorkor and marasmus suggested marked differences between the two forms of protein-energy malnutrition[13]. This was later to be confirmed in community-based studies designed by myself and carried out in Uganda and the Gambia, to achieve a better understanding of the aetiology of the two nutritional disorders.

In Hadden's investigations, plasma insulin levels were low in marasmus but normal to high in kwashiorkor. Associated metabolic studies in children with kwashiorkor also suggested a 'block' at the entry of short chain fatty-acyl-coenzyme-A into the citric acid cycle.

Although these investigations were essentially clinical, and McCance was by nature always very much the experimental physiologist, he nevertheless took a close interest in all the details. His personal research, however, centred on three main topics, the basal metabolic rates (BMRs) of severely malnourished children, the ability of the kidneys of such children to concentrate urine and the responsiveness of the sweat glands to pilocarpine.

Energy metabolism in malnourished children

McCance's work on the metabolic rates of Ugandan children with severe kwashiorkor was carried out in collaboration with Dr John Ablett[14]. For this, a special portable calorimeter had to be designed and built in Cambridge by Bob Spires, and then transported to Uganda. A key finding was that the BMRs of the sick children were subnormal, but rose with treatment, until after a few days they were within the normal range. The reason for the low values was not clear but the results were consistent with those of previous investigations carried out in Cambridge on malnourished pigs.

The authors speculated that specific metabolic pathways could be deranged, or that the turnover rates of the proteins in some organs might be low. Furthermore, the absence of all the normal metabolism of growth must certainly have been a contributory factor. Perhaps the rehabilitation data were the most interesting as they showed that even after a long period of deficiency, the ability to utilise food remained unimpaired. The food conversion ratios, that is the gain in weight per gram of food consumed, were absolutely normal even during early rehabilitation.

Kidney concentrating ability and the functional capacity of sweat glands

These two topics were naturals for McCance to carry out as they followed on closely from interests he had had all his life. In collaboration with Dr Tom Hall and Bob Crown, he showed that, although untreated children suffering from protein deficiency could concentrate their urine above plasma levels, this was never more than twofold and less than half that achieved on discharge[15]. He said this was entirely due to their initially very low intake of protein and the consequent small daily formation of urea. Of more fundamental importance was the observation that neither the treated children, nor their parents, appeared to produce normal urea concentrations, by European standards, in response to conventional periods of water deprivation. However, by manipulating the dietary regime and periods of water deprivation, it was possible to achieve the sort of response typically found in British subjects on their high-protein diets. Furthermore, both the British and Ugandans lost this capacity again when they switched to local Ugandan diets.

From this work, McCance was able to conclude that while the kidneys definitely were physiologically abnormal when the malnourished children were admitted, they had become perfectly normal again by discharge. The apparent long-term functional differences reported by others were thus not abnormal at all but were a natural consequence of dietary differences.

In some ways the philosophical implications of the studies which McCance carried out on the sweat glands of malnourished children were similar. The origins of the investigations were reports in the literature that the response of the sweat glands to thermal stimuli was impaired in malnourished children. At admission, sweat-gland function, in response to pilocarpine, did indeed resemble that found in cystic fibrosis. On discharge, and in apparently healthy Ugandan children, less sweat production was still observed in comparison with

Members of the Department of Experimental Medicine at a weekend gathering in Windsor held in honour of Professor McCance on the occasion of his 'retirement' from Cambridge.

Front row: Left to right: John Walshe, Brian Strangeways, Willy Jonxis, Professor McCance, Cleo Mavrou, Michael Purves, Paul Fourman, Romaine Hervey, Douglas Black.

Middle row: Left to right: Vernon Pickles, Norman Kent, John Dickerson, Mavis Gunther, Dr Widdowson, Elizabeth Hervey, Daphne McDermott (was Learmouth), Lois Strangeways (was Thrussell), Winifred Young, Colin McCance.

Top row: Left ro right: David Lister, John Cowley, David Southgate, Frank Smith, Mr Bland (from Cumberland Lodge, Windsor), Eric Glaser, FW Baskerville, Jan Jonxis.

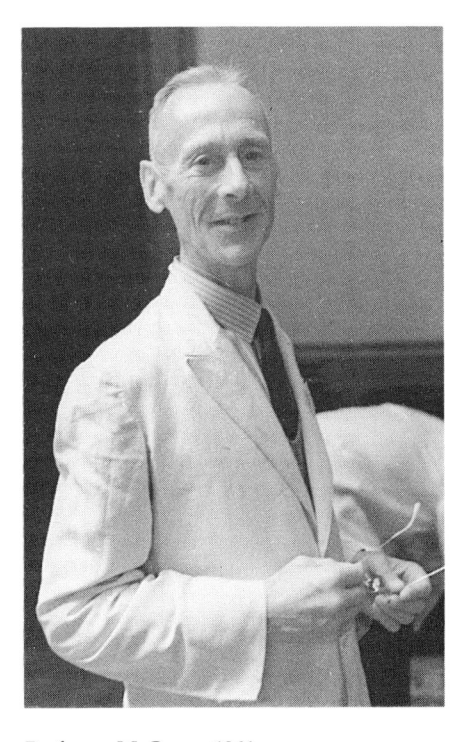

Professor McCance, 1961.

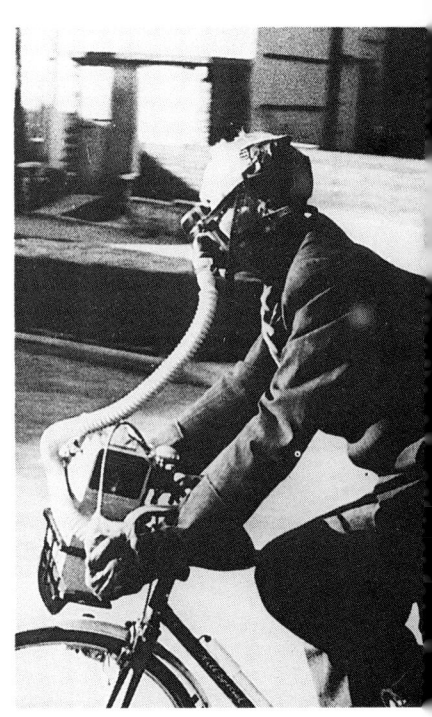

Professor McCance cycling and measuring his energy expenditure, Cambridge, 1954.

Professor McCance in the caravan at Bartlow, with his experimental newborn pigs. Note the bed for the Professor to sleep between measurements.

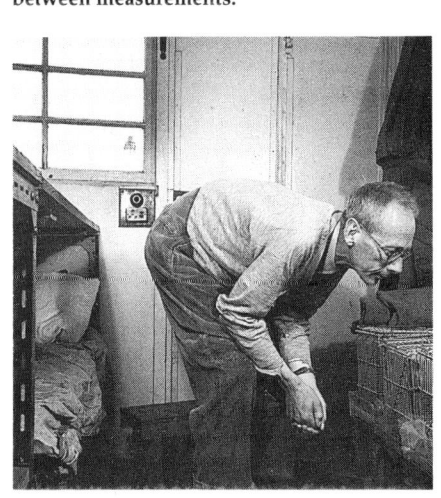

Professor McCance and Terry Cowen at Bartlow with a control animal for the study on undernourished pigs, 1957.

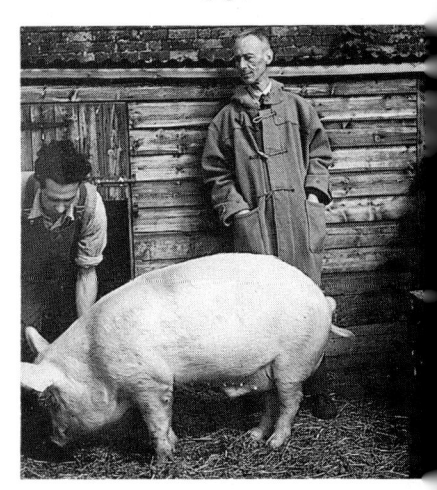

Russell Elkinton's cartoons illustrating the activities of the Department of Experimental Medicine, Cambridge, 1957.

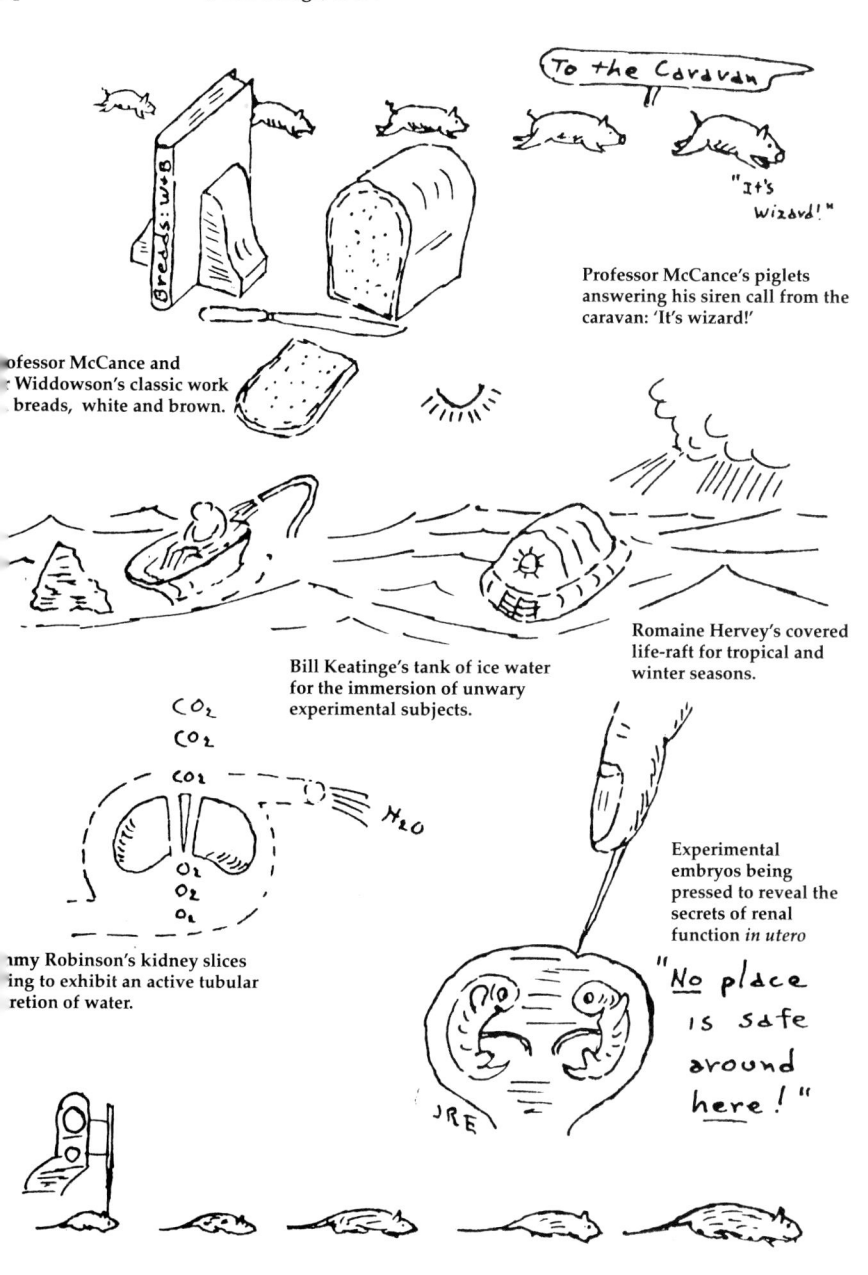

Professor McCance's piglets answering his siren call from the caravan: 'It's wizard!'

Professor McCance and Widdowson's classic work on breads, white and brown.

Bill Keatinge's tank of ice water for the immersion of unwary experimental subjects.

Romaine Hervey's covered life-raft for tropical and winter seasons.

Jimmy Robinson's kidney slices trying to exhibit an active tubular secretion of water.

Experimental embryos being pressed to reveal the secrets of renal function *in utero*

Gordon Kennedy's rats doomed to obesity by experimentally-induced lesions in the hypothalamus.

XI

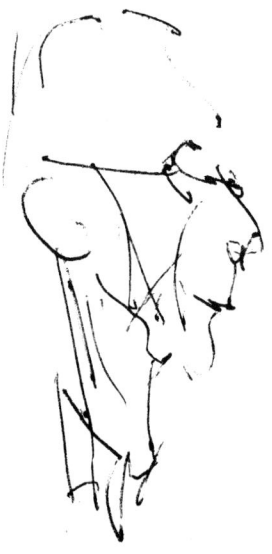

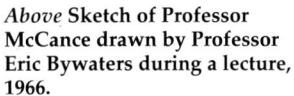

Above Sketch of Professor McCance drawn by Professor Eric Bywaters during a lecture, 1966.

Above right Dr Widdowson with Professor Archie Morrison at Rutgers University Medical School, New Jersey, USA, 1967.

Right Professor McCance with Professor Archie Morrison, 1967.

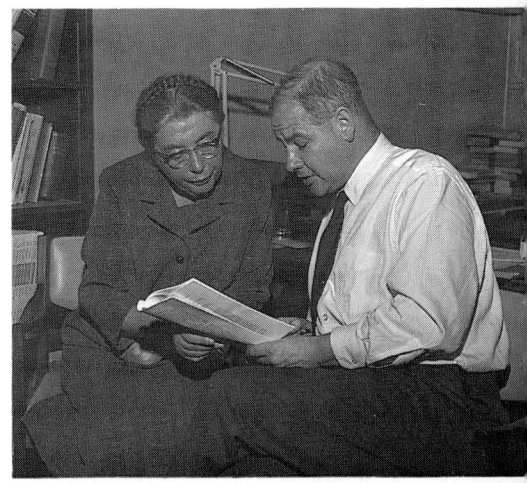

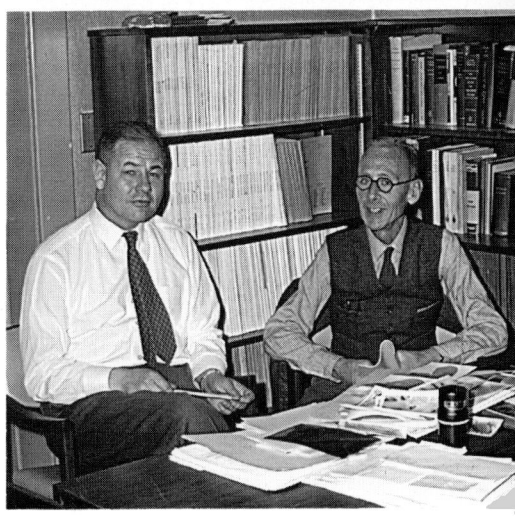

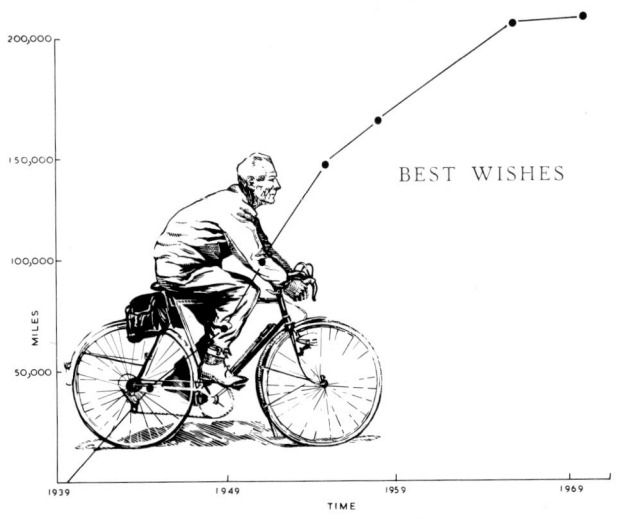

BEST WISHES

Left Professor McCance's Christmas card, 1972, drawn by his daughter Catriona Ogelvy.

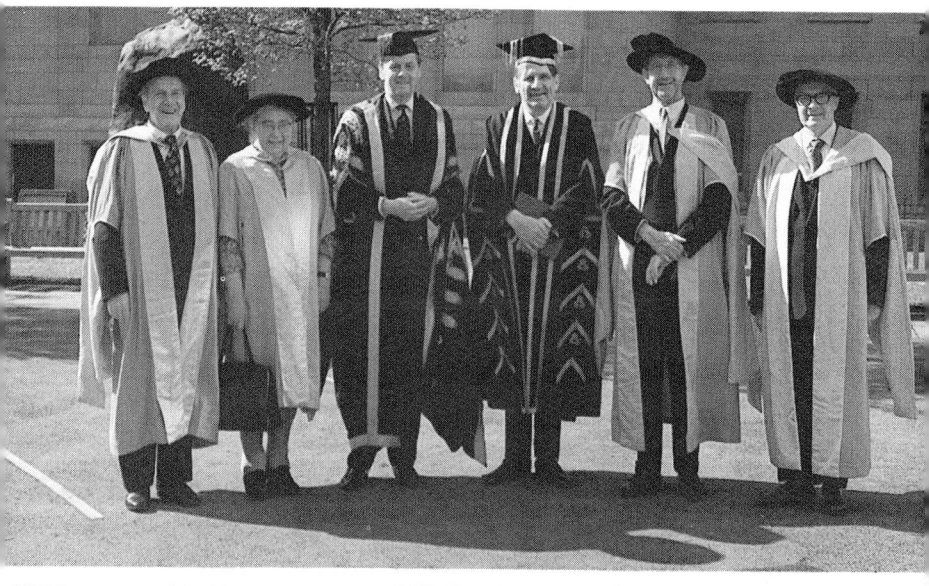

Widdowson receiving her Honorary Doctor of Science degree at Manchester University, 1974. Dr Widdowson carefully positioned herself between Vic Feather, Secretary-General of the Trades Union Congress (on the extreme left of the group) and the Duke of Devonshire.

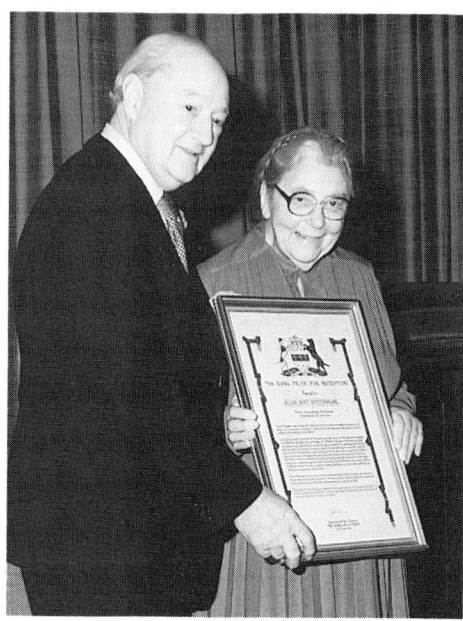

Sir John Davies presenting The Rank Prize Funds Award to Dr Widdowson, London, 1984.

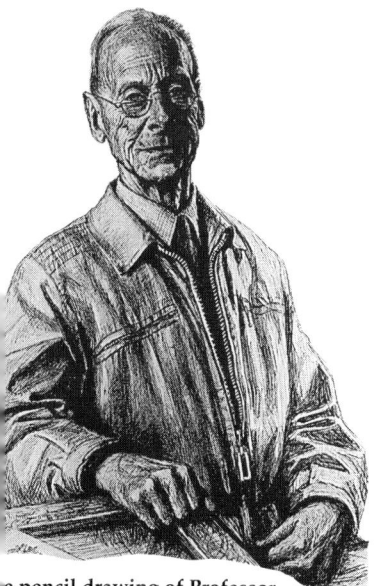

A pencil drawing of Professor McCance by WA Narraway, which was presented to the Professor by the Neonatal Society, 1979.

XIII

Above Dr Widdowson receiving her award for delivering the McCollum International Lecture, Brighton, UK, 1985.
Left to right: Dr Harry Day (Chairman of the McCollum Commemoration Committee), Agatha Rider, Dr Widdowson

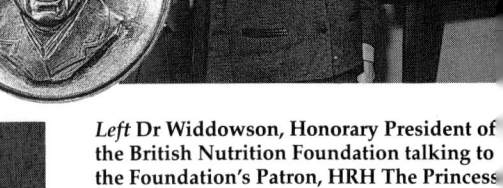

Below Dr Buford Nichols presenting Dr Widdowson with a bronze plaque which now hangs in a Seminar Room at the Children's Nutrition Research Center, Houston, Texas, 1990.

Left Dr Widdowson, Honorary President of the British Nutrition Foundation talking to the Foundation's Patron, HRH The Princess Royal, London, 1991.

Below The first Edna and Robert Langholz International Nutrition Award presented to Dr Widdowson (American Dietetic Association Foundation), Washington DC, 1992.

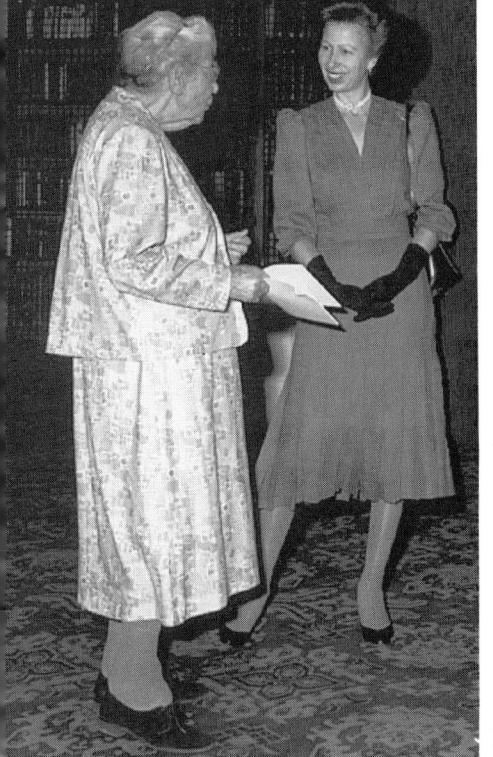

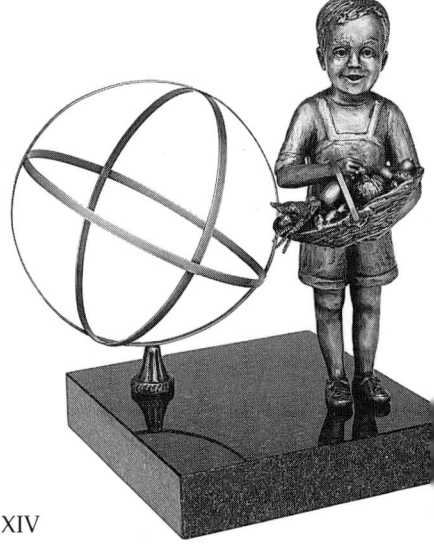

XIV

The Department of Pathology in Tennis Court Road, Cambridge. The Department of Medicine and of Experimental Medicine were housed in this building from 1938 to 1958.

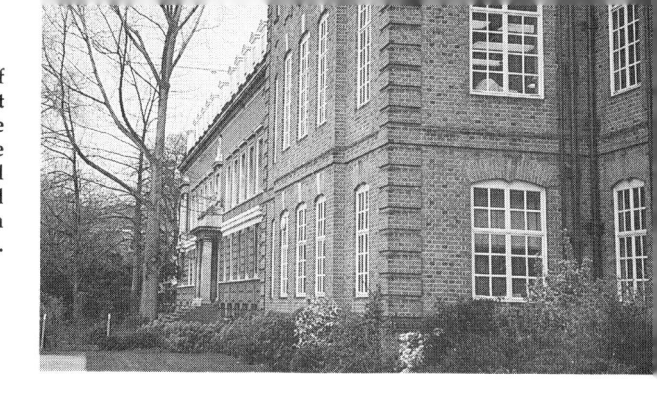

Städtisches Krankenhaus, Wuppertal-Barmen, Germany. The hospital where the MRC team did their clinical work, 1946 to 1949.

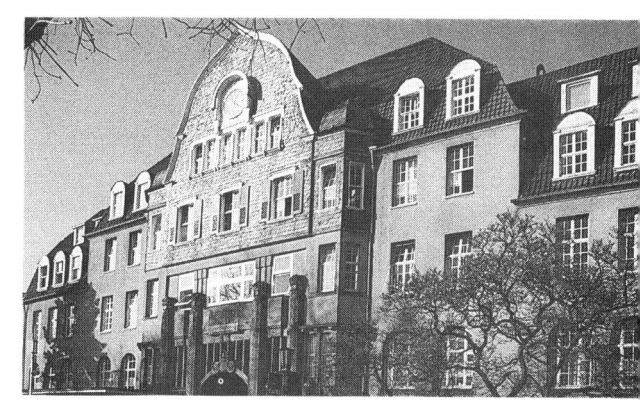

5 Shaftesbury Road, Cambridge. Staff of the Department of Experimental Medicine worked here from 1955 to 1968.

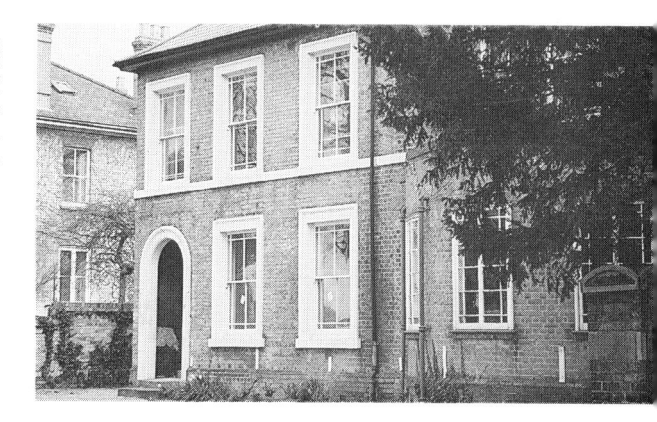

The Dunn Nutritional Laboratory, Cambridge. Dr Widdowson and her team worked here from 1968 to 1973.

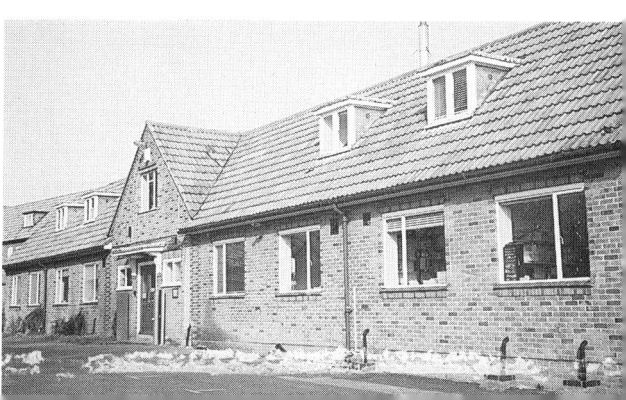

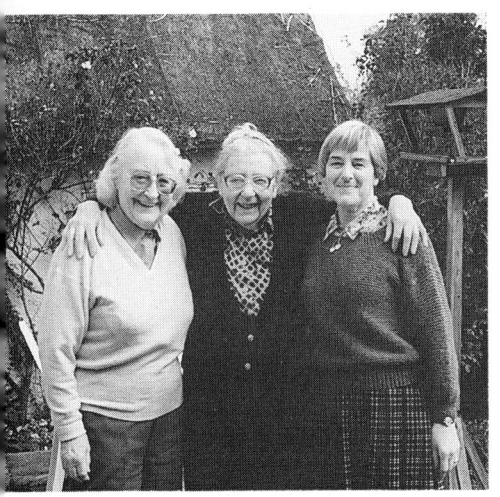

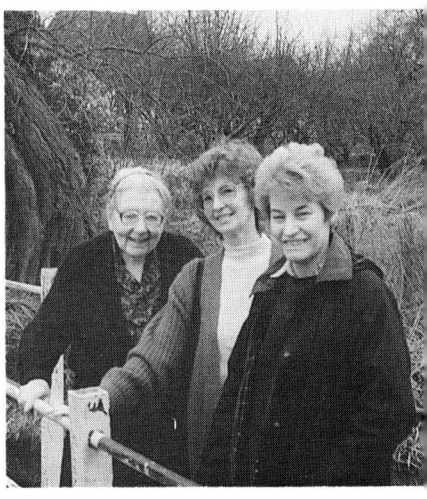

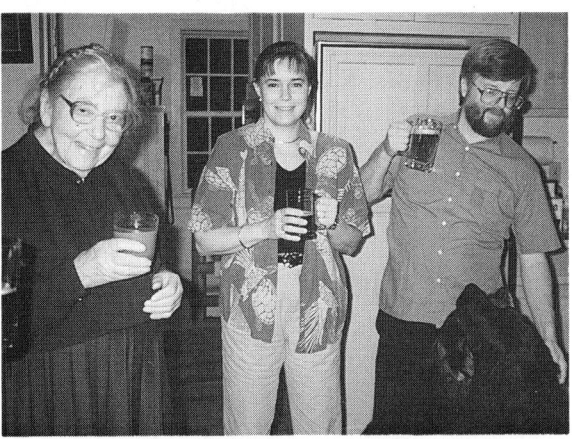

Above left **Dr Dorothy Rosenbaum, Dr Widdowson and Lois Strangeways, Barrington, Cambridgeshire, 1991.**

Above **Dr Widdowson, Dr Janet Kirtland and Dr Margaret Ashwell at the bottom of Dr Widdowson's garden in Barrington, 1991.**

Left **Dr Widdowson with Dr Olav Oftedal and Dr Mar Allen in Olney, Maryland, October 1992.**

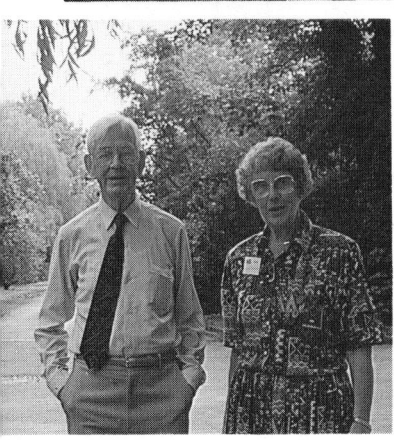

Above **Professors James and Marion Robinson in Cambridge, 1991.**

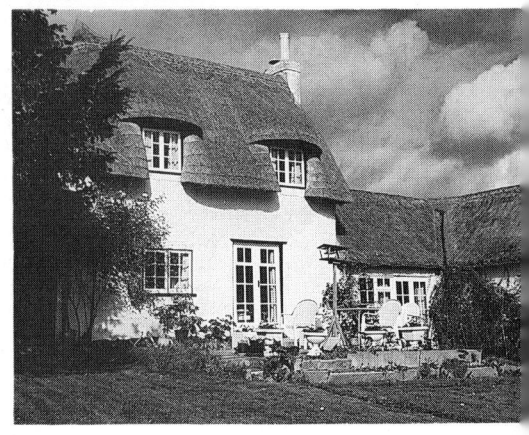

Above **Dr Widdowson's cottage in Barrington, Cambridgeshire…where much of the preparation of this commemorative volume took place.**

Caucasian children. This, however, was shown to be due entirely to differences in the number of functional sweat glands. This is a further example of how McCance's painstaking physiological investigations helped to provide a more satisfactory interpretation of the effects of malnutrition and its response to treatment.

This is just a limited selection of the studies that McCance carried out, or helped to initiate in Kampala. Looking back at the range of activities embarked upon, one is amazed that so much could have been achieved in such a short period of time. What is even more surprising is that this was done by someone approaching 70 years of age. It provides hope and encouragement for us all. There is much that someone who is still young at heart can do to assist the academic development in the Third World, even in retirement.

SUDAN

If all this activity in Uganda was not sufficient, it was at this time that McCance and Widdowson decided to embark upon a major collaborative programme on the response of normal men and women to a large change in their environmental temperatures and ways of life[16]. This was part of the International Biological Programme and involved British and Sudanese men and women being flown to each other's countries at the most extreme times of the foreign climate: the middle of the winter for Cambridge and the height of the hot season for Khartoum. The British temperatures dropped as low as −5.6°C and the Khartoum ones got up to 38.7°C.

A range of physiological and, perhaps more importantly, in collaboration with Dr RT Wilkinson of the MRC Applied Psychology Unit in Cambridge, psychological parameters, was also measured. It was the perceived wisdom of the day that major environmental differences would initially place considerable stress on the mental performance of translocated personnel, requiring a substantial period of acclimatisation before their customary functional capacity would be restored. The results did not support this view, however. To quote, '...no evidence was obtained that the heat in the Sudan was great enough to upset the performance of the British subjects; nor was there any evidence that the Sudanese subjects were put off by the cold of the Cambridge winter, to an extent which made them do their tests worse than they did them later at home'. Once again careful quantitative study was to question widely accepted, but scantily-based beliefs.

To emphasise that there was never a dull moment working with this pair, let me finish with a further anecdote arising from this Sudan study. I was engaged to record the investigation on 16mm movie film. I was assisted by McCance's technician, Dick Luff. During the filming, we were arrested three times! The first was at London Airport. Although we had permission to film on the tarmac, when the Sudanese subjects arrived at Heathrow on a cold winter's afternoon, we were arrested immediately on entering the immigration department. Seemingly not all the staff on duty were *bona fide* immigration officials and the last thing they wanted was for their faces to be recorded on film. It took a lot of time and careful persuasion to get away with the precious film still intact.

The second arrest occurred on arrival at Khartoum Airport. The Sudanese air crew kindly let us off the plane first so we could film the British subjects being hit by the heat and glare of the Sudanese sun for the first time. What no one told us was that it was absolutely forbidden to film in such a potentially strategic place (the 1967 Arab war with Israel had just ended). The final event was in Omdurman market. All of a sudden, Dick Luff and I found ourselves being bombarded with eggs and tomatoes and arrest rapidly followed. This time they thought we were CIA spies. The belief was that if the CIA could not interpret their high-altitude aerial reconnaissance photographs, they sent photographers posing as tourists to fill in the gaps. With our expensive cameras, tripods and lighting equipment, we fitted this bill perfectly. Off we went towards the gaol but luckily one of the Sudanese students who had been with us ran off to alert his boss, who was also a well-known footballer, Nasr El Din. As a footballer, he was about the only person who could have got us off, which he did—and complete with our film!

How did McCance and Widdowson react to the predicaments that they had got us into? Predictably, Elsie showed her typical regard for the welfare of her staff. McCance, on the other hand, seemed more concerned that these adventures had not interfered with the success of our part of his programme. Only after we could reassure him on this point, did he allow himself to acknowledge the drama, and indeed the humorous aspects.

Why do I conclude with this story? I do so because it illustrates the tenacity of purpose McCance has always shown in everything he does, a tenacity which has been with him all his life and which is surely a major reason for his success. One of Elsie's roles has been to provide a moderating effect on any tendency towards excess. As a partnership, they make a perfect pair!

References

1 *Dean RFA.* **Plant proteins in child feeding.** Medical Research Council Special Report Series No. 279. London: HMSO, 1953:1-163.

2 *Dean RFA.* **The treatment of kwashiorkor.** Brit Med J. 1952; **ii:** 791-806.

3   Whitehead RG. **Rapid determination of some plasma amino acids in subclinical kwashiorkor.** Lancet 1964; **i:** 250-252.

4   Whitehead RG. **Hydroxyproline creatinine ratio as an index of nutritional status and rate of growth.** Lancet 1965; **ii:** 567-570.

5   Widdowson EM. Whitehead RG. **Plasma amino acid ratios and urinary hydroxyproline excretions in rats deficient in protein and calories.** Nature 1966; **212:** 683-686.

6   Harland PSEG. **Tuberculin reactions in malnourished children.** Lancet 1965; **ii:** 719-720.

7   Rutishauser IHE, McCance RA. **Calorie requirements for growth after severe undernutrition.** Arch Dis Childh 1968; **43:** 252-256.

8   Wharton BA, Howells GR, McCance RA. **Cardiac failure in kwashiorkor.** Lancet 1967; **ii:** 384-387.

9   Wharton BA, Balmer SE, Somers K, Templeton AC. **The myocardium in kwashiorkor.** Quart J Med 1969; **38:** 107-116.

10 Balmer S, Howells G, Wharton B. **The acute encephalopathy of kwashiorkor.** Develop Med Child Neurol 1968; **10:** 766-771.

11 Staff THE. **Treatment of severe kwashiorkor and marasmus in hospital.** E Afr Med J 1968; **45:** 399-406.

12 Hadden DR, Rutishauser IHE. **Effect of human growth hormone in kwashiorkor and marasmus.** Arch Dis Childh 1967; **42:** 29-33.

13 Hadden DR. **Glucose, free fatty acid, and insulin interrelations in kwashiorkor and marasmus.** Lancet 1967; **ii:** 589-593.

14 Ablett JG, McCance RA. **Energy expenditure of children with kwashiorkor.** Lancet 1971; **ii:** 517-519.

15 McCance RA, Crowne RS, Hall TS. **The effect of malnutrition and food habits on the concentrating power of the kidney.** Clin Sci. 1969; **37:** 471-490.

16 McCance RA, El Neil H, El Din N et al. **The response of normal men and women to changes in their environmental temperatures and ways of life.** Phil Trans Roy Soc 1971; **259:** 533-565.

Day-to-day recollections of life with McCance and Widdowson

Once Professor McCance and Dr Widdowson had given me a long list of various people who had worked with them during their 60-year partnership, my job was a delightful one of helping these people to relive and record their memories. A few were initially reluctant to do this, not because they did not wish to share in the tribute to McCance and Widdowson, but because they felt their own memories would not make a worthwhile contribution to the book. In these instances, gentle persuasion from Dr Widdowson was exerted, and as one contributor confessed, *'As ever, I hasten to obey'*.

A recurrent nightmare for all the contributors to this book was the problem of how they should refer to Professor McCance and Dr Widdowson; and many asked for editorial guidance on this point. In the end, I decided that editorial consistency could not, and should not, be observed and that each contributor should use the names with which he or she was most comfortable. Sometimes contributors have referred to 'McCance and Widdowson' when talking about their early acquaintance in more formal times, and then lapse into 'Mac and Elsie' as formalities have lessened and their relationship has become closer.

Determining the order of presentation of these Recollections was also difficult, but I eventually decided upon a chronological order, based on the contributor's first encounter with McCance and Widdowson.

I hope that the Introduction to each is sufficient to tell the reader what the contributor had done before meeting McCance and Widdowson, and what they did afterwards. One of McCance and Widdowson's many talents was to take in people from a wide range of disciplines, and to send them out to work on a completely different topic from that of their original expertise.

I was particularly keen that this section should not be overburdened by references to scientific publications or by extensive cross-referencing to other parts of the book. If more scientific detail is required, the reader will find it easy to refer to other sections such as the *Autobiographies of McCance and Widdowson* (pages 18 to 44) with the references in their *Selected Publications* (pages 45 to 52), or to the section on *The Scientific Achievements of McCance and Widdowson* (pages 67 to 132).

I hope that these Recollections will be enjoyed for what they are—assorted memories of everyday life with McCance and Widdowson.

MA

Monica Verdon-Roe
(now Mrs JS Ellis)

> Monica Verdon-Roe worked for Professor McCance and Dr Widdowson during their time at King's College Hospital, London (from 1934 to 1938). She helped with the studies of individual diets and the quotes in italics are from her diaries written at the time.

I came down from Cambridge in 1933 with a degree in Natural Sciences. I began work in the Diet Kitchen at St Bartholomew's Hospital, London (Bart's) with Miss Abrahams in the spring of 1934. It was while I was at Bart's that I met Dr Widdowson and later worked for her and Dr McCance at King's College Hospital.

At King's I undertook the preparation of special food for the different diets that Dr McCance and Dr Widdowson needed for their experiments on mineral balances. This was painstaking work, needing careful weighing of all ingredients. The salt-free diet was particularly tasteless and volunteer subjects found it very unpalatable. The equipment in the lab was primitive, with an oven, scales, sink and various essential tools.

Later I was involved with the preparation of cooked dishes, eg cakes, puddings, savouries and meat dishes, for the construction of the food tables. The composition of the cooked foods was calculated from the composition of the listed ingredients and the change in weight on cooking.

In 1937 the individual dietary surveys were started. We investigated pregnant women in various income groups and also a number of children. The women were asked to weigh all food eaten during a week. I had the task of delivering balances to each woman and explaining how to use them. I visited them every day to see how they were getting on. They were Salter Spring Balances weighing up to 2lb in $\frac{1}{4}$ oz increments (I should add that I am still using mine today after 50 years!).

My first group consisted of 20 pregnant women from Bermondsey, the wives of employed labourers. and I visited these women from King's.

At the end of February 1937, I went to Lincoln, and the local doctors arranged for me to meet possible experimental subjects. The husbands of these women were all unemployed. I had ten mothers and 12 children to see every day.

March 6th 1937: *I collected six balances from families who had finished. I* said goodbye to Mrs Clarke this morning. She said she hoped I'd come again and do some more work. She's done her two boys most beautifully.

March 8th: *Dr Widdowson here. We had a party for the children. We measured all their heights and weights. Dr Widdowson did the haemoglobins on some of them and Mr Clarke looked at teeth. I got the nine children into the car, took them and went back for the second lot.*

Later I went to Merthyr Tydfil for two weeks and stayed in a commercial hotel. The Medical Officer for Health and doctors in the clinics were very helpful and gave me the names of 25 women who might be experimental subjects. A district nurse took me round on the first day and I realised that the conditions were fairly bad. The husbands were unemployed miners and the houses were cramped and dirty. However, the women were very willing to help. At the end of the fortnight, Dr McCance and Dr Widdowson came. We had a very funny evening and laughed a good deal at supper. Next day, after Dr McCance had finished visiting the various Medical Officers in the district and Dr Widdowson and I had collected the bloods and taken them for storage in the Hospital, we set off for a walk and a picnic in the Brecon Beacons. This was an excellent occasion and we did not get back to the hotel till after 11pm.

April 27th 1937: *The houses are so poor, so dirty and horrible. One house had coal in one corner of the room—all bare and loose—and children playing on it. I asked one woman if she had any children and she said, 'Yes, six'. She'd already buried eight and had one more on the way.*
  I can't believe that the people whom I visit live in these sort of surroundings year after year, for all their lives. It's ghastly. The children all have colds and wheezy chests and are dirty, dirty.

May 4th: *I saw Mrs Evans today. I told her I'd come for the balances and she said 'Oh, is it your last visit?' I said 'Yes, I'm afraid it is!' 'Oh, I've got so used to you,' she said, 'I should like you to come again.'*

May 7th: *The children are going along so nicely. The mothers are quite sweet and only too willing to help.*

May 8th: *Dr Widdowson and I set off to do haemoglobins. We got 19 women and three children during the morning. After lunch, we went to the school; the little girls were awfully good. We finished at 3.30pm, went to the Town Hall and were taken to the Hospital to put the bloods in the refrigerator.*

In August, I went to Gateshead and here again the women were the wives of unemployed men. The local doctor gave me a list of women and a map of the area and a district visitor to help me start the week. It appears the survey went well and Dr McCance and Dr Widdowson came at the end of the period to collect blood as usual. The only mishap was that for some reason, we had to leave the bloods in the ice chest at the mortuary.

August 30th 1937: *The women seem to me to be very dirty and the children are filthy, wearing no pants in most cases.*

September 2nd: *I have discovered that one woman can neither read nor write and her poor husband has to attend to her meals and the weighing.*

I continued working at King's College Hospital until my marriage in 1938. This was about the same time that Dr McCance and Dr Widdowson moved to Cambridge.

David Whitteridge

> David Whitteridge has known McCance and Widdowson for virtually all of their 60-year partnership. He qualified at King's College Hospital London, in 1937, went back to Oxford and subsequently became Professor of Physiology, first at Edinburgh and then at Oxford.

In 1935 I was a fourth-year medical student at King's College Hospital—better known at that time for the number of its consultant staff who were medical members of the Royal Household, than for its scientific activity. The outstanding exception was Dr RA McCance who was Research Biochemist and Assistant Physician.

Somehow, word reached medical students that McCance wanted volunteers as subjects for a study of pure sodium deficiency. It was known that he always experimented on himself first, and had already used a contemporary, RB Niven, who had survived the ordeal. His success rate was reduced by the next subject who was given an early sample of inulin and had collapsed with a rigour and subsequent anuria for 24 hours. This gave rise to the unusual sight of McCance and Charles Newman themselves pushing a trolley with the supine form of a medical student along King's long corridor to the Private Ward. At the time it was thought that the inulin contained an impurity, but subsequently a pyrogen was held to be responsible. I was the next subject, but was spared inulin; sucrose was used instead to estimate changes in glomerular filtration rate.

The next subject was a female medical student who was unable to lose more than about a litre of sweat in two hours and never became seriously salt-deficient. After sweating, while still naked, she was washed by Elsie with a jet of distilled water to remove any salt left on her skin. McCance always seemed surprised when the resulting lantern slide was so much appreciated by the medical students! Perhaps this experience led to McCance's later work in Africa on sweating rates in men and women. Women never sweated as well as men.

McCance's account of the salt-deficiency experiments in his Goulstonian lectures is so full and clear that I can only add what my own feelings were as 'the toad beneath the harrow'. I remember very clearly lying on a rubber sheet over a mattress on the floor, under a six foot long metal half-cylinder, well furnished with electric lamps. I sweated so freely that pools formed in the hollows made by my elbows. My temperature did not rise above 99.5° Fahrenheit and I felt very comfortable. I gathered that those who sweated poorly had temperatures up to 103° Fahrenheit and felt very miserable. I think I held the world's (unofficial) sweating record until work started on the men who stoked the boilers in the Navy.

During the sweating sessions, I overheard McCance and Elsie Widdowson discussing the design of a new series of nutritional experiments concerned with the welfare of mother and child. Even to a naive medical student, it was clear that McCance was laying out the main lines of the investigation, while Elsie was pinning him down to precise numbers of categories of patients and controls and the number of patients in each group.

The salt-free diet was eatable (just), but I found everything tasteless, even with plenty of pepper. Curried mince rissoles were a moderate success, and salt-free bread and synthetic salt-free milk were reasonably palatable. The last two-hour sweating session was the worst. After it, I felt cold and vomited. I was packed off to the Private Ward where the Charge Nurse took one look at my quite considerable dehydration (the bones at my ankles and wrists were pretty conspicuous), wrapped me in a hot blanket kept on a radiator for patients in shock, and popped me into bed. I have never known anything more comforting than that hot blanket. The nurses, who had even less interest than the medical staff in scientific activity, commiserated over McCance's apparent cruelty to his subjects, a charge which we as volunteers hotly denied.

McCance remarked in his lectures on the torpor that gradually overcame me during the course of the salt-free days. On the first day I read a medical textbook, and on the second I chose some light reading. After that I was quite content to sit in an armchair and do nothing all day. Surgeon Captain Baskerville also remarked on the torpor of severely dehydrated seamen in lifeboats, unwilling or unable to do anything to save themselves. Languor and lassitude are mentioned in the classic descriptions of Addison's disease, but I do not know of any investigation of the cause. McCance himself did not show this picture of torpor when he was salt-deficient, but he was in charge of the experiment, and could not afford to be irresponsibly comatose. He found climbing two flights of stairs while salt-deficient gave him dyspnoea and precordial pain. He was then a fit 37-year old. We all had very viscous venous blood and the increase in total peripheral resistance must have been quite considerable.

Both during and after these experiments we overbreathed for 30 minutes, sufficient to show that when one is salt-deficient, the urine fails to become alkaline, presumably because of a shortage of available base. Once, when McCance overbreathed, he failed to start breathing again and became unconscious. On recovery, he felt ill enough to go home early, but collected his urine samples for the whole period and wrote a short note on the results.

Subsequently, I have spent 29 years trying to run departments of physiology, and although I was labelled as a 'spark physiologist', I felt I had seen enough of 'soup physiology' for me to make sure that the teaching of body fluids and chemical physiology was not neglected. For this, any credit should go to Professor McCance and Elsie Widdowson.

James Robinson

> James Robinson first met Professor McCance and Dr Widdowson in 1938 when he was a medical student in Cambridge; at that time he took part in the **Experimental study of rationing.** *In 1947 he came back to the Department as Assistant Director of Research for ten years, until he went to New Zealand for a year. He came back to Cambridge before returning to New Zealand as Professor of Physiology at Otago University, Dunedin. He retired in 1979.*

In 1938 I was a research student, working in the Departments of Biochemistry and of Colloid Science. I was wondering whether to go off and get medically qualified, and I had consulted Professor John Ryle about this. He thought I should and suggested that I should ask Dr McCance, who had recently come from King's in London to be Reader in Medicine at Cambridge.

McCance received me very kindly, and gazed at me with those blue eyes, as I told my story. I still remember his reply. 'Oh, of course you must; you'll hate it; but you'll never regret it.' In the end I became a medical student, and I have not regretted it; and I didn't hate it either—not even the anatomy. In due course I went off to the London Hospital, but before that, while still in Cambridge doing the anatomy, I got drawn into one of the Department's early wartime activities.

The Professor has always had a persuasive way with him. When the Irish charm is turned on, he is pretty irresistible. He was planning an experimental study of rationing. My part in this was very humble, and very easy. I only had to eat. Incidentally, that experiment left its mark on the Department because, while it was running, wartime rationing was introduced; and in order for the experiment to continue, the Department had to be licensed as a catering establishment, and that was the beginning of the famous lab lunches.

The experimental diet was based on bread, cabbage and potatoes; and although it represented a considerable departure from what we had been eating, it was believed to supply all that was essential, so nobody need fear starvation. Although it was in one sense a strict ration, there was a lot of it. It needed a pretty big stomach to get enough calories.

Nobody came to any harm, although some people thought they felt cold. I think we all felt pretty full after meals. I remember walking about on tiptoe, breathing rather tentatively, after some of them. And the diet had some mysterious influence upon our renal function, or maybe only our bladders, for at times the need to empty them came upon us with an extreme urgency—especially noticeable during collecting periods when we were a long way from our bottles. Professor Ryle, who kept a clinical eye on us (and ate the lunches with us), asked us once if we had wind; and whether it was upward wind or downward wind. The diet was indeed extremely flatogenic.

All things considered, we did very well on this diet. Of course we were pretty sedentary, possibly not active enough to test it properly—except perhaps the Professor. He was sedentary too, after his own fashion; but he did a lot of his sitting on a moving cycle. Anyway, greater physical activity was needed. So a husky Pembroke man, called Cameron, I think, ate with us for a time and stroked the College boat on it. And then the Professor's mother-in-law was borrowed as a representative of an older generation. She found the diet more than she needed, and thrived on it too. A more thorough testing of ourselves on the ration was carried out just after Christmas. We had a magnificent Christmas dinner at Elsie's house in Barrington, made of things that had been secretly saved from the ration for weeks beforehand. And then, two days later, the Professor and I set out on bicycles heading for Langdale in the Lake District. We kept to the ration all the way up the Great North Road, stopping at hotels. We would order soup, double portion of 'veg' and no meat; then we brought out our diary and our spring balance and weighed and entered everything before we ate it.

Elsie, Andrew Huxley and Colin McCance set out later in the car, and came behind to pick up the bits. They caught up with us at Skipton, and we all spent the night there before crossing the Pennines. There was snow on the road for the rest of the way. The motor party gave the 'wheelers' hot drinks somewhere around Kirkby Lonsdale, and they then went ahead and had a fire and a grand lunch ready for us when we arrived in Langdale, a little after noon on the third day. My chief function there was to provide one extreme of biological variation to balance the Professor at the other extreme.

I was new to the hills, although I grew up near them and went to school in Ulverston. However, I was not sufficiently addicted to discomfort to eat my full ration in the open. The Professor could stand on a rock in a snowstorm on the top of a mountain and eat a two-pound loaf of bread. I remember a lovely picture of him, holding his loaf much as a squirrel holds a nut. But I went short on those days, and made up in comfort by the fire the day after.

My first contact with the Department then, was as an experimental animal. Later, after I had qualified, and had three and a half years in the army, I came back to Cambridge in 1947 to look after the medical students at Emmanuel College. The Professor had a University post created for me in 1949. I belonged to the University, though the Department was mostly Medical Research Council (MRC). Not that this mattered a great deal. But I do not think I contributed as much to the mainstream of the Department's work as most other people did.

I may have added something to the atmosphere though, for I was still working under the influence of my time in colloid science, and I got into a chase after water pumps which at one time looked like being quite exciting. The handling of water, and the things dissolved in water, is a fundamental activity of all living cells, and one which has a great bearing on the things that cells do together—in organs like the kidney, or in the body as a whole. And renal function, and the physiology of water and electrolytes, were right at the core of the Department's developing interests in growth, maturation and maintenance of the whole organism, especially at the extremes of life.

To help with the Professor's experiments on survival at sea, we 'borrowed' some sailors from the Navy who very much enjoyed their time. They thanked us by painting the Department (including the bust of Sir Clifford Allbutt) and presenting the Professor with a pair of cycle clips. They had watched the daily ritual of how he would come into the lab at the end of the afternoon and prop up each leg slowly and carefully, so that he could tie a piece of string around the bottom of his trousers. The cycle clips were not really appreciated and seldom worn, probably because the Professor enjoyed his ritual with the pieces of string and the way that it signalled that he was about to go home. The clips would have taken less than half the time to make the same point.

Considering its large output of distinguished publications, the laboratory was remarkably small, modestly equipped and located in a few rooms on the ground floor of the Department of Pathology. In 1939, there was a large common room which housed a gas stove, where lunches were prepared and eaten. There was also a big laboratory of similar size where a handful of technicians carried out the analyses of foodstuffs and end-products—including human and animal material, blood and other offerings from subjects of experiments, and from patients on balance studies in the Professor's beds in the hospital. The only entrance to the Professor's office was through this lab; with this set-up he kept in touch with the action and could also be warned of the approach of visitors.

In 1947, I spent my first year in a room that had housed Professor Ryle's secretary. It had no gas or water. My water supply was a large aspirator bottle on the window ledge, and my sink a carboy on the floor with a large funnel in its neck. But I had a good (though slow) long-beam Oertling analytical balance and a set of Barcroft manometers for metabolic experiments on tissue slices. Two years later, as Assistant Director of Research, I had a laboratory of my own and a single-pan Sartorius balance which speeded things up a great deal. But I still determined sodium by a zinc uranyl acetate procedure, and what was then called 'total base' in tissues, by a complex process which started with digestion with nitric acid, sulphuric acid and hydrogen peroxide in a boiling tube held over a flame, and took more than a day to complete.

The work on the Department of Experimental Medicine, which yielded so many exciting new insights and made many major contributions of an extraordinarily wide variety to physiological knowledge, was achieved with a relatively small nucleus of workers, in surroundings which appeared so modestly equipped that one Japanese visitor came back after the Professor had gone home and pleaded with us to show him the 'real' laboratory. We did our best to assure him that he *had* seen everything, but he did not seem fully convinced. He could not of course see, for they were invisible, the real secrets of the Department's success. These were the responses of a small but loyal and dedicated staff to Professor McCance's innovative thinking and intuition and the superb implementation of the research programmes by Elsie Widdowson.

If I tried to summarise what I gained from close association with the highly selected group of people that the Professor and Elsie gathered around them, I think I could list five things:

First, the constant reminders, which came partly from clinical problems, that cells are parts of people. In these days of increasing abstraction it is more than ever necessary to keep the whole animal in mind. And patients pose problems which are less tailor-made than those we try to construct or isolate in the laboratory.

The Professor was a great man for ideas. He lived 14 miles away and his daily bicycle rides on quiet roads to and from Cambridge gave him two hours every day when he could think, unhindered by visitors or telephones. He also had something of Claude Bernard's genius in choosing the right animal, devising useful experimental approaches to a problem and a tremendous enthusiasm.

He had to go to London to attend many meetings and also to use the library of the Royal Society of Medicine, too often for continuity in bench work. The Cambridge libraries were deficient in many clinical journals, and McCance's reference lists were characteristically remarkably long and complete. But though the Professor spent little time in the laboratory, Elsie more than made up for any deficiencies in supervision. She also had good ideas, and great laboratory skills; above all, she could see exactly what was needed to turn the Professor's ideas into practical reality.

Elsie also had a remarkable capacity to think through the implications of results and ideas and to present them in unusually lucid prose. So she played a large part in the detailed planning of the studies; she directed the laboratory work and took a major share in interpreting the results, which she calculated with the aid of an exceptionally long slide rule. I used to picture her as hanging on to the Professor's ankles and keeping him close to earth when his head got too high in the clouds.

Second, there was the great stimulus that came from the stream of distinguished visitors who flowed through the Department and talked around the lunch table. That was how I first met Eddie Pratt, Daniel Darrow and Homer Smith, to name only three. The lucky guests got invited to the lab lunch and it was probably the existence of these specific times for discussion that made the Professor intolerant of visitors at other times.

As soon as the lunch visitor sat down, he would be faced with the question, 'Hot or Cold?'. Not knowing to what this referred, the usual polite response was, 'Whatever you've got handy'. The Professor would usually reply, 'We've got them both,' and only gradually would the visitor realise that he was being asked whether he wanted hot or cold milk in his coffee.

Third, I gained most of what I now know about setting down scientific results on paper. The Professor's editorial skill was one of his greatest contributions to the education of all who passed through the Department. He could see his way through an idea and Elsie had the ability to see the problem in practical terms. They were both very skilled in writing. The Professor's favourite expressions were 'What are you really trying to say?', and, 'Just say it'. He was a superb editor—very few of his papers required any editorial work once accepted.

It is hard to believe from the polished final versions of his published writings that the first drafts were often written in trains and other odd places, on the backs and insides of old envelopes! Versions of most of the papers that emanated from the Department during my ten years there were critically read, redrafted, reread and rewritten, often many times, by all of us, before a final version went to a journal. And, of course all this was before the days of word processors.

Fourth, I gained a subject for research which lasted me for the remainder of my professional life.

Fifth, I gained a wife.

Andrew Huxley

> Sir Andrew Huxley was awarded the Nobel Prize for Medicine, jointly with Sir Alan Hodgkin in 1963, for his work on the mechanism of excitation and conduction in nerves. After working in Cambridge from 1946 to 1960, he moved to University College London, where he was Head of the Physiology Department from 1960 to 1969 and a Royal Society Research Professor from 1969 to 1983. He was President of the Royal Society from 1980 to 1985 and Master of Trinity College from 1984 to 1990.

I finished undergraduate studies in Cambridge in 1939 and had planned to do research for two years before going to a hospital for my clinical studies. On the outbreak of war, however, it seemed right to start clinical study at once but I had not got a place at a medical school.

There were several other students in the same situation and Professor John Ryle, the Regius Professor of Physic, organised an introductory clinical course for us at Addenbrooke's Hospital, Cambridge. It ran for six months, the principal teachers being Ryle himself and Professor McCance, with assistance from several of the consultants. This brought me into contact with McCance and Widdowson for the first time and McCance invited me to participate in the *Experimental study of rationing*.

I was one of the four people to go to the Lake District to check that we were physically fit, despite the dietary restrictions. I kept my diaries for that period and my daily records (with explanatory notes) are shown here:

December 24th 1939: *Walk am, with Professor McCance. Shepreth and Fowlmere. Walk pm, with Dr Widdowson, Professor McCance and James Robinson to Harlton.*

December 25th: *Walk with Dr Widdowson. Orwell and Wimpole.*

DAY-TO-DAY RECOLLECTIONS

December 27th: *Bicyclists go north.*

December 28th: *Start north. Skipton* (presumably the car party stayed the night in Skipton).

December 29th: *Arrive in Robin Ghyll* (the house in Langdale owned by Dorothy Ward where we stayed).

December 30th: *Scafell Pike with Dr Widdowson, Professor McCance, James Robinson and Professor McCance's son Colin.*

December 31st: *Bowfell—53 minutes—Crinkle Crags etc, with Dr Widdowson and Colin McCance.*

January 1st 1940: *Sergeant Man and Langdale Pikes with Dr Widdowson, James Robinson and Colin McCance.* (Sergeant Man is a hill in the same group as the Langdale Pikes).

January 2nd: *Stake Pass, Borrowdale, Honister, Scarth Gap* (Scarth, not Scarf as in the MRC Report). *Black Sail, Wasdale Head, Boot, Hard Knott, Wrynose, with Professor McCance* (the long walk, not a cloud in the sky the whole day).

January 3rd: *Thirlmere, home over Ullscarf etc, with Dr Widdowson and James Robinson.*

January 4th: *Coniston Old Man and Dow Crag. 43lb rucksack. Total greater than 200lb. With Professor McCance, Dr Widdowson and Colin McCance.*

January 5th: *Stake Pass, Honister Hause, Green Gable, Great Gable, Styhead, Esk Hause, with Dr Widdowson, Professor McCance and Colin McCance.*

January 6th: *To Windermere, pm.*

January 7th: (Sunday) no entry in my diary; no memory.

January 8th: *Ambleside, Fairfield, Grisedale, Helvellyn, Striding Edge, Patterdale.*

January 9th: *Three Tarns, Scafell, Scafell Pike, Esk Hause.*

January 10th: *To London (Windermere 11.15am, Euston 6.36pm)*

The *Experimental study of rationing* was eventually published in the Medical Research Council (MRC) Special Report Series in 1946. I am amused to see that I was described as:

'...a medical student and graduate of Cambridge University who had an excellent academic record and was then just commencing his clinical work. He was physically fit and mentally stable. He was unknown to us till the experiment began, and was invited to participate on the suggestion of a friend. He volunteered to do so without cavil and was with us to the end. He did not take part in the balance experiments.'

All these years later, it is quite satisfying to see that I was described as 'the most perfect subject,' in that I 'was a trained observer,' and that the data given in one of the Tables showed there to be a suggestion of a correlation between my exercise level and my recorded Calorie consumption. On the five days that my exercise was classified as 'light' (including Sunday, January 7th), my average daily consumption was 3872 Calories, whereas on the six days that my exercise load was classified as 'heavy' (including the 36 miles I walked and the 7000 feet I climbed on Tuesday, January 2nd), I consumed an average of 4714 Calories.

The final two paragraphs of the MRC Report were as follows:

'In conclusion, we would draw attention to the value of experiments such as this in planning relief diets for starving populations in stricken areas.
    One experiment can never settle every question. While, therefore, in the meantime we make our deductions and suggestions, with reserve, we feel that we have established one point with certainty, namely, that these problems of national nutrition in times of stress can be tackled by experimental methods. We do not expect our studies to have provided more than a first approximation to the truth. Other experiments, however, can easily be designed to cover, to check, and so to confirm or refute every statement we have made.'

I consider myself very fortunate to have been one of the people involved in these pioneering studies and that, to this day, I am still in contact with two great scientists, Professor McCance and Dr Widdowson.

Jan Jonxis

> Jan Jonxis has known McCance and Widdowson for more than 50 years. He met them first in 1939 when he was spending a year at the Molteno Institute in Cambridge. He returned to the Netherlands just before the outbreak of the Second World War, and was paediatrician in a Rotterdam hospital throughout the war years. No communication was possible between the Netherlands and England during that period, but the friendship was renewed in March 1946, when Professor McCance and Dr Widdowson went to Rotterdam en route to Germany for an exploratory visit. Since then, they have visited each other frequently, both in their homes and places of work. Jan Jonxis retired as Professor of Paediatrics in Groningen in 1977, and is now investigating the nutrition of old people, and the metabolism of vitamin D, in Curacao and the Netherlands.

To write on a personal level about contact with Mac and Elsie seems easy, but with further thought, the picture is more complicated. To draw an accurate picture of two scientists who have worked together throughout 60 years and have regularly made important contributions, when science has progressed so unpredictably, is a different task. I shall try to write mainly as an old friend and to focus the influence of their work in The Netherlands.

Even in Western Europe, the way in which biologists of different nationalities approach questions and try to solve them, differs according to their cultural background. One has only to read papers on the same subject, but written by German, French or British investigators, to appreciate this. So, even in this developed part of the world, differences in culture still exist. Let us hope that they never vanish. I hope that I am right in considering the approaches of Professor McCance and Dr Elsie Widdowson as typically British. The friendship my wife and I enjoy with both of them may, to a certain extent, reflect the fact that we, like so many Dutch people, feel ourselves more at ease in England than in either France or Germany.

In 1938/39, I spent a year in Cambridge in the Molteno Institute working on fetal haemoglobin. Being a paediatrician, I thought it instructive to pay a visit to Professor McCance, some of whose papers I had read, for a discussion on infantile nutrition. My first impression of the Department at Tennis Court Road, was the presence of many books, boxes and parcels, but hardly any apparatus. Everything looked as if it had been got ready for an expedition. Professor McCance soon put the shy young man, whose English was not too good, at ease and we started a discussion about the problem of vitamin D deficiency and calcium and phosphorus metabolism in young children. His questions were direct, to the point and stimulating.

Half a year later, I returned to Holland with an appointment as a paediatrician in a newly opened hospital in Rotterdam. With our discussion still very much in my mind, I started to work on the prevention of rickets. That morning at Tennis Court Road is one of the reasons why very few children in Rotterdam got rickets during the War.

When the War was over, but Rotterdam was still in ruins, Mac and Elsie came to visit us on their way to Germany for their studies on undernutrition. My wife collected them from the poorly repaired station and took them to our house, where we continued our discussion on rickets, exactly where we had left it six years before.

After that, we met quite often, either in Cambridge or Rotterdam. I learned much from Mac and Elsie about malnourished German children and their recovery. During one of their visits, a young medical student asked me to introduce him to Professor McCance; he was writing his doctoral thesis on starvation of elderly people in Holland in the last months of the War. I did so, but I had some doubts because I hardly knew the student. Mac made it very clear that the data the young man had collected were muddled and that his conclusions were wrong. I though it wiser to leave the room. I never did learn whether the doctor-to-be had really understood the reason for Mac's criticism; he told his colleagues only that he had spoken with the famous Cambridge Professor.

In the post-War years, we took many excursions together in our car (a Morris 10) into the Dutch countryside. Mac and my wife used to sit in the back seat discussing their strict Protestant upbringing; Elsie and I talked about gardening, especially about vegetables. Our children loved their visits and still keep in touch with Mac and Elsie.

Once I was back at my old University at Groningen, our contacts remained as close as ever. Members of my staff eagerly accepted the opportunity to take part in our discussions, especially those with Dr Widdowson on infant nutrition. I now believe that Mac's talks were often too remote for a man or woman whose future was to be paediatric practice in a small town, but a Cambridge Professor who brought his bicycle and cycled from Groningen to the Hook of Holland (200km) could not fail to make a deep impression on everyone.

Elsie gradually extended her research on the human newborn to include that of the newborn of those animal species whose way of life has highly specialised aspects. She collaborated with American and Canadian colleagues, who had made expeditions to Canada to study the nutrition of the young seal during its first days after birth on the ice off the Labrador Coast, and to study the baby bear and its hibernating mother. It was always fascinating to listen to her, talking about the resulting findings. The adaptations of those newborn animals to survive under extreme circumstances is striking. Darwin, I suppose, would have liked this work.

Let me conclude with a few remarks on the influence of both Mac and Elsie on paediatrics and nutrition. By their regular visits to The Netherlands, they have stimulated research on neonatology and infant nutrition here. Until recently nutrition was mainly taught in Wageningen, the Governmental Institute of Agriculture. By training members of staff of the Section for Human Nutrition of that Institute, Elsie, in particular, is very well known.

Just as in the late 17th and early 18th centuries, the second half of the 20th century has been a period in which British science has had a major influence on that of my country. Mac and Elsie played a very definite role in that influence.

Barbara Alington
(now Mrs Barbara Cassels)

> Barbara Alington went to the Department of Medicine in 1940 to take charge of all the catering and cooking for the studies on 'mineral metabolism on white and brown bread dietaries', and was also one of the subjects in these experiments. She continued in this role during the later studies on bread, till the time of her marriage, when she left.

I left the Dietetic Department at Bart's in 1940 to join the Department of Medicine in Cambridge. I looked after the cooking and catering for the various 'bread experiments' and I was a subject in the first and longest of them. My salary was £200 per annum. Because the experiment took place in Wartime, I had to ask for the ration books of the people on the experiments. I also had to apply for extra ration coupons because one-fifth of the amount each person had eaten was set aside in a closely covered aluminium bowl, to be used as a duplicate diet for analysis. At least 40-50% of the calories had to come from bread, which worked out to a 1lb loaf each day for women, with an extra ½ or 1lb loaf for men. The flour came from Foster Mills Ltd of Cambridge, and the bread was baked at the village bakery in Barrington where Dr Widdowson lived. We got through 15 loaves a day, which she brought in her car. Some of the flour was used for pastry, steamed puddings, scones and plain cakes.

I can certainly remember the embarassment of the urine and faeces collections during the three-week experimental periods. I was courting at the time and had to take all the bottles and bowls with me on each date, without the benefit of today's improved packaging devices. This must have been very off-putting to my boyfriend at the time, though he did marry me!

Once the samples were returned to the lab, Professor McCance usually took total responsibility for the homogenisation of the faeces and then he and Dr Widdowson performed the analyses. They were assisted by a lab technician called Haynes, although I remember that Haynes was often in trouble when the Professor suspected that he had got the results wrong. The analyses for most of the minerals relied on colorimetric methods and the Professor, Dr Widdowson and Haynes spent many hours matching colours by eye using the 'Lovibond' visual Colorimeter. After that, it was back to me, to work out the intakes of nitrogen and minerals from the many columns of figures, with no help from a calculator or computer!

Amicia Melland
(now Dr Amicia Young)

> Amicia Melland was one of the subjects in the experiments on the absorption of minerals from different varieties of bread. She worked in the Zoology Department at the University of Cambridge from September 1939 until she left for a British Council post in Chile at the beginning of 1942. Dr Melland settled in London in 1944, undertaking a succession of voluntary/paid jobs which all contributed to her development of editorial, publishing and administrative skills. Remarried in 1950 (widowed in 1975), she has a married son who lives in London, providing her with three grandchildren to keep her actively interested in the present.

Dr Widdowson and I spent hours picking the fruit (plums, greengages, apples and damsons) in her orchard, oblivious of the air-raid warnings around us. Fruit consumption was encouraged in the 'bread experiments', once some initial studies had shown that the variations in calcium balance, produced by alterations in the intake of fruit, were 'quite trifling compared with the differences produced by a change from white to brown bread'.

One of the subjects on the experiment (Dr Steiner) had a somewhat excessive consumption of fruit. Not only did he eat the flesh but he ate the cores and all, thus giving us the dilemma of whether we should extend our analysis to the pips of the apples.

I kept detailed diaries during that time and have picked out some entries (and added some extra notes) which give some idea of what life was like as an experimental subject:

DAY-TO-DAY RECOLLECTIONS

July 12th 1940: *Start weighing our food.*

August 5th: *Today I bicycled to Grantchester with a friend and told her about the diet while drinking a cup of coffee at the Orchard. Suddenly realised what I'd done as we left, and got them to give me half a cup of coffee in a beer bottle (for duplicates). As I had no milk or sugar in the coffee, I was forgiven when I confessed next morning in the lab.*

During the experiment, we had to provide half measures of all that we drank for analysis. For food, we had to give up one-fifth for analysis. So if we ate chocolate, we had to give up one square for every five squares we ate. We tended not to eat such rationed luxuries for the duration of the experiment.

We are all finding the white bread (plus calcium phosphate) a terrific effort—it seems to accumulate all day and doesn't leave you perpetually ravenous as does the brown. We're going to have to repeat the phosphate brown because we ate too much.

That awful bloated feeling! It made me realise why prisoners can *look* well-fed on a diet high in bread.

September 14th: *McCance ate the equivalent of five times my amount.*

December 18th: *The guinea pigs have their Christmas dinner: goose and accompaniments, with Christmas brandy on it, as well as 2s 6d worth (12½ pence nowadays) of silver in it. Rather hard to go back and cook buck rarebit for evening meal with Bassadone (one of the other guinea pigs).*

January 3rd 1941: *Meat ration reduced to 1s 6d and to include offal and pork—actually only 1s 1d in Cambridge this week, and off-ration stuff (eg rabbit) unobtainable or impossibly expensive. Saw some onions on a cart outside Fitzbillies and bought a pound (not daring to ask for more) for the guinea pigs.*

In summarising the calcium balance experiments on the white and brown-bread diets, Professor McCance described my calcium balance as *most consistent* (in spite of some irregular dieting practices, partly due to severe dysmenorrhoea). According to the published paper, even on the brown-bread diet I was only in negative balance to the extent of 26mg/day, whereas the Professor himself had a negative calcium balance of 150mg/day. Unfortunately, this has not helped me to escape the advanced osteoporosis and osteoarthritis which now afflicts me 50 years later!

The results from this series of bread experiments were published in 1942 and the subjects who had participated were duly acknowledged:

'The present work really represents the united efforts of the ten subjects, BA, CB, EB, KB, NK, AM, RM, PS, EW and RW. The authors have merely had the pleasant task of committing the results to paper.'

From my own experience, the authors (RM and EW) couldn't have found the experimental conditions too easy either, but their mastery of the understatement shines through clearly in the final sentence.

Romaine Hervey

> Romaine Hervey first met Professor McCance as a student in 1942. In 1949, after qualifying in Medicine, he was seconded from the Navy and took part in studies on survival at sea. He remained in the Department of Experimental Medicine and, in 1952, began his work for a PhD in the field of experimental obesity. He left in 1957 to go to the University of Sheffield. In 1967, he was appointed to the Chair of Physiology at the University of Leeds. He retired in 1989 and now lives in Somerset.

In my first term as a medical student in Cambridge, I responded to an advertisement asking for volunteers for experiments on survival at sea. Little did I know how this would influence my career. It was the beginning of a lifelong interest and eventually led to my succeeding Professor McCance as Chairman of the Royal Naval Personnel Research Committee (RNPRC) Survival at Sea Sub-Committee, and to my appointment as Civilian Consultant in Physiology to the Royal Naval (RN) Medical Service.

The survival-at-sea experiments illustrated Professor McCance's particular talents and idiosyncrasies. Some years previously, Ambard and Papin had introduced the concept of 'urine obligatoire' which stated that, however extreme the deprivation of water, urine volume does not decrease below a minimum volume. Professor McCance wanted to know why. To find out, the volunteers drank sodium chloride, sodium bicarbonate and urea solutions as well as being subjected to varying levels of water deprivation.

The results from these studies led our team to discover the principle of osmotic diuresis, which was a major factor in elucidating the mechanism of water reabsorption in the kidney. We published a note in *Nature* and an abstract, but left it to Rapoport's team in the USA to complete and publish a full investigation. I also constructed a micro-method for determining freezing-points that, had we made the right use of it, could have given us a breakthrough in this area. McCance had the knack of putting his finger on important things: his instinct nearly always proved to be right, but only some of the opportunities his insights created were actually followed through.

I think Professor McCance first established his standing by pioneering in this country 'do-it-on-yourself' methods to study what appeared to be clinical problems. This work was well described in his Goulstonian lectures of 1936. He was aware of Gamble's work in the USA—both were paediatricians and introduced 'do-it-on-yourself' methods—but their ideas were derived independently. McCance did much to put the body sodium and water state on the clinical map—an immensely important contribution.

I joined the Navy as a Surgeon-Lieutenant at the end of 1949, and Professor McCance got the Navy to agree that I should spend much of my time on researching survival at sea under his direction. My initial assignment was to test the new tented Naval life raft, working immediately under Dr Eric Glaser. The raft had already been designed and it was our job to test it in realistic trials in Arctic, tropical and temperate environments. The numerous sea trials, in all sorts of interesting locations, including Tromsö Fjord, the Johore Straits and mid-Atlantic in rough weather, were a marvellous experience that I would not have missed for anything.

Eric Glaser was the victim of an unfortunate incident when we returned to Invergordon in Scotland after one of the Arctic expeditions. The press were aware of the trials and had intended to meet our ship when it docked. Unfortunately, they missed us. One reporter though, caught up with us when we were changing trains at Glasgow and saw his opportunity for a scoop. Sadly for him, the sailors, released from their duties as guinea pigs and having had time to refresh themselves rather liberally, started to 'rag' him. The poor reporter got his story, but it was Eric who suffered in the end. He turned up for his tutorial class in Cambridge, only to be greeted by his students brandishing a copy of a popular newspaper with the headline, 'Cambridge doctor gives sex talks on rafts'.

The temperate experiments were done in the Physiology laboratory in Cambridge. There were no thermal problems here, and we concentrated on finding the most efficient rations. Since death from total deprivation is due to lack of water, it had been assumed that all storage space should be devoted to water; but a carefully controlled crossed-over experiment showed that it was worth devoting some space to sugar. The metabolism of sugar not only generates metabolic water but spares protein, and so decreases the formation of urea, which is excreted and carries water with it. A daily ration of 100g barley sugar improved water balance by 200g, making it well worthwhile including it. Our recommendation to this effect has been followed ever since.

We became involved in controversy in studying whether castaways should drink sea water. Alain Bombard, a likable but lunatic Frenchman, had gained much publicity in advocating that they should. He had survived a short Mediterranean cruise in a raft doing this, but I felt certain he could not have been telling the whole truth about his subsequent raft crossing of the South Atlantic. He was also much at fault in making his voyages on temperate waters and then claiming that his 'system' would enable people to survive anywhere in the world. Our controlled experiment showed that drinking any amount of sea water, however small, always increased plasma hypertonicity and must accelerate death. The work was published by Professor McCance and myself in The *Proceedings of the Royal Society.*

Another important area of research for the Navy was into remedies for seasickness. We tested various drugs at sea and on artificial waves. It must have been disappointing to the drug companies when hyoscine, a well-known and non-patentable drug, emerged as the most effective.

This work was commissioned by the RNPRC (which later became a Medical Research Council Committee). Professor McCance was Chairman of its Survival-at-Sea Sub-Committee and during this period Frank Golden was 'talent-spotted'. We had been aware for some time that the RN Air Medical School at Hillhead, near Portsmouth, in southern England, had a unique facility of a tank—effectively a small swimming pool, whose temperature could be controlled almost down to freezing point—and we were anxious to see this used for research on hypothermia. We then learned that Frank, as a Surgeon-Lieutenant routinely appointed to the School, was doing such research on his own initiative.

The Committee arranged for him to spend much more of his career at the Institute of Naval Medicine (which absorbed RNAMS) than would have been customary. He later took a PhD, joined the Survival-at-Sea Sub-Committee, and became a world expert on immersion physiology and pathology. We were in fact taking some risk with his Naval career, but things turned out happily and Frank is now the Surgeon Rear-Admiral based at RN Hospital, Haslar (near Portsmouth).

The Professor not only had the knack of getting good people onto his Committee, but was also a good Chairman because he could focus on the important issues and keep things moving. Of course, this Committee was more of a Working Party to get research done and to publish the results. I'm not so certain that McCance would enjoy chairing present-day Government Committees which seem to exist simply to generate papers, rather than getting actual work done.

One of the Professor's great talents was the way he practised 'Lifemanship' in a charming way. In all circumstances, he had the habit of taking the standpoint of someone who was just a little bit removed from the assembled company. If he was among nutritionists, he would call himself a physiologist; if he was among endocrinologists, he would call himself a paediatrician, and so on. In this way, he would always appear to have 'something extra' to say on the subject under discussion.

The only description that was not appropriate to Professor McCance was that of an experienced laboratory worker. His love of DIY physiology did not arise from his love of experimental methodology. He rarely appeared in my laboratory in the Department. On one occasion when he did, I remember him saying to me, 'Hervey, don't fiddle,' as I was trying hard to standardise an old-fashioned 'wet' analysis accurately.

It was the Department's interest in energy balance that formed the basis of my PhD work when I left the Royal Navy and started working full-time in the Department of Experimental Medicine in 1952. Professor McCance was interested in the control of energy intake and the physiological role of the body fat content in this respect. One thing that was known was the central role played by the hypothalamus. Lesions in this area of the brain could cause rats to become grossly obese. This technique had been developed by Anand and Brobek in the United States, followed by Gordon Kennedy working at the National Institute for Medical Research at Mill Hill in London.

McCance suggested that I attempted to make pairs of 'parabiotic' rats, ie, rats that were surgically united so that the blood circulated freely between both members of the pair, who were effectively 'Siamese twins'. Then if one rat was made to become obese by hypothalamic lesioning, the effect on the other should show the effect of any blood-borne message that was being generated. I have to admit that McCance and I expected results opposite to those we found. When the lesioned rat became obese the other member of the pair became thin. So it appeared that, as body fat increased in one rat, a blood-borne messenger caused the other to reduce its food intake. I have since shown that the same effect occurs when the obesity in the first rat is produced in a number of different ways, and that the second rat does indeed stop eating. I therefore interpret the experiment as demonstrating feedback control of food intake.

The project is an example of whole-animal, 'systems' physiology centred on feedback control. While in no way denigrating the achievements of cell and molecular physiology, I have always seen this as 'real physiology' (it was Claude Bernard's approach). In McCance's Department in the 1950s there was no problem in undertaking such an investigation, albeit with primitive methods. I continued the work, but quantitative study of the control system had to wait for microcomputers to control tube-feeding and measure voluntary feeding round the clock.

As time has gone on, it has become ever harder to get grant support and I had to abandon the project unfinished. Investigation of a control system with a time-constant measured in weeks is bound to be time-consuming. In today's climate of pressure for quick results, I fear that to embark on such an investigation would almost be academic suicide. It may be a long time before the control of body fat content is elucidated.

A year later Gordon Kennedy came to work in the Department of Experimental Medicine. I was rather taken aback at the time because this could have been seen as a threat to my position in the field; as time has passed I have come to have more and more admiration for the quality of Kennedy's thinking. His disabling illness and early death were tragic.

I never worked directly with Elsie Widdowson but I remember her mainly in her role as an 'interface' between McCance and the outside world. She was the great 'soother of nerves' in the Department and was intensely loyal to the Professor. Once I was getting hot and bothered about some slides I was making for him. 'The Professor must have a good set of slides to take with him to the United States,' she remarked, as if to emphasise the importance of the task I had been given and at the same time to flatter me on my slide-making ability.

I finished my PhD in 1955, and after two years on a scientific staff appointment with the Medical Research Council, I decided to pursue a university career in Sheffield. I could have stayed on in Cambridge with its name and its kudos, but a move to a University post—and to the North—seemed right for me at that stage. I have never lost the very special relationship I enjoyed with McCance and Widdowson, and, for good or ill, my time in 'The Department' shaped the rest of my scientific career.

Douglas Black

> As a medical student Douglas Black learnt that well over half the body was body fluid. With typical pragmatism he thought that this might be a good thing on which to work. McCance's three Goulstonian lectures, published in 1936, confirmed his interest and showed how problems of fluid metabolism could be tackled in the human subject.
>
> In 1942, he had the privilege of taking part in a study of water deprivation in the Department of Medicine in Cambridge. Although he was only there for a few months, he was able to apply the lessons he learnt to studies of potassium metabolism which he later described in his own Goulstonian Lectures in 1953. He had, meantime, joined the Department of Medicine in Manchester, where he spent 26 years, ending up as Professor. During that time he also practised general medicine, with a special interest in kidney disease.
>
> From 1977 to 1983, he was President of the Royal College of Physicians and he became a Knight Bachelor in 1973.

The Department of Medicine was a rather 'cheeseparing' outfit. I had been having a soft time of it at the Nuffield Department of Medicine where the technicians did all my mineral analyses, but Mac believed strongly in scientists doing their own analysis. I recall Elsie having her own array of individual crucibles instead of a muffle furnace.

I was in the Department when Isaac Harris opposed Mac's scientific evidence for adding calcium to bread and wrote a booklet called *The calcium bread scandal*. Harris had the simplistic idea that having extra calcium in the diet would cause chalking up of the arteries. Mac used to rage about Harris and about the millers who didn't want to add calcium to the flour and Elsie would have to calm him down. I remember how scathing Mac was of a volunteer who dropped out of the 'bread experiments', having struggled through three months. 'I always knew she was a poor subject,' was the scant sympathy from the Professor.

I was an experimental subject myself in one of Mac's water-deprivation experiments. I remember the difficulty of eating dry foods such as oatcakes and shortbread, blowing out clouds of crumbs and foaming at the mouth, and of seeing *Gone with the Wind* during the three-day experimental period. One day, I visited Elsie in Barrington. I asked if there were any jobs that needed doing and she asked me to water the garden, forgetting that the sight of water would drive me mad! After Mac and I had done the experiment for three days, he and Elsie decided that the next person would suffer four days.

Because it was Wartime, I remember Elsie bringing in potatoes from her own garden for the famous lab lunches. In fact, the lunches consisted mainly of bread and vegetables. Not that Mac had more than a cup of black coffee for lunch during the War, although he apparently had a banana with his coffee for his pre-War lunches. The Professor was a marvellous conversationalist. He was extremely good at bringing people out and getting them talking.

Mac's evening meals in Sidney Sussex College were a different matter entirely. He was known to have six helpings of potatoes and to beg those from his neighbour's plate. One night that I spent with him at his home at Bartlow, we had half a chicken and half a plum pudding each. I don't think that Mac's eating habits had any nutritional basis—otherwise he would have had experimental volunteers testing them out. Rather, his eating habits reflected his general desire to show his eccentricity in all ways. I'm not certain whether Mac habitually took a small or large breakfast. Once, when staying with us, he went out for a long walk before breakfast and then only wanted half a grapefruit without sugar on his return!

On one occasion, because of Mac's absence, I had written up quite a chunk of work by myself. On Mac's return, I was praised for my spontaneous effort but damned for my failure to plan. Mac had a very broad knowledge and he was very imaginative. Later in his life, he found it difficult to escape from the things he had done in the past. When he was well into fetal development, he got annoyed if people questioned him about his work on bread and his views on the National Loaf.

Maureen Young

> Maureen Young took her first degree in Physiology from Bedford College for Women in London in 1938. At the beginning of the War she spent two years at a London Blood Transfusion Unit. She rejoined Bedford College in 1941, as a demonstrator in Physiology. After the War she was one of the first women lecturers on the staff of the Physiology department at St Thomas's Hospital Medical School, London. She stayed there for 36 years and during the last 19 of those she had a small unit in the Gynaecology department that concerned itself with the placental mechanisms of fetal nutrition.
>
> Professor Young also enjoyed fruitful collaborations in Hungary through Dr Julius Mestyan and Dr Gyula Soltesz. Her personal title of Professor in Perinatal Physiology (1977) was the first of its kind in England. She was one of the founder members of the Neonatal Society and was President from 1984 to 1987. She is now retired and lives in a Cambridgeshire village very close to Elsie Widdowson's village of Barrington.

Bedford College for Women was evacuated from London to Cambridge at the beginning of the Second World War, and the Physiology Department became the guest of Professor ED Adrian in his laboratories on the Downing Street site. The senior lecturer in our Department, Margaret Murray, always wanted her students to know of the latest research work, and no opportunity was missed to send them to the large variety of Cambridge lectures—as well as their own!

The two people who had the most influence on us were Sir Joseph Barcroft—Joe—and Professor McCance—Mac. The former was writing his book *Researches on Pre-natal Life,* a record of his last new line of enquiry, which was to be a great stimulus to us all. He started the work when he was 64 years old and, at 74 he was still asking questions about the initiation of labour and of the first breath, and inviting us to help with his experiments on lambs delivered with their umbilical cords intact, with the ewe lying in an enormous warm saline bath!

With very crude apparatus and very shrewd observation, Barcroft, and his many collaborators, had shown that the fetus had a different metabolism from that of the mother and that the rate of development of the circulatory responses differed among the species. Further, he introduced the ideas of critical periods for organ development and the possible interaction of a nutritional, as well as a genetic framework for fetal growth. He would have been the first to appreciate the imaginative and detailed extensions of these ideas, and their rigorous experimental proof, provided by McCance and Widdowson in the years after the War.

Mac was a great admirer of Barcroft and his experimental approach, so the atmosphere in Cambridge was a most appropriate one for himself and Elsie to flourish in, with their insatiable curiosity and diversity of interests. We were all fascinated by stories of the activities in their laboratory at King's College Hospital; for instance—naked medical students being salt-depleted by sweating at high temperatures! By the time I got to know them in Cambridge, they were already engaged in their *Experimental Study of Rationing*.

Others may recount stories of Mac's idiosyncrasies, especially his dietary habits, but I remember especially the liveliness of his lectures and the twinkle in his eye as he told a good story. Once he described a visit to Madrid (on behalf of the British Council during the War) and the wiles of a lady who wanted him to buy cigarettes on the black market; her husband was in charge of cleaning the drains, but kept one quite dry for her stores! Mac's forthrightness was also legendary; a young man who gave a poor paper at a meeting was told to go home and do some more experiments.

Mac has always been known as a medical physiologist, but Elsie is often thought of as a nutritionist and has, indeed, been closely associated with the Nutrition Society since its beginning in 1941. In my opinion, however, she is also a most original physiologist, using changes in nutrition to gain an understanding of function in the fetus and newborn. She and Mac helped to lay the foundations of our knowledge of the importance of the timing of nutritional factors in fetal and neonatal growth: age and size were separated and they showed that different organs responded differently to the plane of nutrition.

Elsie made studies on the chemical composition of the body during development and growth, and used a variety of unique experimental approaches. She and Mac provided quantitative values for the differences between fetuses and adults in their anatomical, chemical and physiological characteristics; between the fetuses of different species and their varying speeds of adaptation to a new environment during the neonatal period; and during growth to maturity. As the knowledge of perinatal physiology grew, so an intercollegiate course unit in the subject started in London University, and it was to Elsie and Mac's papers that we directed our students' reading. Elsie's thinking was beautifully put together in her Sanderson-Wells lecture, entitled *Harmony of Growth*, given in 1970.

The beginning of the 1960s were halcyon days for the universities, and a University Department of Gynaecology was started at St Thomas's Hospital Medical School in London; it was provided with a unit of physiology as well as endocrinology—exceptional for those days. Because the clinical problem of the infant who is born small for its gestational age, and considered to have been undernourished *in utero*, was becoming of increasing importance, we started to look into the maternal to fetal placental transfer of nutrients, particularly the amino acids.

One day in 1972, Elsie said quite simply, 'I wonder why the fetuses of my undernourished guinea-pig mothers are small?' I suggested that we should look at the placental transfer of amino-isobutyric acid (AIB), a nonmetabolisable amino acid, very popular for transport studies because it has minimal fetal to maternal backflux. Elsie's laboratory in Cambridge looked after the guinea pigs and I travelled up from London by car to inject the mothers with radioactively labelled AIB when they were near term, and returned with the tissues for analyses at St Thomas's.

Two experimental diets, one deficient in energy and the other in protein, retarded fetal growth and led to smaller litter numbers and smaller fetal and placental weights in comparison with the well-nourished controls. In the energy-restricted animals, the relationship between the fetal and placental weights was similar to the control animals, and the placental function and fetal uptake per unit weight was similar in the two groups. Feeding a low protein diet, however, increased the ratio of fetal weight to placental weight and enhanced both placental and fetal uptake per unit weight, suggesting the possibility of adaptation in animals whose energy supply is adequate, but whose protein supply is reduced. In human pregnancies the fetal to placental weight ratio is usually quite high, making the low fetal to placental weight ratios, now found by epidemiologists to be associated with the greater likelihood of adult hypertension and cardiovascular disease, even more interesting.

The paediatricians joined in the great expansion of investigative medicine during the years following the Second World War but the British Paediatric Association meetings became too large and did not provide the right forum for those interested in the newborn and in animal physiology. Simultaneously, fetal physiology, which had been stimulated by Barcroft and Huggett, was growing in many university departments, including Geoffrey Dawes' group at the Nuffield Institute in Oxford, and investigators needed to discuss their results at a smaller forum than the Physiological Society. McCance and Widdowson's work on the newborn kidney and that of Kenneth Cross on infant respiration formed important links between the laboratory and the nursery. Mac describes the birth of the Neonatal Society in its first Handbook. The 'womb' was a dismal room in the 'pelvis' of the Royal Hotel at Scarborough where the British Paediatric Association was holding its annual meeting in 1958. A group of about 36 investigators agreed to form the Neonatal Society and both Mac and Elsie were founder members.

Mac was the first President, for a period of six years from 1959 to

1965, and Elsie was President from 1978 to 1981. The meetings were always informative and lively; investigators from Europe and the Americas were invited to give papers and lectures and many became members and honorary members. The Society has thrived and the membership now stands at over 300. Sadly, the old links between the laboratory and the clinc have loosened because of changing interests in physiology departments and the increasing numbers of academic paediatric units; there are few established posts for someone like Elsie who can range freely among the newborn of species from mice to bears, via the human infant! The main vigour of the Society now lies almost entirely with the clinicians.

Finally, I remember Mac shining as a clinician as he described a case of neonatal diabetes, during a speech which he gave at the Neonatal Society's dinner held in Sidney Sussex College, Cambridge, on the occasion of his 80th birthday in 1978. The Society was holding a symposium in his honour entitled *The development of fetal and neonatal physiology in the United Kingdom*, and many of his papers were reproduced in a volume entitled *Studies in Perinatal Physiology*. At the dinner he was presented with a pencil drawing by WE Narraway: the portrait was commissioned by the Neonatal Society, and this gift from his many friends and colleagues now hangs in Sidney Sussex College.

Christine Walsham
(now Mrs Christine Spray)

> *Christine Walsham joined the staff of the Department of Medicine in 1944 at the same time as Betty Wilkinson; both had recently obtained degrees at Bedford College, London. They had been evacuated to Cambridge and taught by Maureen Young. They took part in the same metabolic balance experiment on* The digestibility of English and Canadian wheats with special reference to the digestibility of wheat protein by man. *Christine subsequently spent a few months with the team in Wuppertal before she left in 1948 to get married.*

What do I remember of my time in the Department of Experimental Medicine? Let's see: Mac cycling in from Bartlow to Cambridge every day, in all weathers; Elsie arriving with baskets of apples from her lovely orchard cottage; lunches every day conjured up by Mrs G from Wartime rations and ingredients (but Mac ate nothing more than two apples each day); an endless stream of distinguished people coming to those lunches in the laboratory so that even I, the youngest and greenest of the research workers, could listen to, and join in their discussions; seeing Mac examining the first of the severely undernourished prisoners-of-war who had arrived in Addenbrooke's Hospital; going to the National Institute for Research in Dairying in Reading to borrow a rat-milking machine, then coming back to the laboratory and actually milking rats.

These are just some of the memories of that time between 1944 and 1948 that I treasure, but perhaps the most vivid memory I have of working in the Department is of the smell! When we spent days boiling different parts of different 'animal' bodies in acid, the resulting odour was bound to be potent and pervading. I dissected and weighed the pieces, covered them with hydrochloric acid and left them in large vessels to soften for days, perhaps weeks, eventually getting them into solution for chemical analysis. Looking back now, I am quite amazed at what I did…but then it was all in a day's work.

The wheat protein digestibility experiments bring back memories of great camaraderie and competition among ourselves. The team of six guinea pigs would vie with each other. Who could get the highest percentage of their calorie intake from the bread we were eating that week? It was always Mac. He achieved 93% while the rest of us averaged about 80%. Who could save their treat of the day until supper-time? Who could get the carmine marker through their body quickest at the end of each experimental period? I think the poem that someone wrote at the time says it all:

IF
(with apologies to Rudyard Kipling)

If you can eat with only bread, as master;
If you can drink with weak tea as your aim;
If you can chew the 'English' faster, faster;
Then up it comes, and round and round again;

If you can get your vol up to four litres
With uric acids dropping down like dreams;
If you can get your nitrogens quite perfect,
And keep off coffees, chocolates and ice creams;

If you can keep your fat while those around you
Are using theirs and blaming it on you;
If you can keep your treacle tarts and shortbread
When all the rest have only bread in view;

If you can recognise your friends by faeces,
Use both sides of the paper on the roll;
If you can separate your carmine clearly
And never, never, use the wrong fruit bowl;

If you can keep it going for a fortnight,
Then come up smiling when the feast is done;
Your name will evermore be wrapped in glory,
For you're the perfect guinea pig, my son.

Small wonder that we became such good friends after being so closely involved in each other's lives for weeks on end. And almost 50 years later, five of that team of six guinea pigs are still in touch with each other.

Of the work that went on in Germany, at Wuppertal and Duisburg, much has been written by others. I was there for only a few months but I lived for years on the reflected glory of having been part of the team that discovered how very good a food is bread of any colour. In some ways it was like being at a prolonged house-party, but it was a deadly serious one with lighter relaxing times of outings, opera, music-making and so on, to ease the burdens.

Those were stimulating and exciting days and I still feel immensely proud to have played a tiny part in them.

Betty Wilkinson
(now Dr Elizabeth Tayler)

> Betty Wilkinson was a PhD student in the Department of Medicine from 1944 to 1947 and she has a particular reason to remember her role as a 'bread guinea pig' for she married a fellow bread-eater.

I was a student at Bedford College, London, in the early 1940s, when the College was evacuated to Cambridge. I went to the Department of Medicine after I had taken my degree in Physiology and Biochemistry in 1944. The Physiology Department of Bedford College worked in conjunction with both Cambridge schools, so as well as my excellent tutoring, I was part of both Part II Courses.

Because of the War, most young people were in the forces, but there was brilliant work being done by refugees. I was taught by Professor Keilin about the discovery of the cytochromes, and by Feldberg about the nature of nerve transmission at the synapse. Partition chromatography had still to be devised and the structure of DNA had yet to be discovered.

Much routine analysis went on in the Department, particularly all the work on composition of foodstuffs. By chance, I became a guinea pig in the experiment on the availability of protein in bread made from different extractions of English and Canadian wheat.

Both types of wheat were extracted to different levels. The guinea pigs—assorted humans—lived on 'biblical diets' of bread and water for 40 days. We consumed a weighed quantity of bread made from each extraction of wheat for 10 days and the nitrogen intake and output were measured. It was no hardship to live on bread alone in the summer of 1945. Food was strictly rationed anyway.

I remember the time very clearly because it produced a marvellous result for me. I was very surprised to find that I was not destined to be a scientist, but I discovered a lifetime partner with whom I have raised a family of five doctors, who have now produced 14 grandchildren. When people ask us 'How did you meet?' I have the perfect reply: 'We ate bread together for 40 days'.

Lois Thrussell
(now Mrs Lois Strangeways)

> *In 1945, Professor McCance went to the Medical Research Council (MRC) and said he must have a research nurse. This was quite a new idea at that time; the MRC did not employ research nurses, had no idea how much to pay them and knew nothing about them. The Professor persisted in his usual way and he got his research nurse—Lois Thrussell.*
>
> *She arrived from University College Hospital, London, about a year before Professor McCance and Dr Widdowson went to Germany, accompanied them there and stayed for the entire three-year period. She remained in the Department until she married a colleague, Brian Strangeways, in 1953.*

I was training as a midwife in 1945 when I decided I really wanted to do research. A colleague mentioned that she had been offered, but not taken, a job in Cambridge that might still be available. She persuaded me to write and apply for the job; she composed the letter, and I merely copied and signed it.

The job turned out to be with McCance and Widdowson. I was invited to my first lab lunch after my interview. I agonised long and hard the previous evening about whether or not I should wear a hat. Meeting one's future in-laws and taking one's driving test were easy after that ordeal.

After Professor McCance and Miss Widdowson returned from their preliminary trip to Germany in 1946, the Professor asked me if I would like to go back there with them. He was somewhat taken aback when I readily agreed. So, in 1946, I went out to Wuppertal with the Professor, Miss Widdowson and Rex Dean.

We all had to wear uniforms. The men wore army uniforms and the women wore 'Control Commission' uniforms, with very short tight skirts. I spoke no German, but somehow, with the aid of a dictionary, I managed to do whatever was wanted. If the Professor said that he wanted something done, it was up to me to do it. I felt rather uncomfortable sometimes, as a British woman making measurements of Germans so soon after the end of the War. The only ones I couldn't do were the Basal Metabolic Rates at 6am, because we lived at Wuppertal-Elberfeld some way from the hospital and there was no transport so early in the morning. Dorothy Rosenbaum did these because she lived on site.

Living together in the same house was rather like being in an Arctic sub-station—the inhabitants just had to get on with each other. We all ate together at the evening meal; the Professor always had a whole bowl of vegetables to himself. Our only free day was Sunday and we often went on outings and picnics then. Miss Widdowson sometimes joined us but the Professor usually went walking on his own, often taking photographs, Wuppertal was too hilly for cycling. I once joined the Professor on one of these excursions but I got so cold waiting for him to take a photograph of a sunset that even my handkerchief was frozen solid. He was known in Germany as 'Herr Professor' or 'The Funny Professor'.

My most vivid memory was the study involving the two orphanages in Wuppertal. I lived on the premises and did all the measurements necessary for the energy and mineral balance studies. In one orphanage, the very strict *Hausfrau* would not let me do these inside and made me work in a hen house in the grounds. Unfortunately, the hen house had whitewash on the walls that was prone to flake off and ruin the calcium balance measurements. I mentioned my dilemma to Miss Widdowson who somehow found me a beautiful piece of cretonne to drape over the walls. I can now claim to be the only woman in the world who has mashed, by hand, 12 salad bowls full of faeces in a cretonne-lined hen house!

I mentioned to Miss Widdowson how the impossibly strict *Hausfrau* used meal times to scold the children in public for their latest misdemeanours. In fact, if it hadn't been for me weeping on her shoulder about this, the reason for the low-weight gains of the orphanage children might never have been explained.

When we returned to the UK in February 1949 I helped the Professor to write up the results from Germany. We spent hours with the slide rule; the research nurse had turned scientist! I looked up hundreds of references about hunger oedema in the University Library, and found a poem in medieval French about bread. I checked figures, drew graphs, sorted out pictures and generally acted as a universal handmaiden. All wonderful training for subsequent years helping children with their homework.

Accompanying both Rex Dean and Professor McCance on their ward rounds, I remember having to soothe the patients down sometimes if the Professor inadvertently upset them. He had an unfortunate habit of standing by a patient's bed and announcing, 'We'll try such and such—though I don't know if it'll do much good!' At least my help was always acknowledged. In one particular book, the Professor and Miss Widdowson thanked me because I had 'bestowed much labour on them'!

I remember the Professor as a charming man who could be rather unpredictable at times. On one occasion, a group of students *en route* for Greenland visited Cambridge. I think they were probably pressing McCance for some scientific objective for their expedition and he quickly thought up something one of his PhD students might be able to use. The students were asked to collect blood samples and to keep them below a certain temperature at all costs.

Some months later, the students returned with their cherished blood samples, telling stories of how they had kept them cold by digging holes in the snow and how they had persuaded the ship's captain to store them in the limited space in the refrigerator on the return voyage. They were somewhat taken aback when the Professor insisted that he had no recollection of asking them to collect the samples, let alone go to such great lengths to keep them cold. His brain was always seething with new ideas so it was hardly surprising that he forgot the occasional one!

Miss Widdowson provided the charm and the empathy. The Professor would always be demanding 'results' from her. Once he had his 'seed corn' for an idea, he would leap on his bike, ride off and think about the implications of the result. Thus the 'seed corn' was developed into a hypothesis.

Let me try to pick out things I learned in the Department of Experimental Medicine which have proved useful to me since:

The *first* thing I learnt was to keep calm in totally unfamiliar, sometimes frightening situations. Dealing with the urgent needs of a toddler when stuck in a traffic jam seemed easy after some of the situations I had to cope with in Germany.

The *second* thing that impressed me, coming direct from the rigid hospital hierarchy, was that *everyone's* opinions and ideas were considered worth listening to, and might even be proferred unsought. This has proved very useful whenever two or three parents and teachers have been gathered together, and perhaps it is this that has made our children such assertive talkers and interrupters.

The *third* thing I learnt was to treat nothing as routine, but constantly to bear in mind the purpose of whatever I was doing and to modify methods accordingly. This has certainly contributed to simplification, and even abandonment, of some household tasks.

These, I suppose are some examples of McCance and Widdowson's influence upon subsequent thoughts. What about subsequent work? From the practical point of view I learnt that any old kind of bread is good, provided you eat something else with it; that too much vitamin D is not a good thing for your baby; that there is no particular virtue in obliging your milk-hating daughter to force it down, or make any child eat something greatly disliked, however nutritionally desirable. But all the same, I got wild when mine wouldn't eat the good meals I had cooked for them!

I learnt quite a lot of German, some of it useful for talking to *au pair* girls, but most of it too medical for polite conversation, I fear. I got used to working erratic hours rather than to a timetable, and to coping with all kinds of excretions in all kinds of containers, in all kinds of places.

I think this is enough to show that my time with Professor McCance and Miss Widdowson had a very favourable influence upon my subsequent work and thought. In fact, one begins to speculate upon the desirability of such a preliminary to marriage for every bride. No doubt, a proper study should be made first, but there is plenty of material, as many people have married from the Department and in some instances, like mine, both partners had worked there.

Those eight years were the most stimulating of my life and widened my horizons immeasurably. What I should have missed had I not been approved at that first lab lunch, and how grateful I am to the Professor and all in the Department for the memory of many interesting conversations and not a little laughter.

Finally, I should like to emphasise that though Professor McCance and Miss Widdowson have such different personalities, they both inspired great enthusiasm, great loyalty and much affection. I owe them much gratitude for many kindnesses shown to a young newcomer to the strange world of research and later on for the trust they both placed in me to carry out their requirements.

Dorothy Rosenbaum

> Dorothy Rosenbaum became a doctor in the Städtische Krankenanstalten in Wuppertal-Barmen in 1936. She had a German father, an English mother, spent the First World War in London, and the Second World War in Wuppertal, and was brought up to be completely bilingual. Her first schooling was in London, followed by grammar school education in Germany, where all her medical training also took place.
>
> She first met Professor McCance and Dr Widdowson in the Spring of 1946, and has maintained her friendship with them ever since, visiting Dr Widdowson's home in Barrington frequently for over 40 years.

One day in the summer of 1946 my boss, Professor Heilmeyer, and I, were asked to show a visiting group of English doctors round our hospital. We decided to show them a museum converted into wards for convalescent patients, as we feared confiscation of our main hospital. I therefore received them rather coolly in the museum and spoke with a German accent.

Looking round I overheard Dr Widdowson say to Professor McCance, 'This doesn't look like a hospital, I'll have a look upstairs'. Without thinking I called out in my usual London English, 'Here, you can't go up there!' Dr Widdowson was startled, 'Wherever do you come from?' Once we had established that we both came from South London, I risked the question, 'Why do you want our hospital?' Very relieved to hear they wanted to do research work, I took them to the real hospital and introduced them to Professor Heilmeyer, who knew their names well from their publications on iron metabolism.

They went back to England; I heard nothing from them and I thought I should never see them again. However, several months later, in the summer of 1946, they came back, having decided to work in Wuppertal, and to investigate the effects of undernutrition in the German population.

I was at that time employed as 'Oberärztin' (Head Assistant) on the hospital staff, but found time to help Professor McCance, Dr Widdowson and their team to establish an out-patients' clinic twice weekly to see people suffering from hunger oedema. It was a somewhat tricky job for me, as the German patients had applied for extra rations and they were naturally suspicious of the English doctors interfering. Being bilingual and binational, with loyalty to both sides, I managed somehow, and as time went on, the outpatients' clinic was a happy gathering for all of us.

Very soon Dr Widdowson and I became good friends, so from then on, it was 'Elsie and Dorothy'. Both Professor McCance and Elsie enjoyed visiting my parents and heard about the difficulties of life in Germany during the War, and afterwards in 1946. They always came with very welcome little gifts to supplement our rations, and we were pleased to be able to offer fresh peaches out of our garden. I can still see Professor McCance picking and eating a luscious peach. He also enjoyed listening to stories about 'hamstern'. I am using the German word, a verb derived from hamster, the name of the animal. People went to a lot of trouble, travelling miles in overcrowded trains, sometimes on the buffers, to get into the country to barter textile goods for farm produce, to preserve and store for the winter. I used to go 'hamstern' myself at weekends and was very surprised (and embarrassed) when Professor McCance met me at the station with his camera to take a photograph of the 'Hamsterer'.

When the effects of undernutrition had been established, Elsie decided to see how these people would respond to unlimited food. I remember driving around with her, visiting the chosen patients in their homes, and persuading them to join the experiment. Elsie's natural kindness helped a lot, the German people trusted her and nearly all volunteered to come into the ward set aside for them for nine weeks. I chose a very competent ward sister to overlook the food that was weighed and eaten: Schwester Maria, having been a believer in Hitler, would not take a morsel of food for herself from the British! At the end of the experiment, she and the English nurse, Lois Thrussell, were the best of friends. Helping Professor McCance and Elsie during those years was a very happy experience for me, the first time I had come into contact with dedicated research workers; my part in medicine had always been on the clinical side.

I think it was Professor McCance's and Elsie's friendly approach to their German patients that helped to overcome difficulties. I had the opportunity to notice that not every member of their team had this attitude and it necessitated a lot of diplomacy on my part to persuade patients to allow themselves to be investigated. In fact, I can truly say that it was only the kindness of Professor McCance, Dr Widdowson and Nurse Lois Thrussell, that made this research work in Germany at all possible so soon after the end of the War.

DAY-TO-DAY RECOLLECTIONS

Eric Glaser

> In March 1946 Professor McCance and Dr Widdowson went to Germany to find somewhere to establish their Medical Research Council Unit. They stayed overnight at an army mess in Clausthal-Zellerfeld; the officer in charge of that mess was Eric Glaser. The outcome was that Dr Glaser joined McCance and Widdowson in their unit in Wuppertal. He stayed there for six months and then went to the Department of Experimental Medicine in Cambridge. There he dedicated himself to work on survival at sea. He left Cambridge at the end of 1951 to go to Singapore as Professor of Physiology. He returned to become Professor of Physiology at the Medical School of the London Hospital. After that, he spent several years working in the pharmaceutical industry. Sadly, he died in December 1992.

In the Spring of 1946 I was in charge of a small medical unit in the Harz Mountains of Germany when I got a message from Divisional Headquarters that two English scientists were in the region. Would I look after them over a weekend? Mac and Elsie duly turned up on a Saturday. There was nothing frosty or pompous about them and they were easy guests. Food among the German population was very scarce and army rations were modest, but bread and potatoes were not difficult; so Mac was no problem, and Elsie's frugal needs were met easily enough. The evening went quite well and this encouraged me to say that I had planned a long walk through the Harz Mountains on Sunday, so would they mind if the other doctor in the unit looked after them? Mac immediately responded that he would enjoy a long walk and Elsie said that she would appreciate a quiet day.

The walk was a great success. Mac expanded upon his plans for a Medical Research Council (MRC) Unit and explained that he was looking for somebody in the Army who would maintain liaison with the Military Government, preferably with a little understanding and experience of research, and be able to lend a hand to the work. Though my total experience was limited to a year at the Hammersmith Hospital, leading to one paper in the *Lancet* and a communication to the Medical Research Society, I met the specifications to a certain extent, and by the end of the walk, we had agreed, to my joy, that the MRC should ask for my secondment to the new Unit in Germany. Mac and I also became lifelong friends and established a habit of occasional long walks together.

I did not do much administrative work when I joined the Unit in Wuppertal. By the time I was transferred at the end of June 1946, most of the administrative arrangements were working smoothly due, I think, to Elsie's energetic efficiency. I was more interested in getting back into research and I got two small papers in the Wuppertal book (as well as a chance to apply for an MRC grant in Cambridge). In retrospect, I failed to fulfil my side of the agreement and only stayed for six months. If Mac and Elsie resented this, they never gave a hint of it, and this also tells us something about them. Possibly they decided that my contribution made little difference.

Elsie had a group of friends in Wuppertal, the nature of whom threw an interesting light on Elsie's personality. On Sundays Elsie often disappeared for a while to see some German acquaintances and take them gifts of clothing, soap and other unobtainable items that had been sent to her from England for them. There was little interest in who these acquaintances might be, but as Christmas approached, we were all invited to meet them. They turned out to be a fundamentalist Christian Group (much disliked, even persecuted by the Nazis), and quite unlike other Germans we met. Most Germans were obsequious, some still arrogant, many understandably still suspicious, and none friendly. These were simple straightforward good people. If I remember right, we enjoyed their simple hospitality and sang carols that were common to England and Germany.

It was clear to me on our first walk that Mac was a truly remarkable man; it took longer and a more gradual understanding to realise that Elsie was no less remarkable. Like most people who were in any way associated with Mac and Elsie, I was often asked what was the nature of their collaboration and who was the dominant partner. It took me some time to conclude that both contribute equally to their phenomenally successful partnership, though each provides different aspects of their work. There is no remote relevance in such suggestions as 'Elsie does the work, Mac does the talking,' or at the other extreme, 'Elsie is a good technician dragged along by Mac's genius.'

The remarkable thing is that the talents of Mac and Elsie are entirely complementary: as in a resolved crossword puzzle, each word has a significance of its own, but also forms part of other words, so each of their abilities reinforces the other's abilities. The result is a perfect blend of their talents in which the effect is far greater than a mere summation of their skills. I wonder whether there has ever been such a continued and effective partnership between two scientists of genius?

Ability is of no avail if it is not supported by suitable personality. Mac and Elsie's personalities also seem to reinforce rather than match each other. To an outsider, it looked as if the relationship were based entirely on mutual courtesy and respect. It would have been improper to speculate, but I never saw any evidence of the occasional hurt look or irritable word that is not unusual, even among the best of friends.

Daphne Learmouth
(now Daphne Tabor)

> Daphne Learmouth (subsequently McDermott and Tabor) worked for Professor McCance and Dr Widdowson in several places in Cambridge: the Department of Experimental Medicine in Tennis Court Road (from 1946), the house in Shaftesbury Road, the Dunn Nutrition Unit in Milton Road (from 1969), and finally the Department of Investigative Medicine in the new Addenbrooke's Hospital (from 1973). She has now retired and lives in Burnham Market, Norfolk.

I had a rare bone disease in my teens and was in Wolverhampton General Hospital under the care of Dr JH Sheldon. He asked a friend of his, Professor RA McCance, if he would take a look at me. He offered to have me in Addenbrooke's Hospital, Cambridge, and I went there in May 1945 for calcium balance investigations. I was Lois Thrussell's first patient. The measurements showed that I was excreting excessive amounts of calcium. Professor McCance decided to give me very large doses of vitamin D_2. He told me some time later that he did not know what it would do to me. Fortunately, I did begin to get better, but it was only after I had a tumour removed from my femur that I made really rapid progress. The Professor used to refer to my recovery as 'one of his most successful experiments'.

I came out of hospital in the spring of 1946 and, because the Professor wanted to monitor my progress, he found me part-time jobs in the Department of Experimental Medicine and in the Pathology Laboratory. At the beginning of 1947, the Professor asked me to be his full-time secretary. This also meant dealing with the administration and personnel for the whole Department, ie doing the wages, the book-keeping, looking after the library, filing and recording the reprints that came to the Professor and Miss Widdowson.

In the early years, Miss Widdowson was still in Germany so I did not get to know her well until she returned to the Department at the beginning of 1949. I became her secretary in 1966 when Professor McCance retired from Cambridge and went to Uganda for two years.

I was very fond of the Professor, although I will admit that there were times when he was difficult. It was often the trivial mistakes which made him cross, rather than the major ones. He didn't turn a hair when I invited the wrong person for lunch (I didn't know there were two Dr Dicks in the University!) but he was furious with me when one of the research nurses went on holiday without telling me, or anyone. I was so upset that I took my lunch and ate it in a room that was seldom used. He looked everywhere and asked if anyone had seen me. He was quite relieved when I turned up again mid-afternoon and we continued our work as if nothing had happened.

In the early days the lab lunch was taken at two tables. The Professor, Miss Widdowson, the scientists and their guests sat at one table, and the rest of us sat at the other. At one time, the Professor insisted on making the coffee for the people at both tables, and we used to sit and wait until he had poured it for us. Once, when he was not feeling too happy he looked across at us and said, 'Look at them sitting there, like sparrows waiting for the crumbs!' Some of the lunches were extra-special because we had roast pork. We knew that the meat was left over from one of the experimental pigs, but it never seemed to worry us!

When parcels arrived, I never cut the string but always untied it as the Professor used string to tie up his trousers for cycling, and he kept it in a little bag. When I was clearing out a drawer before I left the Department, I found the bag containing the neatly rolled string.

The Professor was also particularly frugal with paper. There were many times when I typed out scientific papers that started life written on the backs of envelopes in his small neat writing. If that space was insufficient, the writing would spread all around, or be intertwined with the address on the front. If he wasn't using envelopes, he would write on the back of drafts of old manuscripts. I still find myself doing the same thing and I will never use brand new paper for making rough notes!

The Professor's writing was more difficult to read when he was on train journeys; he never wasted time and always made certain he had paper. He enjoyed going to the States by sea because it gave him more time and he once wrote a whole paper on the *Mauretania*. He hated flying and used to confide in me that he thought he would never come back.

Because the Professor was such a perfectionist and his papers were meticulously composed, typing them out was quite a trial in the days before word processors. Very often, whole pages had to be retyped for one minor correction. Once photocopiers were available, my life became a little easier and I could do a cut-and-paste job.

Most of the McCance and Widdowson papers were the prime responsibility of one of them. The prime author would write the first draft, consult the co-author, and then continue to process the drafts alone. Miss Widdowson could work from handwritten drafts, but the Professor liked to have each draft retyped. Because so much attention was given to scientific detail and the papers were so well written, there was never too much rewriting needed in response to editorial comments. I only remember one paper, on chickens, being rejected.

The Professor and Miss Widdowson always shared an office. His desk was always left tidy with neat piles of papers that no one dared to touch. Her desk was strewn with papers—but she always knew where to find everything.

Working for Professor McCance and Miss Widdowson from 1946 to 1987 meant that I acquired a certain amount of nutritional and physiological knowledge. Although I found certain things, like renal physiology, more difficult than others, I was always aware of the experiments going on around me.

My first memory of meeting Miss Widdowson was of seeing her grinding up baby rats with a pestle and mortar. The only experiments that really upset me were Rex Dean's studies on dogs. Years later, at the height of concern about vivisection, I told the Professor how I had felt about those experiments; he was surprised that I had not mentioned it to him before.

The Professor and Miss Widdowson were known to all of us as Dad and Mum. I still get former members of staff writing to me and asking whether I've seen 'Mumsy' recently. I think I have been very lucky to have worked in such a happy Department for such eminent scientists as Professor McCance and Miss Widdowson, and to have contributed in my own small way to their success.

Marion Harrison
(now Marion Robinson)

> Marion Harrison left Dunedin, New Zealand, in 1948 to work under Professor McCance for her PhD. She married James Robinson in 1951 and they both left Cambridge in 1957 to return to New Zealand. Professor Marion Robinson retired from the Department of Nutrition, University of Otago in 1989.

Anyone coming from afar expects everything in the United Kingdom, and particularly in Cambridge, to be so much better than one has had at home. I don't think I shall ever forget my surprise when I was shown the big lab in Tennis Court Road, and was given a three foot square of bench space with a solitary drawer beneath it. Maybe the pioneering spirit of my forefathers still flowed in my veins, for soon I had increased my area of occupation. The accommodation was so like what I had left behind in New Zealand. There I had a basement room where I did countless fluoride estimations.

My time in the lab in Cambridge was invaluable for me. I never ceased to wonder during those lunches in the late 1940s and early 1950s, when large-scale experiments were being planned, how

Professor McCance and Dr Widdowson could disregard the inessentials and focus the whole experiment on ways to find out what they wanted to know.

I finished my PhD in 1951. I felt I might have blotted my copybook early on by discovering that the Professor's own method for measuring sodium was measuring potassium as well; they were both precipitated out because the refrigerator was running at 0°C instead of 4°C. It was distinctly embarassing for an overseas research student to start her career by finding a snag in the Professor's special technique!

Looking back, I was even a greater disaster when it came to having children. Knowing I was expecting twins, the Professor was looking forward to me producing boys. My twin girls did not have the correct 'plumbing' to be suitable experimental guinea pigs for his experiments on infant physiology. I did not have too great a sense of guilt, though, because I knew the Professor was already a grandfather to twin granddaughters of his own.

The Professor's wife, Mollie, was a very warm person, but also long-suffering. Though she appeared to be in the background, living in the Dower House at Bartlow, she was very active behind the scenes, not least as a transport officer who regularly shifted the Professor's books and various other items between home and the lab by car. He rarely drove, and the bicycle had, of course, a rather limited carrying capacity. We visited Bartlow one day for Sunday lunch and I remember the famous bike sitting majestically in the hall. The Professor carved a beautiful joint, but,of course, ate none of it himself.

At the evening meal though, the Professor had a great capacity to eat potatoes. Soon after Mollie died, he came with Dr Widdowson to have dinner with us in Cambridge. We threatened our daughters with dire penalties if they showed any reaction to his large serving of vegetables. In the event, all went well until he picked up the potato dish and emptied *all* the potatoes onto his plate; that really was too much for them!

I arrived just when the Department's staff were preoccupied with the return to Cambridge from Germany. So it was not until Dr Widdowson had settled back into the Cambridge scene that I discovered just what a friendly and hospitable person she was. She introduced me to the Cambridgeshire countryside, and took James and me on many visits to local churches from her lovely thatched cottage at Barrington.

One of my most vivid memories of Elsie Widdowson's extraordinary skills in lecturing was when she addressed the Cambridge Women's Research Club. Her topic was announced as *White and Brown*. Little did the audience know that she was going to talk about bread, not about race! Her account of the Department's comparative studies and experiences led to a discussion which unleashed from this educated, intelligent group a host of prejudices and anecdotal testimony, underlying their own widely divergent views on the attributes of white and wholemeal breads.

Dr Widdowson showed James and myself great kindness when she realised that we were becoming fond of each other. She has always been generous with time in meeting us at airports and docks etc. We were thrilled that she could be the Guest of Honour at my retirement in 1989 and that she gave the Muriel Bell Lecture. Even when she was in New Zealand, Dr Widdowson would ring the Professor at his flat in Cambridge to make certain that he was looking after himself and eating properly. 'Have you had that?' she would say, checking he had not overlooked some delicacy she had left with him.

Terry Cowen

> Terry Cowen worked as an animal technician and looked after the experimental pigs at the animal out-station of the Department of Experimental Medicine in Bartlow from 1949 to 1973. He joined the staff at the Dunn Nutrition Unit in 1973 and left in 1988. He now runs a hotel near Bournemouth, on the south coast of England, looking after people, rather than animals.

Not many people can claim they had their job interview in an apple orchard on a Sunday in spring! When I arrived at Professor McCance's house by arrangement at three o'clock on this particular afternoon, I was told that the Professor was 'somewhere in the garden'; the only problem was that the garden covered about ten acres (four hectares).

I eventually found the Professor perched precariously on top of a rickety pair of steps, pruning his apple trees. After initial introductions, I was asked how old I was, then which piece of tree should he cut next, and then did I like animals? Suddenly, I had to grab the steps as the Professor lost his balance trying to cut a piece of branch slightly above and behind his head. The interview continued like this for the next half an hour.

I didn't hear any more from the Professor for nearly a month until he called at my home one day. He said it was about time I started work. 'When?' I asked. 'Thursday sounds a good day,' he said. So my first week was only two and a half days, for which I received 30 shillings (£1.50 now).

Dr Widdowson and Professor McCance were very kind in different ways. One day I gave the Professor some notes about a particular animal. On reading them, he said, 'I don't think you spell diarrhoea that way'. He said he was unsure himself how to spell the word, so he thought we'd better go to the library and look it up. On finding it, he said, 'There, now we have both learnt something today'. I knew all the time that he knew how to spell the word but was just being kind to me.

Although Professor McCance was a very busy person, he always had time for other people. Every Sunday afternoon when he was at home during the blackberry season, he would call on my mother and ask for a basket. He'd then spend all Sunday afternoon picking blackberries for her. He was generous in other ways too, although sometimes his forgetfulness added to the generosity.

We had an old chap working with the animals called Ernie Freeman. One Christmas the Professor said that he would like to give Ernie something and decided on a ten-shilling note (50p). The following Christmas, the Professor asked me how much he had given Ernie for the previous one. I felt sure he really remembered, so I said £1. The Professor thought he had better give him 30 shillings (£1.50). The next Christmas, I was asked the same question; I said £2, so the Professor gave Ernie £3. Thankfully for my guilty conscience and the Professor's bank balance, Ernie retired before the following Christmas.

Not surprisingly, a lot of my recollections involve stories about the pigs that I looked after at Bartlow. We restrained our large and breeding pigs by an electric fence. When they had cleared the grass in one area, we moved them to another. To do so, we would switch off the fence, remove it and then move the pigs out. This was sometimes very difficult as the pigs had worn down the ground inside the fence, so they could tell where the fence used to be and would not pass on to the new pasture. The best way was to entice them out with food. One day, one pig refused to come out. We tried all ways, even pushing her out with the Land Rover. We removed all the huts, just leaving one drinking trough. Just before going home, we tried to move her again without success, so we left some food and water, gave up and went home. The next day was the same. On the third morning, I was driving to work, approaching the Bartlow crossroads, when I saw a very large pig fast asleep in the middle of the road. I picked her up, drove her to the farm and put her in her rightful pen. Later that morning, an irate neighbour came charging into the yard saying he had just laid a new lawn and one of our pigs had dug it all up. I told him he should have kept his gate shut, and luckily we never heard any more about the matter.

On another occasion, I had just delivered a pig to the lab in Tennis Court Road and was driving along Hills Road at the end of Brooklands Avenue. A glance in the driving mirror showed the trailer I was supposed to be pulling was vanishing up Brooklands Avenue. At first, I didn't want to stop as there was a lot of traffic about and I didn't dare to imagine all the damage the trailer had done. Eventually I found somewhere to turn round, only to find a man parking the trailer on the footpath and a lady getting out of a car, wiping her brow with a handkerchief. She said that the trailer had been coming straight for her, but suddenly it had spun round in the middle of the road and stopped. I thanked them both, hooked the trailer onto the Land Rover and quickly drove away, hoping no one had taken my number.

The incident that was the talk of the Department for many years to come, was the story of the pig called Houdini. Professor McCance and Dr Widdowson called at the farm at Bartlow one day to collect a 10-week-old pig to take to Cambridge. It was secured firmly in a wooden box and put into Dr Widdowson's trailer, so that if it escaped from the box, it would not get out of the high-sided trailer. About 45 minutes later, I had a message from Cambridge saying that there was no pig in the trailer. After phone calls to the police, it came to light that the pig had been found trotting along the footpath in Abington by, of all people, the local butcher. When I called to collect the pig, I had great difficulty persuading the butcher to let me have it. He obviously had other plans for it! Although it was a female, there was only one name for her—Houdini. We kept her as a pet at Bartlow. She eventually produced lots of litters but we never had an opportunity of finding out whether they had inherited their mother's powers of escape.

Ashton B Morrison

> Ashton (Archie) Morrison joined the Department of Experimental Medicine in September 1952. Five years earlier, after qualifying in Medicine at the Queen's University of Belfast, he had been a Demonstrator, first in Biochemistry and then in Anatomy, and also gained a PhD. He had a travelling fellowship from Queen's and Professor McCance helped him find a suitable laboratory in Germany, where he spent time before joining his Department. In September 1955 he left the Department, and since then has held academic appointments in the USA.

On my first day in Cambridge I turned up at Tennis Court Road at 8am to find there was no one about. A little after 9am, a small dark-haired lady (Daphne) arrived, and told me Professor McCance would not appear for at least another hour. Sure enough, around 10.15am, the thin figure of the Professor, perched on a large racing bicycle with low-slung handlebars, wove into the area. It appeared much too large for him, and ever afterwards, I always felt, when I saw him riding it, that he was not really in control.

He told me that he did not have time to see me until after lunch, and even then it seemed to me he had not thought much in advance about my duties, except that I would be in charge of his hospital patients. I felt a little like Alice in Wonderland—quite alone in a place with fairyland qualities where almost anything was liable to happen.

Over the next few weeks, I discovered from Brian Strangeways who everyone was, what they were doing and, more importantly, what my precise duties were. I came to know the interesting people who made up the small Department. Two were clearly central figures: Elsie Widdowson, who worked closely with the Professor, and seemed to know more about what was supposed to go on than any of the rest, and James Robinson, the Assistant Director of Research, a University title with a full University appointment.

James Robinson was an outstanding physiologist with, even then, an international reputation. He was very kind to me and gave me guidance on the University of Cambridge and the relationship of the Medical Research Council (MRC) Unit to it. This was important to understand, for my salary was paid by the MRC and I was a member of its staff. Ian Holman, a chemist who worked closely with Elsie, was from South Africa and I became friendly with him. Romaine Hervey was there on my arrival, and stayed for some years after my departure.

Of all the people in the Department, Romaine, in my view, represented best the Englishman of legend. He was absolutely and completely dependable in every conceivable situation. Joe Cort, an American visiting fellow, who had graduated a year before from Yale Medical School, was just completing work with the Professor and left shortly after I arrived, to take a job at Birmingham University. John Dickerson was also there, and worked with Dr Widdowson in immediate charge of all the chemical work in her laboratory. Bob Spires was the head technician and laboratory steward and an endless source of help with equipment and technical know-how.

A year or so after my arrival, Gordon Kennedy joined us from the National Institute of Medical Research at Mill Hill in London. I was greatly impressed with Kennedy's abilities and his wellspring of ideas. I carried out some work with him, and he helped and guided my own project with the Professor. I am sure he would have had a reputation of the order of McCance, had he not died so tragically early, of Parkinson's Disease.

About the same time as Kennedy came to the Department, there arrived from the University of Buffalo John Boylan, who was a member of their faculty, and held a fellowship from the USA. An American of Irish background, John, his wife Jean and his family, found their way into our hearts. I admired and liked him and was to have an ongoing friendship until his death in August 1991. John was a master of the spoken and written word, and his papers have a literary style unusual in the literature of scientific medicine.

While the Professor wanted me to decide what area of research I was to work in, clearly it was to be something ongoing in the Department. He hoped that I would follow up on work already started by Marion

Harrison but I was not drawn in this direction. I felt she had taken the idea as far as it would go at that time, so I turned to another area.

As it happened, the Professor had long been interested in the matter of survival at sea by castaways, and the problem of drinking sea water. A recent voyage by Bombard, who claimed to have made an Atlantic crossing, taking some sea water as well as squeezed fish juice, had raised the whole question again. The Bombard hypothesis was contrary to all the work already done by Professor McCance, and he and I set out to use an experimental model, in the Professor's words to, 'Nail this Bombard nonsense down'.

We used the five-sixths partially nephrectomised rats as our model. The remaining piece of kidney in these rats could not produce, as did the whole kidney, a urine more concentrated than sea water. In them we could test the effect of varying the concentrations of salt in equal aliquots of drinking fluid to measure the effect on the rat's body fluids.

As I worked, it became clear to me that these partially nephrectomised rats could be animal models of chronic renal disease in man. I tried to get the Professor interested in this idea but he never took it up. For him, they were a means to analyse the physiological mechanisms in which he was interested, and the analysis of the pathological mechanisms in chronic renal disease, as a disease process, did not interest him.

I continued to work on this animal model in the United States and established it as the prime experimental model of chronic renal failure. It took me 20 years to show that the progression of chronic renal disease results from the increase in single nephron glomerular filtration rate in these animals. The work has been confirmed extensively by others, and it is now recognised that a similar mechanism may occur in chronic renal disease in man, and that a reduction in protein intake may slow the process. Considering the length of time expended in establishing the idea of the partially nephrectomised rat being a model of chronic renal disease, perhaps the Professor's reluctance may have been justified.

I have always believed that the Professor missed a great opportunity by not studying the morphological and physiological and other consequences of renal disease upon the various organs, by using these animal models. He never seemed to have much interest in disease as such—he was always more interested in the physiology and biochemistry of diseased states. It was always difficult to work on projects which held little interest for Professor McCance.

The only occasion that I worked with Dr Widdowson was when she showed much more interest than the Professor in a certain project of mine. We injected Dextran intravenously into dogs, as a means of increasing oncotic pressure, and showed that a reduction in serum protein level took place, along with a change in the distribution of the various proteins as measured electrophoretically. I then realised Dr

Widdowson's tremendous abilities were of the same calibre as the Professor's, but she was more modest about them.

One day, one of the experimental pigs at Bartlow died of a kidney infection. Dr Widdowson appeared on my doorstep at seven in the morning and told me that the Professor wanted me to perform an autopsy on the animal. I drove her in the Departmental truck out to Bartlow, taking my wife along. Terry Cowen, the animal technician, was already with the pig, which proved to have an acute purulent pyelonephritis. We took some samples back to the lab for histologic studies and bacterial analysis. Then the Professor and I took the pig's carcase to Linton, where we persuaded the local butcher to hang it in his cold room. Soon afterwards, Dr Widdowson got a phone call from the irate butcher who had just realised that he had an infected animal on his premises. I think poor Terry got the task of removing the offending carcase and dealing with the angry butcher.

Another incident I can recall involved Peter John when he first became Professor McCance's patient. Peter had a severe problem with his weight and various physicians had failed to help him lose his excess fat. The Professor's first idea was to let Peter eat 'ad lib' and to measure his total energy intake—it turned out to be about 7000 Calories. He asked me if I had any suggestions for weighing Peter; the regular hospital scales could not accommodate someone whose weight exceeded 160kg (350lb). I contacted a local dealer in farm scales, and came up with the idea of using two sets of scales, each weighing up to 230kg (500lb). When this plan worked, the Professor could weigh his patient.

Peter was asked to put one foot on each scale and then the two weights were added together. I received a rare accolade for my idea. The Professor turned to me with one of his favourite expressions and said, 'Archie, that's wizard'. The idea was not all that original, for it figured in James Cain's novel *Galatea*. I always took an interest in the Professor's subsequent attempts to slim Peter. After I left Cambridge, I was particularly pleased to receive a photograph of Peter wearing *my* old white lab coat to demonstrate what progress had been made.

In the era of Stephen Potter's 'one-manship', there was a lot of 'McCance-manship' at lunch. One day, the Professor claimed to have seen a rare bird—a marsh harrier—as he cycled in from Bartlow. Someone remarked that it was quite a way from its natural habitat but the Professor retorted that, 'the high winds prevailing today may have blown it in'.

Professor McCance had an extraordinary knack of picking up facts and giving them a relevance which few others would have recognised. He listened, asked questions, and questioned the answers. He was always eager for new, and preferably bright, ideas. A favourite remark of his was, 'You are not going to make any money in the stock market if you just ride into the City with the rest of the stockbrokers, reading the *Financial Times*. You've got to do something absolutely different like standing on your head, preferably in the middle of the road'.

On the occasions when I worked closely with Dr Widdowson, I quickly recognised an original and inquiring mind, with a great depth of knowledge in every area related to the activities in the laboratory. She never let her bright ideas run ahead of her as the Professor sometimes did. She also seemed to be the one person capable of deciding which of his ideas were the brightest, and might actually pay off in satisfactory scientific work. At the same time, she kept the Department running smoothly.

The Professor was never a diplomat, and was capable of making the most critical, but often accurate, remarks about his colleagues. Worse still, he sometimes made them rather directly. My overriding memory of Professor McCance was of a very brilliant man who could, at times, be difficult. He had a certain winning charm and, like all outstanding people whose contributions have been of the greatest magnitude, he is always the subject of reminiscence among former colleagues. Dr Widdowson, fortunately, worked closely with him and was always there to keep things going and to act as an arbitrator. Together, they made a wonderful partnership.

John Dickerson

John Dickerson joined the Department of Experimental Medicine at the end of August 1952, after he had received an External London University BSc. He gained his PhD in 1959 for his work on aspects of body composition during normal development, and as a result of undernutrition. He left the Department in 1965, just before Professor McCance retired, and went to work with John Dobbing in Professor Tanner's Department at the Institute of Child Health in London.

In 1967 he became a Reader in Human Nutrition in the Department of Biochemistry at the newly formed University of Surrey, and in 1973 he became Professor of Human Nutrition. Professor Dickerson retired in 1988 and was later appointed an Emeritus Professor.

I have very warm memories of Professor McCance's interest and support during my time in Cambridge. He was always keen to know what I had been doing, and his almost daily visits to the Department in Shaftesbury Road were something for which one had to be prepared. These were always friendly visits, with the Professor keen to hear what one had to say. At times questions and comments were rather more probing than usual and one was inclined to get a little exasperated but, almost always, one reaped benefit from such experiences.

Mac had a sharp mind, coupled with real physiological understanding and insight and an excellent memory. These attributes enabled him to think clearly about problems, even while riding his bicycle; it was not uncommon for him to stop at a telephone kiosk while on one of his cycling meanderings, in order to communicate his latest thoughts on the interpretation of data. These gems were known as Mac's 'cycling thoughts'. His preference for string, instead of trouser clips, worn even when making visits to his patients in Addenbrooke's Hospital, will always be part of 'The Professor'.

Anyone who worked with Mac could not help but be impressed by his mastery of English, both written and verbal. He could write a letter to which there could only be one answer.

I have warm memories of Mac's interest in my family. This was often one of the main topics of conversation during my many visits to his flat in Sidney Sussex College. He once severely reprimanded me for working late, telling me that my wife needed me. When my wife started making wine, we soon found a very appreciative recipient of it.

I got to know Elsie Widdowson very well. It was always a pleasure to work with her, as well as an education. While valuing all the help and encouragement that Elsie gave me in my work, my wife and I also appreciated the very real interest that she took in our children. They, with us, have warm recollections of her visits to us and also of our visits to Barrington. Elsie loved children and gave her own china doll to our daughter.

In the mid-1960s, Mac and Elsie were very involved in setting up the nutrition course at Surrey University. It started as a dietetics course, but I was keen to produce graduates in nutrition rather than dietetics and our first students graduated in 1968. The nutrition course at Surrey was just one of several that benefited from advice freely given by Professor McCance and Dr Widdowson. She acted as our external examiner for a number of years.

Peter John

> Peter John met Professor McCance when he was referred to him as a patient in 1955 by Dr Leonard Simpson in London, in the hope that the Professor would find some endocrinological defect to explain why Peter weighed so much. He did not, but by reducing his food intake considerably, Peter's weight gradually came down.
>
> Peter became a laboratory technician in the Department of Experimental Medicine, Cambridge, in 1956 and remained there until 1968, when he was transferred to the Dunn Nutrition Unit. He retired in 1991, and the speeches on that occasion demonstrated how much his willing help had been appreciated by all those with whom he had worked.

I remember Professor McCance in a dual role—as my doctor and my employer. As a doctor, he gave me the support and motivation to reduce my weight from 225kg (550lb) to 76kg (168lb). I suffered none of the humiliation that I had done as a patient at St Mary's Hospital in London, when I had to be taken by ambulance to be weighed on Paddington Station. Once I had lost a lot of weight and had become more mobile, the Professor invited me to do some odd jobs in the Department of Experimental Medicine. I was offered a junior technician's post in December, 1956 and acted as an apprentice to John Dickerson. I worked mainly at the Shaftesbury Road Annexe and John encouraged me in my career. I spent months doing phosphorus measurements using a spot galvanometer, manually winding a wheel to read the endpoint. There were two young girl technicians—Greta Humm and Rosemary Still. Professor McCance and Dr Widdowson had a policy of taking technical people straight from school because they preferred to train them themselves.

One of my special techniques was the preparation of rat bones and skins for subsequent chemical analysis. I became very good at shaving rat pelts with a scalpel. After John Dickerson left, I taught Peter Adams the calcium and parathyroid hormone assays.

When I first joined the Department, it was housed in the Pathology block in Tennis Court Road under sufferance from Professor Dean, the Professor of Pathology. We had five to six labs, plus office space. Later, we acquired some huts on the Peterhouse site to give us more room. Dr Widdowson and the Professor shared an office in the Department at Tennis Court Road. Dr Widdowson always had her own office in Shaftesbury Road with an enormous desk and a large window looking on to the garden. The Departmental Secretary, Daphne, and her husband lived upstairs—he was the caretaker.

There was a very happy atmosphere in the lab; the technicians were always introduced to visitors. Over the years I met, and helped, quite a few overseas visitors, some of whom stayed for some time. Everybody worked till 12.30pm on Saturdays, but we were allowed one Saturday off per month as a gift from the Professor (although he was always happy to accommodate special requests to go to weddings and other 'occasions').

The Professor and Dr Widdowson were referred to as 'Father' and 'Mother'. I think this all started one Sunday when we were working in the labs and were worrying about missing our lunch. The Professor knew that Dr Widdowson, being well organised, would cater for everyone, so reassured us that 'Mother knows best'. Their relationship was almost like a married couple. Dr Widdowson would say, 'Yes, you can do so and so, providing the Professor agrees'. She always called him 'The Professor'. He called her Miss Widdowson, Dr Widdowson and, occasionally, Elsie.

I was involved with some of the metabolic studies going on in the Department, together with Jack Booyens, who later became a Professor in South Africa,. We did some activity studies that involved collecting samples of expired air in a football bladder attached to a portable gas meter. I remember seeing the Professor cycling past the hospital, wearing a mouthpiece attached to the meter, always being keen to try out experimental equipment on himself. The Professor's bicycle was a very lightweight machine with thin high-pressure tyres and he used to keep it in the lab near his office. Sometimes he asked me to check the tyres for flints etc, because he had a fear of getting a puncture on one of his cross-country rides.

When Professor Wilkinson did operations on Professor McCance's pigs, Professor McCance acted as anaesthetist, dropping ether from a bottle on to the pig's nose. Every so often, the Professor would 'nod off' momentarily when the anaesthetic got to him as well as the pig. I used to provide the transport between the Department and the pigs at Bartlow, and went with John Dickerson to the slaughterhouse when the biggest pigs were killed. Once I was asked to dry some newborn pigs to constant weight. I took a short cut and used a spring balance instead of pan balance with weights. Dr Widdowson told me that it was not very scientific and never to do it again. I didn't.

In later years, when the Professor was officially retired, he and I worked together quite a lot, tidying up the long-term work on some of the pig experiments. He got into the habit of telephoning me at home with some problem or idea that had occurred to him. On one occasion, he rang before breakfast. I was speechless and had to tell him that I would ring him back when I had collected my thoughts and calmed down. Sometimes he thought I spent all my free time worrying about the scientific problems, as he did.

J Russell Elkinton

> Russell Elkinton spent a sabbatical six months in the Department of Experimental Medicine in 1957. He had received his MD from Harvard in 1937 and spent three years as resident physician at the Pennsylvania Hospital in Philadelphia. From 1940 to 1948 he had been in the faculty of Yale University School of Medicine where much of his research was directed to body-fluid problems related to the Second World War. In 1948 he joined the Department of Medicine at the University of Pennsylvania.
>
> In 1960, he was appointed by the American College of Physicians as Editor of the **Annals of Internal Medicine,** which evolved into a full-time post. He retired in 1971 and the next year he came back to the UK with his English wife, Teresa. They lived in Herefordshire before returning to his native USA in 1984.

I have many memories of that happy sabbatical of six months spent in Cambridge more than 30 years ago. RA McCance, Professor of Experimental Medicine, together with his partner-in-science, Elsie Widdowson, made many major contributions of an extraordinarily wide variety of physiological and nutritional knowledge over long years. These included studies of body composition, infant and fetal physiology, undernutrition, and many other subjects. Their experiments were always simple, clear and decisive; many of them were conducted on themselves as experimental subjects (as well as on their colleagues). For me, it was a privilege to work, however briefly, with Mac and Elsie.

Their laboratory was indeed a stimulating place to be; the range of interesting people and ideas was tremendous. In a letter written at the time, I tried to give a verbal picture of the laboratory atmosphere and scene:

'Every week there are visitors from all over the world, and every day the midday meal is a unique Departmental event. Vera, the full-time cook, serves up a hot dinner for the whole Department, cooked right in the lab and composed of meat and vegetables produced on the farms of McCance and Widdowson. Picture, if you can, a long table set down the middle of a large lab room. There is the Professor (Mac), long, lean and tanned, in white coat, sitting at the head of the table nursing his only share of the food — a tall mug of black coffee. He very definitely is master of the occasion, fixing each member one by one with penetrating eye and still more penetrating questions, but withal a keen conversationalist with a wry humour.

Here is Elsie Widdowson around the corner on his left, rotund, jolly and 50 - ish - looking maternal and anything but the famous chemist and nutrition scientist that she is. Hers is the guiding hand behind the scene that makes the whole organisation function smoothly. MCance and Widdowson for 20 years have been, and are, the brains, heart and soul of this laboratory.

But what of the others? Next we have Jimmy Robinson, biochemist, physiologist, physician, keen of mind and gentle in manner, scholar and bibliophile (he it was who introduced me to the delights and temptations of Heffer's, the fabulous Cambridge first- and second-hand bookstore). He is endeavouring to prove, in the face of world opinion, that kidney cells actively pump water as well as salt. Jimmy is leaving this summer, with his family, to take the Chair of Physiology in Dunedin, New Zealand. And here is Gordon Kennedy, younger, a North-Countryman, bristling with ideas as well as a large moustache, endocrinologist and hypothalamic physiologist; he can convert an idea into an experiment before you can say 'Jimmy Robinson'.

Next there is Romaine Hervey, another younger North-Countryman, environmental physiologist, part-designer of the new inflatable, covered life raft now standard in the Royal Navy. He personally tested this raft, his brainchild, in winter seas off Norway and in summer seas off Singapore. He is the chief protagonist of the Cambridge school of the belief that it is fatal for the castaway to drink sea water (the Frenchman, Bombard, notwithstanding); Hervey and McCance are right, in my opinion. Next we have Bill Keatinge, young naval doctor, master of a large tank full of very cold water, into which he thrusts such human subjects as he can capture, seeking the cause of sudden death on jumping into the icy waters of winter seas.

In succession, we have Margaret Stanier, charming young Oxford-trained biochemist, late of the nutritional lab in Uganda; Cleo Mavrou, Greek paediatrician from Athens; Jack Booyens, Afrikaner physiologist from South Africa. Nor must we forget some of the technical staff who make the wheels go round: Elizabeth Colbourn, research-trained nurse, equally adept at handling difficult elderly patients, helpless baby ones, or newborn rats; Bob Spires, provider of any possible kind of equipment that you can dream up; Peter, technician, tall, slim youth of 175lb, who, two years ago when a patient, weighed 582lb — now, on 800 Calories per day, is less of a man but a happier one. And our key secretary, Daphne, who is the only recorded case of vitamin-D resistant rickets (now happily cured). So you see, all in all, this is a fascinating place'.

Those lab lunches were unforgettable occasions. We had many interesting foreign visitors and the Professor kept a very tight control on how it went. His system was simply Machiavellian—15 minutes with himself immediately before dinner, then public extraction of the visitor's relevant information, then pass him on for successive postprandial interviews down the Departmental totem pole.

I have another memory of Mac. Occasionally, he would accompany me on his bike as I rode back to the house in which we were living. I remember one very hectic afternoon when we were riding down Trumpington Street in the middle of the rush of traffic: Mac riding along serenely next to the gutter, I riding between him and the swiftly passing lorries and trying to keep from being annihilated by them on one side and from bumping the Professor into the gutter on the other—and all the time he was quietly discussing the renal tubular reabsorption of bicarbonate!

Mac rode everywhere on his bicycle, which had been built especially to his physiological specifications. Each morning, he rode 14 miles from his farm into the lab and each evening, 14 miles home again. By the time of sending out his Christmas card in 1972, he had cycled, in more than 30 years, well over 200,000 miles (typically he presented this as a graph on his card). He was proud of this and liked to boast that on the day he became a grandfather, he cycled 120 miles (admittedly on a level dyke in Holland with a following wind). Finally grounded by the passage of time, he still, in his late 80s, walked everywhere in his beloved Cambridge.

In conclusion, if I can come to any conclusion, it seems to me that McCance and Widdowson's contribution has been this: that in addition to the wealth of new physiological and medical knowledge they brought into the scientific world, they have drawn together and stimulated a marvellous fellowship of workers, younger and older, over the years; that they have always been fellow workers, keen critics, provocative collaborators and real friends of those who have participated in the fellowship. All of us who have had the privilege of working with McCance and Widdowson will never forget, will never lose, the scientific mark of those days with them both in Tennis Court Road. Those were dandy years, those were wizard years!

Vernon Pickles

> Vernon Pickles spent a sabbatical year in the Department from 1959 to 1960. He came from the Department of Physiology in Sheffield and later went to the Chair of Physiology in Cardiff. He retired in 1981.
>
> These recollections are based on Dr Pickle's contribution to the meeting held in 1966 to pay tribute to Professor McCance before he left Cambridge for his two years in Uganda.

In 1941 to 1942 Professor McCance had in his Part II class an undergraduate in whose memory two things at least remain firmly fixed: one was a very distinct reluctance to swallow stomach tubes in the cause of medical education; the other was a particular lecture with the title *Menstruation and all That*. In this lecture, the Professor introduced us to the classic work (I am sure it merits that word) of McCance, Luff and Eva Widdowson (Elsie's sister) in the *Journal of Hygiene* (1937), entitled *Physical and Emotional Periodicity in Women*. He also referred us to a paper published in 1934 by DI Macht and RS Lubin, which showed that almost every accessible fluid taken from a woman during menstruation, contained a substance or principle that was toxic to growing plants.

Here I recall quite vividly some further words of the Professor's. He told us that myths concerning this type of phenomenon were fairly prevalent in many parts of the world, and persisted to this day in Yorkshire and places like that! Later I spent 18 months or so in general practice in Wensleydale, and we had a domestic servant from Coverdale, which was then a very remote side of the valley of Wensleydale. She told us that menstruating women were not allowed to make cheese—not because of any odour they might impart—but simply that the process did not work properly.

Macht's later work showed that menstrual extracts potentiated the stimulating effect that adrenaline had on the vas deferens of the rat, a rather unusual preparation that he happened to be using at the time. This was a simple statement one could check. I repeated his experiment and it was strikingly positive.

Now this takes me back to the *Physical and Emotional Periodicity* paper. It was apparent from this that there were certain phenomena associated in point of time with the period of menstruation itself, rather than with the changes in oestrogen and progesterone that are so prominent in the control of the cycle.

From this observation, it was a very short step to postulate that the endometrium produced a smooth muscle stimulant, which was released when the endometrium disintegrated, and was partly absorbed in some way, passing to the myometrium, causing contractions, and in part lost in the menstrual fluid.

During a privileged sabbatical spent in the Department of Experimental Medicine in Tennis Court Road investigating this problem, HJ Clitheroe and I extracted the lipids from many hundreds of what we euphemistically called 'specimens'. We concentrated the active substances and separated them by countercurrent-distribution, chromatography, and various other methods, and we eventually came up with three components of the menstrual stimulant. We established that these were probably long chain fatty acids, with additional polar substituents that were most probably hydroxyl groups, but we could get no further than that by amateur chemical means.

During this sabbatical year, I also collaborated with Professor McCance, unusually by taking up work which had been done 30 years previously. The original records for the *Physical and Emotional Periodicity* paper of 1937 had been assembled in the 1930s and were still in existence, methodically wrapped up in brown-paper parcels on a top shelf in his office. I knew that these contained records of the subjects' bowel movements, which had been included in order to persuade them to fill up the form every day and not leave it to the end of the week or month; this part of the records had never been analysed. I obtained permission to do this, and found that there was a very small but quite definite intestinal hurry during the menstrual period. This accords with other evidence that the menstrual stimulant spills over into the bloodstream, and affects smooth muscle throughout the body, though to a smaller extent than it does the uterus.

There came another of those odd, apparently accidental occurrences that really had a profound effect. A friend in a drug firm, knowing our interest in this field, sent a copy of a British Patent specification taken out by S Bergström, the Stockholm chemist, then at Lund, who was doing some magnificent work on the chemistry of prostaglandin, which was a physiological principle described by von Euler in 1935, and occurring mainly in seminal plasma.

Well, if a prostaglandin could be patented, why not a menstrual stimulant, which we knew was broadly of the same nature? I referred this to the Medical Research Council, who passed it on to the National Research Development Corporation, who financed what was for them quite a small, but proper chemical investigation. After two years of work, which was generally collaborative because neither the chemists alone nor the physiologists alone would have cracked this problem, we got part of the answer. Our menstrual stimulant substances were the same as the prostaglandins described initially by von Euler and chemically identified by Bergström and his colleagues in Stockholm; but they were present in different proportions, accounting for certain differences in physiological function.

In a way it was a disappointment to find that the menstrual

stimulant substances had already been described, even though only known to a very select group at the time; but in retrospect I am much less disappointed, because it immediately gave me friends and colleagues in various parts of the world who share my interest in prostaglandins.

Among his very varied interests, Professor McCance would, I imagine, list *Menstruation and all That* under the heading 'Miscellaneous', and as a very minor item even there. However, I hope I have been able to show how the scientific study, against considerable sociological difficulties, of this rather untouchable subject, led me right into the centre of one of the growing points of physiology and medicine. I would like to express my very obvious indebtedness to Professor McCance, and to Dr Elsie Widdowson for her encouraging interest in the work.

Jana Pařízková

> Jana Pařízková obtained her MD at Charles University, Prague in 1956 and her PhD and DSc at the Czechoslovak Academy of Sciences in 1960 and 1977, respectively. She has been employed as Senior Research Officer at the Biomedical Centre at Charles University since 1956.

In the late 1950s, I was preparing my PhD thesis at the Laboratory for the Physiology and Pathophysiology of Nutrition in Prague. My first reaction to the announcement that famous professors from England would be visiting the laboratory was one of panic. We were all expected to tell them something about our work. In English, of course. I was scared.

Then they appeared—Dr EM Widdowson and Professor RA McCance. The programme was fortunately quite fully booked by older and more experienced colleagues. At the beginning, I waited anxiously. Then I started to feel better and could observe our guests more carefully. My overwhelming feeling was that Dr Widdowson was an extremely kind person, understanding and very interested in other people's work. By the time I was fearless enough to present my very modest results, the show was over. My turn never came! Nevertheless, my memory of this first meeting was pleasant and full of hope that in the future there would be another opportunity to meet this famous, and very kind scientist again.

Fortunately this has happened many times—first in Czechoslovakia and then at various scientific meetings. At the 1963 Symposium on *Diet and Bodily Constitution* in London, Dr Widdowson kindly listened to my contribution to the discussion in a rather unusual place, because I did not dare to say what I thought in public. Then, there was soon another opportunity to participate and present a lecture at the International Symposium on *Human Body Composition*. How proud I was to lecture at the same meeting as Dr Widdowson—but how uncertain and scared I felt. Again, she gave me words of encouragement.

Another occasion was in the castle of Liblice belonging to the Czechoslovak Academy of Sciences at a Symposium on *Growth and Development*. There were stimulating lectures from both Widdowson and McCance and photographs from this meeting still hang in the castle as a pleasant reminder.

Then there was the International Congress of Nutrition in Prague in the critical year of 1969. It was just one year after the 'brotherly help' (as it was officially defined) from the Soviet Union in August 1968. Some scientists did not dare to visit Prague, but Dr Widdowson came readily, and showed her appreciation of the efforts of the organisers who had not had an easy time under the circumstances.

In 1974, in the historical Burg Wartenstein near Vienna, a small group of scientists participated in a symposium on *Nutrition and Malnutrition*. The programme was very interesting, but strange things started to happen. One by one, several of the participants suddenly left the meeting looking pale and uneasy, returning later mumbling about having a headache. The illness didn't hit me until the last day, but it was quite devastating. Fortunately, my room was next door to Dr Widdowson's in the tower of the castle. I could not have had better assistance with my troubles during that day.

But most of all, I appreciated the kindly help of Dr Widdowson in 1981 at the 12th International Congress of Nutrition in San Diego. Some time before this Congress, I lost my mother unexpectedly under quite tragic circumstances and I was still feeling very upset during the Congress. Dr Widdowson consoled me with all possible comprehension and feeling—at that time her own mother was still alive; she could understand well what such a loss meant to me.

In Geneva, Dr Widdowson participated in a World Health Organisation (WHO) meeting on *Principles for Evaluating Health Risks from Chemicals during Infancy and Early Childhood*. It was organised partly by my husband, Dr J Parizek, who acted as a Co-Secretary and also opened the meeting. We welcomed Dr Widdowson at the airport and very much appreciated having the opportunity to treat her as our guest in our Geneva home. I tried to be an adequate cook, more than at any time before, and she was again kind and appreciative. It was probably not possible for her to be otherwise.

I also enjoyed sampling Dr Widdowson's hospitality in her own home. After the 13th International Congress of Nutrition in Brighton in 1985, I went to Barrington, the village in Cambridgeshire where she has a charming, comfortable cottage and spent an unforgettable weekend. We had a pleasant little walk along the River Cam, visited Cambridge and met other friends from the USA. But the special honour—in addition to all the lectures which I had had the opportunity to listen to during so many years—was to be offered delicious meals, prepared personally by Dr Widdowson; I also took home a large jar of her marmalade. Of all my photographs, the one of Dr Widdowson in her own kitchen is very special.

Another photograph of Dr Widdowson hangs in my office. Somebody once asked me whether this was my mother. 'Well, in a way,' I said, 'Yes...my spiritual mother'. Hopefully she would not deny me this thought.

John Cowley

> John Cowley joined the Department of Experimental Medicine in 1962, coming from the University of Natal. He stayed for his sabbatical year and then left to go to the University of Aberdeen (1963) and to Queen's University, Belfast (1968 to 1975). Since then, he has been Head of Department and Professor of Psychology at Hatfield Polytechnic (now University of Hertfordshire) and more recently (1990) an Honorary Research Fellow at University College, London.

Although I had written to ask Professor Oliver Zangwill of the Department of Experimental Psychology in Cambridge if he would accommodate me while on sabbatical leave, my reply came from Professor McCance, who said he would be very glad to give me what facilities he could.

On my arrival in Cambridge I walked the length of Tennis Court Road for a building of a size similar to those of the other sciences, before finding my way to a conglomeration of huts, well-concealed behind an attractive row of terraced houses. McCance was away and my first meeting with Elsie Widdowson was enlightening. I think we both talked at cross purposes and I remember wondering whether the conversation was taking the particular form it did, so that she could remind herself as to who it was that had turned up in the Department.

The Department seemed a bit like a termites' nest, with a number of small groups, and sometimes single individuals, carrying out their own thing but foraging collectively at lunch time. Lunch was prepared by an expert cook, but there were few departures from British cooking and the fare remained much the same even when VIPs were present.

At Christmas, a key was produced which opened a gate at the back of the Department and gave easy access to the Little Rose public house in Trumpington Street; so avoiding the eagle eye of authority.

I shared a room with two PhD students, Hamad Elneil and David Lister. I was struck by the diversity of research going on in the Department and only gradually appreciated that there was a coherent theme. Dr Gordon Kennedy, working on rats, was making lesions in hypothalamic centres associated with food intake and activity. Dr Walshe was preoccupied with changes in copper metabolism in Wilson's disease, and patients who were being treated with Penicillamine; I was much taken with the alleviation of a marked stutter in one of his child patients. The hut also accommodated Hilda Bruce who, while working with Dr Parkes at Mill Hill, had shown that pregnancy in mice could be blocked by exposure to a strange male. In the other main hut, Dr Lawn was unravelling problems associated with the development of a model placenta.

There was much shuttling between Shaftesbury Road and Tennis Court Road, and my own visits were to use the calculator. Bartlow was another centre of Departmental activity—it housed the pigs that provided a wide range of tissues for analysis; the diversity of brews would have been the envy of *Macbeth's* witches. Like the PhD students, I found myself visiting Sidney Sussex College to acquire something of the language necessary for extending one's own thoughts and enjoying the hospitality that accompanied the wide-ranging discussions with Professor McCance.

I had come to the Department with an interest in the effects of undernutrition as a factor in modifying the behaviour of the indigenous people of Africa, south of the Sahara. We had fed rats on a diet of low protein composition and the results showed that the malnutrition of the mother was instrumental in modifying the growth and behaviour of the offspring—including problem solving—and all in a generation-dependent manner. Elsie, in characteristic fashion, took upon herself a study using the same test of animal intelligence to establish whether rats malnourished from weaning, from birth or from conception, and fed diets of low protein, low energy or a control diet, differed in their performance on the test. The malnourished animals (both low protein and low energy) performed poorly on the test as adults and the same was true of rats rehabilitated on the control diet. Generally, the low protein animals made more errors than the low energy ones.

My recollections about Mac in the early 1960s centre more on visiting him at his rooms in Sidney Sussex College, and walks along the river and across the Commons of Cambridge. Mac rarely came into my laboratory at Tennis Court Road, although on one occasion he came along to watch me test rats. It was not until some years later that I was able to watch him exercise his own laboratory skills in collecting blood from squealing piglets. My impression was that he regarded laboratory tasks as a necessary part of research, but had no great love for involving himself in such routines; his contribution to science lay elsewhere.

Indeed, Mac was a naturalist and had acquired a feeling for nature during his early childhood in the woods and open spaces around his home in Woodbourne near Belfast. He was an observer and a participant in nature—his knowledge of birds and their behaviour reflected this. The snowbound winter of 1962 made cycling well-nigh impossible but it was a good time for walking along the frozen Cam and seeing the effects of the low temperatures on the water fowl and migrant birds. The temperatures were evidence in themselves of the extraordinary internal adaptations that ensured the birds' survival—thoughts that were ever present in Mac's mind and were particularly expressed in his research on survival at sea.

Sidney Sussex College was where much of Mac's serious work took place and, when he later moved to Arbury, and more recently Shelford Lodge, he would recreate the atmosphere of his Sidney flat. The living room of the flat in Sussex Street looked onto the open shopping arcade but it was the unusual non-rectangular shape of the room and its treasured furnishings that gave it character. Mac worked and entertained in the part remote from the entrance and it was here that he had his patterned carpets, the rotating and glass-fronted bookcase, the picture of Iona (painted in different shades of blue), and the photographs that reflected his mountaineering exploits.

There was a comfortable chair for the visitor with a small embroidered mat placed alongside to protect the furniture from the glass of refreshment. Diagonally opposite was the settee where Mac sat (and worked), inevitably partly taken up with a pile of papers. Mac was clad in the inevitable white laboratory coat and wore heavy rust-coloured trousers and, when required, the golden-framed half-lens spectacles of the National Health Service. Mac's talk would centre on ongoing research, papers heard at meetings or read in selected journals. He was good on detail and he would provide an exact account of physiochemical factors involved—catecholamines were then much to the fore. The same meticulous appraisal could be evoked when discussing the health hazards of asbestos (on which he had been consulted by industry) or the implications of dire political events.

The year I joined the department (1962) was notorious, not only because of the weather, but also because it marked the height of the cold war, with Russian missiles in Cuba providing much food for thought. Mac's pleasure in intertwining history with science has always been much to the fore and *Breads, White and Brown* (published jointed with Elsie) and *Food Lore from Nursery Rhymes* (as well as many other publications) reflect his interest in the history of food.

The links between changes in environmental conditions early in life and the subsequent growth and behaviour of rats, was the theme for the study that Elsie and I undertook at the time of my joining the Department. Elsie's work on children in two orphanages in post-War Germany raised questions about the importance of relationships between carers and the growth of children. The replication of such studies would be difficult and unacceptable on ethical grounds, but newborn rats made a good model. They are entirely dependent on their mothers for food during first weeks of life and the mother licks the ano-genital region to facilitate the release of urine and faeces. We provided additional tactile stimulation by stroking rats for half a minute every day; either from birth to two weeks, or from three to nine weeks of age. Handling increased the rate of motor development and activity in the 'open field' test at nine weeks, but the rats grew at the same rate as their unhandled littermate controls.

Working closely with Elsie in the laboratory provided the opportunity of getting to know her, the way she responded to other people and how she set about conducting experiments. A person of enormous patience, she would elicit the participation of the animal technicians in her work while emphasising the importance of the information she was collecting herself in pre-prepared log books, details not only of the animals in the experiment but also of their mothers' growth history.

The pleasure of working with someone with a commanding knowledge and understanding of the biology of growth was stimulating; ideas acquired then have continued to exercise my own thinking and research. Elsie suggested that the 'handling' results should be presented at an International Nutrition Congress in Edinburgh. I had arranged to meet Elsie at her hotel prior to the meeting, to read the draft presentation. I did not have the name of the hotel but could recall that Mac said it was near the station. Edinburgh suffers from a surfeit of hotels and the two main railway stations are sited at opposite ends of the city centre. I assumed correctly, as it turned out, that it was more likely to be Waverley Station and soon tracked them down in The Darlings—an appropriate name to describe those whose relationship we commemorate.

In July 1968, I moved from Aberdeen to Queen's University, Belfast, just prior to the first marches that were to herald the start of the continuing ongoing conflict. For Mac, when he visited us, it was not unknown country and I was able to see something of his early childhood haunts and where he and his two brothers had explored and hunted in the local woods. Holidays from St Bees, when he was at school, represented a return to that world of nature and adventure. The medical school at Queen's was delighted to have him visit and the University subsequently honoured his contribution to science and medicine with the award of an Honorary Doctor of Science.

In 1971, my family moved into a small terraced cottage in Newnham, just outside Cambridge, and with my frequent visits to Cambridge, I was once again to see more of Mac. I would call at Sidney or pick him up at Elsie's cottage in Barrington where he would often have spent the day gardening. The weather seemed to make little difference to these activities and he would relate how, with the use of a chair, he would move along the onion rows, or whatever needed to be weeded. The naturalist was in his element participating in the varied but ordered activities that the seasons determine.

Lavoisier and, more particularly Claude Bernard, have always been strong influences in Mac's experimental approach to medicine. Perhaps the exception to the experimental rule was his 1937 paper on *Physical and Emotional Periodicity in Women*. The women filled in questionnaires and kept a day-by-day diary for a period of six months, recording their bodily functions and the accompanying subjective experiences associated with them.

With the collaboration of Elsie's sister, the information was analysed by statistical methods that corrected the data for individual variations in menstrual-cycle length. The records were well-kept by the women and the questions posed reflected Mac's interest in linking biochemical and physiological levels of explanation, with those at a behavioural level. The diaries provided details of social relationships, giving a wealth of information about the way the women perceived and explained their own behaviour. In other words, Mac produced a survey of sexual attitudes that anticipated the more extensive surveys of Kinsey and others. The Wellcome Foundation has accepted the diaries so they will always be available for scrutiny by scholars.

The drawing together of disparate threads and enjoyment in reading about the contradictions in the behaviour of historical and contemporary people is still much to the fore in Mac's conversations. His life in Uganda and his visits to Sudan and South Africa, where he had friends, provide additional common ground in our friendship. What he reads is a challenge to be put into some historical perspective and provide a coherent story to show there is order in the world that will match that of the *milieu interieur*. Mac was born in (and is part of) the last century—a pioneer in flight in the First World War and of medical and scientific advances in the Second, that were of national importance. As he straddles the centuries, so he has integrated the advances of 19th-century physiology with those of biochemistry and neonatal physiology in the 20th century.

Hamad Elneil

> Hamad Elneil, from Khartoum in Sudan, was in the Department of Experimental Medicine between 1962 and 1965. He worked under Professor McCance for his PhD, studying the response of newborn pigs to high temperatures, such as those endured by babies in Khartoum. After returning to Sudan, he continued to work with Professor McCance and Dr Widdowson on an experiment investigating temperature acclimation of students.
>
> After leaving Cambridge, he worked for the World Health Organisation (WHO) in Tanzania, then in The Congo, Nigeria, Zimbabwe, Ethiopia and Switzerland. In 1991 he retired as Director of Emergency Relief Operations for WHO in Geneva, and now lives in Cambridge.

I first heard about Professor McCance when Dr Olive Dunbar arrived at the University of Khartoum in Sudan in 1960. She suggested that I should work for Professor McCance but was rather hesitant as to what reply she would get from him; she worried that he was still cross with her because she delivered a manuscript late to him when he was collaborating with her Department in Scotland! I also heard about Professor McCance from the British Consul in Khartoum who had been a graduate at Cambridge. His reputation with the students was such that I was warned I would be 'eaten alive'.

I arrived in Cambridge at the same time as David Lister. We immediately became great friends and gave each other moral support during our student years. The Professor was very demanding of his students and suffered fools badly. Despite this, I found the whole experience very enjoyable, possibly for two reasons: first, the Professor mellowed with age and secondly, the time he had spent in Uganda had made him sympathetic to the African cause.

David Lister and I had to visit the Professor once a week in his rooms at Sidney Sussex College. He kept a special bottle of sherry for postgraduate students which I initially declined because I don't drink. Eventually, the Professor persuaded me to take the sherry because it was too much bother for him to get orange juice specially for me from the college steward!

My main memory of the lab lunches in the Department was the amount of homework I had to do before many of them. The seat to the left of the Professor was always reserved for Dr Widdowson and the one to the right was kept for visitors. If the visitor was anyone from Africa or the Middle East, I always had to sit next to him or her and had to be an 'instant expert' on all matters African, be they about physiology, archeology or geography. I spent many hours reading up all these subjects; this task was more exacting than my project at times! I did it because I didn't want to let the Professor down, but I often envied David Lister sitting at the end of the table who was not asked to take the seat next to the visitors nearly as often. Years later, though, I realise how much this helped to boost my confidence.

Professor McCance gave me several important 'pushes' in my career. He pushed me to work for a short period at the Department of Physiology at the Royal Free Hospital on new techniques in radioactive isotopes. He also pushed me onto the podium at my first Neonatal Society Meeting. His particular talent was his ability to bring people from many different disciplines into the Department and send them out again, reorientated in some cases. He was a nucleus for all clinical problems and everyone who worked with him departed a stronger person, if they were prepared to see the link between clinical science and basic physiology.

Professor McCance and Dr Widdowson sat at a low bench behind the windows in a room at the end of the lab. This meant that it was easy for us to tell if it was convenient to interrupt them—*and* they could always see who was coming and going outside. The Professor always rehearsed his presentations to his students and asked for their comments on his slides. What's more, he used to accept their advice and make changes accordingly The Professor and Dr Widdowson worked wonderfully together. He provided the *breadth* for any project and she provided the *depth*. He would never have needed a computer because Dr Widdowson was always there with her wonderful memory and her card index when that failed! The fact that Dr Widdowson was so devoted to the depth of the science allowed Professor McCance the freedom to look at broader aspects, such as biological adaptations. They would write papers with great speed. Because of their insistence on a prewritten skeleton, experiments were finished one afternoon and the paper completed the following morning.

Professor McCance was always called *The* Professor, even though he asked me and other people to call him Alec. There was no doubt who was meant by *The* Professor even when there were other professors around. The Professor and Dr Widdowson would work in the Department at Tennis Court Road in the morning, and go to Shaftesbury Road every afternoon, she by car and the Professor always by bicycle.

After I left Cambridge, I went to work for WHO in Tanzania. Professor McCance was, at this time, shuttling back and forth between Cambridge and Uganda and took the opportunity to visit me for a week. My wife was very apprehensive about feeding him, because she had only ever seen him eat potatoes, apples and bananas. Apparently the Professor told her to, 'cook what you normally cook', and during the week's visit, he felt at ease and put everybody else so, and fully enjoyed Sudanese food.

One evening, we invited some friends to our house to meet the Professor. He was not keen on the 'honoured guest' role and insisted on giving out the drinks with me. Professor McCance could never quite get used to the Sudanese custom of forcing more and more food on to their guests. When my wife tried to persuade him to have an extra portion of gateau (of which he was not fond) by saying that it wasn't fattening, he replied that she was the only person in the world who would dare lecture him on his nutrition!

I have been very lucky to be a student of the Professor and am so pleased that I have remained in contact with him and Dr Widdowson for so long.

Kelvin McCracken

> Kelvin McCracken worked for his PhD in the Department of Experimental Medicine, Cambridge, from October 1964 to October 1967. Subsequently he joined the Department of Agriculture, Northern Ireland (DANI), to undertake research on pig nutrition. He is now a Principal Scientific Officer in DANI and Reader in Nutrition at The Queen's University in Belfast.

My first memory of the Department was turning up for my interview full of trepidation and then being surprised that my acceptance into the Department seemed to be a foregone conclusion!

However, during the 'interview' I began to get an insight into the wide range of work in which McCance and Widdowson had been involved for the previous 25 years and also of the close working relationship that existed between them.

In 1964, Professor McCance was Director, Dr Widdowson was Assistant Director and David Southgate and John Dickerson were both on the staff. David Lister was just finishing his PhD at the time. There were three animal-house staff, including Pat Pledger. There were two nurses in the Department—Felicity McSwiney and Dorothy Smith, who soon learnt that they would have to handle rats as well as premature babies. After some initial squeamishness (and screamishness) they became adept at handling my little furry friends.

When I joined the Department, Dr Widdowson was my supervisor, but the project was largely based on the Professor's hypothesis that children with kwashiorkor were burning off excess energy by invoking futile cycles. I set up a rat model, buying *matoki* (green banana) brought in from Uganda, to see if we could produce the symptoms of kwashiorkor, and built a respiration chamber, similar to the one used in London by Gaston Pawan for mice. Around this time,

Professor McCance decided that a respiration chamber should be built for use with children in Uganda. Indeed, he suggested that I take up this project, but being 18 months into a PhD with little by way of results, I firmly declined. I think it took the Professor a little while to digest the fact that someone had dared say 'No' to him!

Daphne was the secretary in the Department. She was extremely loyal to 'Prof' and to 'Mum', as Dr Widdowson was affectionately called (behind her back!). I believe that Daphne felt that she owed her health, and possibly even her life, to Professor McCance.

I am reliably informed that, in his heyday, 'Prof' engendered a degree of fear in staff and students alike with his outspoken remarks (no doubt attributed to his Irish blood), piercing wit and occasionally violent outbursts. However, behind the somewhat fierce image, I eventually discovered a kindly man, when I felt that I had broken through the protective shell. But he did not suffer fools gladly. Perhaps his most important attribute as a scientist and lecturer was his ability to write and to edit other people's efforts. He believed that one should be able to write a paper, setting out the hypothesis and experimental details (and perhaps even the discussion), leaving appropriate blanks for the results to be filled in later.

'Mum' was much more of a peacemaker and played a very complementary role to the 'Prof'. I feel that her own leadership qualities only became fully appreciated when 'Prof' retired and she became Director of the Unit at Shaftesbury Road.

Apart from the opportunity of having spent three marvellous years in Cambridge, I can identify how some of McCance and Widdowson's enthusiasm for critical, analytical research rubbed off onto me. I will always be grateful that I had the chance to participate in the life and work of the Department of Experimental Medicine.

Alison Paul

> Alison Paul went to the Medical Research Council's (MRC) Dunn Nutrition Unit in 1969, on secondment from the Ministry of Agriculture, Fisheries and Food, to work with David Southgate on the fourth edition of **The Composition of Foods**. On completion of the revision, she became a member of the MRC scientific staff at the Dunn.

My initial introduction to *The Composition of Foods* was in the first week of my nutrition degree course at Queen Elizabeth College, London University. One of our lecturers, Anne Brown, saw each student in turn. 'You will be needing one of these,' she said, reaching to a pile of third editions, so I dutifully bought one for £1 10s (£1.50 now). It became an absolute standby during the course, but little did I realise then how involved I would be in its future.

A few years later, while working as a junior nutritionist at the Ministry of Agriculture, Fisheries and Food in London, one of my tasks was to take the minutes of a committee meeting concerned with revising the third edition of *The Composition of Foods*. A new post was to be created in Cambridge, in Dr Widdowson's department, under David Southgate, and I was fortunate to be appointed. Thus started my life in a laboratory environment, yet not doing laboratory work; this was rather unusual, but very stimulating, and an ideal way to be undertaking the revision.

Professor McCance and Dr Widdowson kept a close interest in the work, yet did not stand in the way of changes we proposed. It could have been difficult revising such a famous book with the original authors leaning over our shoulders, but it never was. Being in the laboratory, I absorbed the rigorous discipline necessary to compile accurate tables. My inexperience showed when I remarked at an internal seminar that it would be easier to analyse the foods than to compile values from the literature. Dr Widdowson firmly advised I should do some analyses myself to see if this were true. Time did not allow this, but I never forgot the advice. Compilations are undoubtedly *easier* than analyses, but the latter are much more worthwhile.

I always regretted not being able to help, when asked, with recording and weighing samples from one of the experiments on malnourished pigs. I had to be away elsewhere on the one weekend when this had to be done.

So many other interesting studies were going on in Dr Widdowson's Infant Nutrition Research Division while the food tables were progressing. Keith McCullagh was just finishing his work on atherosclerosis in elephants. Helen Chan was analysing numerous fetal samples, requiring stringent purity for trace elements. She also worked with Bob Bradfield measuring energy expenditure in nearby primary-school children. Dorothy Smith was collecting data on feeding and growth in Cambridge infants. David Southgate was developing methods for analysing 'unavailable carbohydrate', in spite of it being voted by dietitians as the least used constituent in the third edition of the Food Tables. Fortunately their views were ignored when planning the fourth edition.

Equal thoroughness was applied to other activities, most memorably the organisation of the first European Nutrition Conference, which was held in Churchill College, Cambridge in 1973. It was only planned about six months ahead, but it was still extremely successful. Working with Dr Kodicek as well as Dr Widdowson and Daphne Tabor on the administration, especially the social programme, gave me invaluable insight into the many facets that are involved in holding such meetings. Never have I been so pleased to see coaches as when they turned up at the scheduled time.

My association with Dr Widdowson's work in the early 1970s was to stand me in good stead for my subsequent move within the Dunn. While this meant no more direct involvement with the preparation of the Food Tables, having been so closely concerned with the fourth edition really means that they will always remain as one of my prime interests. They are, after all, used in so many studies.

Infant nutrition and growth was to become my main area but an added bonus arose from my connections with Dr Widdowson. I had noticed an interesting graph published by Dr Widdowson, on the growth of breast-fed babies. It turned out that this was derived from the data collected by Dorothy Smith and others in the late 1960s and early 1970s. Dr Widdowson has now given us all the original record cards and meticulous tabulations—all done before the age of computers. The data are specially valuable as few people were measuring babies at that time, which was precisely the period when there was a great tendency to overfeed infants, with subsequent obesity. Perhaps it didn't seem as attractive to be doing such work then, in contrast to the resurgence of interest in infant feeding and growth which has occurred in recent years.

Many are the times I have referred to studies by McCance and Widdowson; their findings of many years ago are still so relevant today.

Joy Dauncey

> Joy Dauncey was a PhD student with Dr Widdowson at the Medical Research Council's (MRC) Dunn Nutrition Unit from 1970 to 1973. Subsequently, she became a member of the MRC scientific staff and carried out modern pioneering studies on energy regulation in man, as one of the founder members of the Dunn Calorimetry Group at the Agricultural and Food Research Council (AFRC), Institute of Animal Physiology (IAP), Cambridge.
>
> With Philip James, Joy Dauncey then helped to establish the Dunn Clinical Nutrition Centre at Old Addenbrooke's Hospital, before obtaining an appointment at the IAP in 1979 to work on the mechanisms involved in the regulation of growth and development, particularly at the cellular and molecular levels.

I finished my BSc in Nutrition at Queen Elizabeth College, London, and was encouraged to pursue a career in research, rather than dietetics. I wrote to Dr Kodicek at the Dunn Nutrition Unit and was welcomed as one of the first students on the Postgraduate Diploma in nutrition course, which had just been set up with Kenneth Carpenter. Dr Widdowson suggested that I did a project on the *Effect of Hard and Soft Water on the Prevalence of Heart Disease*. She had become interested in this subject after talking to Gerry Shaper and Margaret Crawford—an example of how she picked her projects more by an opportunistic approach, rather than by planned policy. The original intention was that this could then be expanded into a PhD topic.

The project involved assaying urine samples from people living in both hard and soft-water areas. Dr Widdowson was very good at 'fixing up' contacts for her students. In this case, she fixed me up with 80 postmen in Glasgow—a notorious soft-water area, with a high incidence of heart disease—via a contact who was a medical officer at the Post Office. London was chosen as the hard-water control area. The original analyses were for calcium and magnesium but these did not produce very clear-cut answers. It was Professor McCance who suggested later that the samples should be reanalysed for sodium/potassium contents. This was more rewarding and the results were written up for the *Lancet*. The Professor was a stickler and checked that I had read every reference in the list for that paper.

He was a perfectionist in other matters too. I had recorded the body weights of my subjects in indoor clothing. The Professor insisted that I made allowances for the average weight of a pair of trousers and had me estimating this from among the Dunn's staff.

Dr Widdowson's group at the Dunn was small. It was the only food/nutrition-orientated group in a very biochemistry-orientated Dunn under Kodicek. Although Professor McCance had officially retired, he was always popping into the lab to work on papers with Dr Widdowson and to do some experimental work.

By Christmas 1971, I realised that there was no way that I could expand my project into a PhD, and after discussions with Dr Widdowson, I set off on a second course—looking at the nutrition and development of pre-term infants. This was arranged through two more of Dr Widdowson's contacts—Douglas Gairdner in Cambridge and Jonathan Shaw in London. Cambridge University agreed that I could submit my PhD thesis in two halves, but in the event, the premature-baby project made up the whole. One of the important advances at this time was the realisation that data on either pre-term or term babies could not be lumped together. At any age, they had to be subdivided into AGA (appropriate-for-gestational age) and SGA (small-for-gestational age) groups. Jonathan Shaw's major interest was in mineral balance and my data showed that pre-term infants were as much in need of copper supplementation as the previously recognised iron supplementation.

Douglas Gairdner's main interest was in following the developmental status of pre-term babies, to find an explanation for why they looked 'toady' at term. I performed standard anthropometric measurements on term and pre-term infants and used adipose tissue biopsies to measure cellularity and fatty acid composition. I well remember being the guinea pig when Douglas wanted to practise his biopsy technique! The biopsies from the babies were so small that the only way to prepare slices for cell sizing was to freeze the samples in solid carbon dioxide (dry ice) and slice them by hand in a Petri dish. The increases in fat cell size, let alone any increases in cell number, could easily account for all the increase in body fat acquired during the first year. Thus I provided a vital piece of evidence against the theory of the critical period of fat cell development, as put forward by several groups at that time.

Another example of Dr Widdowson's opportunism was when she arranged with Professor Jonxis from Holland for me to analyse some samples of fat from Dutch babies, so that I could compare their fatty acid composition with that of UK babies. Dutch expectant mothers were being encouraged to increase the polyunsaturated fatty acids (PUFA) in their diet, and Dutch babies were weaned onto infant foods with much higher PUFA contents than their UK counterparts. The fatty acid composition of the fat from newborn babies reflected the maternal diets, thus proving that polyunsaturated fatty acids could cross the placenta. The fatty acid composition of the infant formula had an even more dramatic effect.

In her role as my supervisor, Dr Widdowson worked on a 'sink or swim' policy. She certainly did not spoon-feed her students and we needed to be pretty independent. She always stressed the importance of answering well-defined questions, rather than spending a lot of time on developing new techniques.

The relationship between Dr Widdowson and Professor McCance can best be described as a 'close to ideal' collaboration between two remarkable people. McCance had considerable scientific insight and was a respecter of excellence rather than rank. Dr Widdowson was the perfect partner because, in addition to her considerable intellectual ability, she had the diligence and application to see their ideas through to the end. From them, I learnt the importance of considering the whole animal when studying cellular mechanisms. I believe this was a very vital lesson which I have carried through my research career.

Michael Gurr

> Michael Gurr's research career began in Biochemistry with Alistair Frazer at Birmingham University in 1960 and continued with Unilever Research. During this time, he was encouraged into nutrition and met Dr Widdowson and then Professor McCance in the early 1970s. Later, his career progressed through the National Institute for Research in Dairying, the Agricultural and Food Research Council's Institute of Food Research and The Milk Marketing Board. He now acts as a private consultant.

Recollections

I did not know Professor McCance nearly as well as Dr Widdowson, but I have two short anecdotes about him:

I once went to a lecture organised by the Cambridge Students' Nutrition Society held at Sidney Sussex College. Michael Crawford was the speaker and the meeting began at 6pm. Professor McCance was Chairman or President of the Society and sat in the front row alongside the young club secretary. The speaker was in full flight approaching 7pm. There was evidence of agitation in the front row. Anxious sign language from Professor McCance to the young secretary, followed by subdued (but clearly visible) conversation between them. Shortly afterwards, the embarrassed secretary asked the speaker if he would kindly draw to a conclusion. Professor McCance's facial expressions made this an imperative!

Madame Secretary wound up with a very brief thank-you speech to the speaker and the meeting closed as the clock struck seven. I was mystified as to the significance of all this, but detective work soon elicited the fact that Professor McCance's lifelong habit was to eat his one meal a day punctually at 7pm and he wasn't going to let any speaker, however eminent, interfere with his routine!

The other occasion was at a Nutrition Society Symposium in the mid-1970s. Dr Reg Passmore and Professor McCance were sitting together in the front row. There was some discussion about the potential benefits of 'nibbling', as distinct from 'gorging', for weight maintenance. Professors McCance and Passmore remarked more or less simultaneously that they didn't think that the 'nibbling' or 'gorging' hypotheses were very helpful. Both of them were as thin as beanpoles but they pointed out that Professor McCance consumed all his daily intake in a single large evening meal whereas Professor Passmore consumed a very similar intake spread among seven separate meals.

My first encounter with Dr Widdowson was after her publication of *Full and Empty Fat Cells* in the *Lancet*, when I was working at the Unilever Research Laboratory at Colworth House. I wrote (with some trepidation as an unknown nutritionist to a world-famous one) to say that our work with pigs fitted well with her concept. Would she be interested in our results and in a meeting to discuss them? (I half expected either no response or a rather terse one—however, I didn't know Dr Widdowson!) I received a most charming letter (which I now wish I'd kept) to say how delighted she was that other people were interested in this.

That was the start of a friendship that has lasted 20 years. I am usually somewhat intimidated by people whose intellectual capacity is way above mine but Dr Widdowson always makes you feel an equal (or even a superior), even when you are not. Soon after this contact, we met face to face and the impression gained from that letter was confirmed. A little later, the Unilever management decided it would like to have the services of an established nutritionist as consultant. I mentioned Dr Widdowson's name and the suggestion was accepted. I was given the job of asking her to visit the Colworth Research Laboratory to talk to the management and to give a more general seminar.

Eminent though she was, I worried that few of the Unilever people would have heard of her. I therefore put together a short biography with material gleaned from various publications, such as *Who's Who?* Before circulating it, I sent Dr Widdowson a draft copy for her approval, in case I'd made any embarrassing blunder. I received this concise response:

```
Dear Dr Gurr,

I couldn't have written a better obituary myself!
No modifications needed.

Yours

Dr Elsie Widdowson
```

Years later, I regularly visited Dr Widdowson in her room in the Department of Investigative Medicine at New Addenbrooke's Hospital, Cambridge. Professor McCance was often sitting there working and we had brief chats, although I didn't find them too easy. Once, we had sent a paper on fat cells to a journal of which Professor McCance was an editor. I well remember spidery annotations in the margin in pencil such as, 'What does this mean in real English?'

On one occasion, I rang Dr Widdowson to say I'd be in Cambridge next Tuesday and asked whether I could pop in to see her. She told me that she was only in her room on certain days now, since she had to stay home on some to care for her mother. I enquired, conversationally, 'How old is your mother?' She replied, 'Oh, she's 101.' A moment's pause, then I asked, 'And how *is* the old lady?' There was a rather longer pause before the reply, 'Oh, she's not so spritely as she used to be!'

As my career has progressed over the last 20 years, Dr Widdowson has been a constant source of encouragement and inspiration and has given me a friendship that is deeply valued.

Marta Fiorotto

> Marta Fiorotto is an Assistant Professor at the Children's Nutrition Research Center (CNRC) in the Department of Pediatrics at Baylor College of Medicine, Houston, Texas. This is one of six human nutrition centres funded by the US Department of Agriculture/Agricultural Research Service. The Center's mission is to define the food requirements that ensure good health in pregnant and lactating women, infants, children and adolescents. The Center was founded in 1978 by Buford Nichols and has developed with the guidance of the Council of Scientific Advisors, an external review group of which Dr Widdowson has been a member.

I was a postgraduate student at the University of Cambridge in the Department of Applied Biology from 1972 when Dr Widdowson was one of my primary lecturers for the courses leading to the Diploma in Human and Animal Nutrition. This was the last year in which that particular degree was awarded. I continued my close relationship with Dr Widdowson during subsequent years when I was working for my PhD degree at the Dunn Nutrition Unit. She is one of the finest teachers I have had, and it was her influence, almost exclusively, that guided me towards continuing my research career in pediatric nutrition, particularly with regard to the effects of early malnutrition on growth and development. It is in this field that I am still working.

I will always remember her enthusiasm for all aspects of nutrition, her wealth of personal experiences in conducting nutrition experiments, and her straightforward approach to analysing and solving problems.

We invited Dr Widdowson to join the Council of Scientific Advisors to the Children's Nutrition Research Center in 1986, and so our relationship was re-established when she began to visit the CNRC on a regular basis. In addition to her thoughtful evaluations of the animal and human studies conducted at the CNRC, she has made an invaluable contribution of approximately 3,000 reprints, and numerous books from her library, to the CNRC Historical Archives.

Her significant contributions to our understanding of the role of nutrients in human growth and development was recognised by the CNRC when a bas-relief was commissioned and dedicated in her honour in 1989. It now adorns the wall in one of our seminar rooms to remind us of our favourite British scientist.

Olav Oftedal

> Olav Oftedal was born in Norway in 1949, and graduated in Biology from Harvard College, USA, in 1971. After graduate work in international nutrition at the Massachusetts Institute of Technology (1973 to 1975), he obtained a PhD in Animal Nutrition from Cornell University (1981). In 1978 he became the nutritionist at the National Zoological Park (the first such position in the USA), and has been in the Zoo's Research Department since 1980. He is a member of the Committee on Animal Nutrition of the National Research Council, US National Academy of Sciences.

I first met Dr Widdowson in 1975 when I was at Graduate School at Cornell University. I was interested in comparative aspects of milk composition and the nutrition of neonatal animals inspired by the McCance and Widdowson paper in *Mammalian Protein Metabolism*. When I heard that Dr Widdowson was coming to Cornell University to give a seminar in the Division of Nutritional Sciences, I asked if I could meet her plane.

As it happened, this was a very brave offer. Dr Widdowson experienced difficulties in flight connections and her plane arrived at Ithaca airport well after midnight on a cold midwinter night. She was extremely surprised that anyone had waited, but I explained that I was determined to meet her, because I felt she was the only person in the world who was interested in what I was doing.

In 1978, I moved on to the Zoo of the Smithsonian Institution and I gradually got more involved in studying seals and going on long, expensive offshore expeditions to take physiological measurements of them. When Dr Widdowson visited Washington in 1981 to receive the Bristol Myers Award, I asked her advice about the projects I was doing on hooded seals found off the coast of Newfoundland. The hooded-seal pups are fully weaned by four days, having been suckled on milk with an extremely high fat composition (60%), and having gained in weight from 25kg to 45kg. Until then, our measurements had been confined to those of body weight and thickness of blubber (subcutaneous fat). Dr Widdowson persuaded me to take a look at the composition of the individual tissues. In turn, I persuaded her to come back to Washington and help us to do this.

So, in 1986, Dr Widdowson joined our team of four people to start the dissection of the frozen seal pups. She volunteered to do the most difficult dissection—the digestive tract—and we worked extremely hard throughout the week. On the Friday night, I suggested we should call it a day and reconvene on Monday. This did not suit Dr Widdowson, who saw no reason for stopping, and suggested we continued the dissections all over the weekend. The same thing happened the following weekend. In the end, Dr Widdowson wore us all out. Although we were all tough men who were used to gruelling conditions on freezing windswept islands collecting the seal pups, we were not tough enough to stand up to the drive and stamina of an 80-year-old woman who was thrilled to be doing experimental work once more!

Apart from her experimental prowess, I also remember Dr Widdowson's stimulating discussions about some of the scientific issues. Why does the hooded seal have such a short lactation period? How does it gain so much weight (almost all fat) in four days? How can the pups digest so much fat (5-6kg fat per day from milk with 60% fat in it)? Her interest in this latter point was largely responsible for inspiring one of my PhD students to continue her studies of gastric lipolysis in the seal pups.

Dr Widdowson was also fascinated that hooded-seal pups have the capacity to shed their whole fur coat 'in utero'—reflecting their advanced state of maturity. A little hair was found in the pup's gastrointestinal tract, but much more, tightly interwoven, in the amniotic sac. Dr Widdowson thought there were two possible explanations: either it was formed in the stomach and regurgitated or it was formed in the amniotic fluid.

In pursuing the answer, Dr Widdowson stirred seal-pup hair with water, to see if the balls formed, but they didn't. Once she got back to the UK, she was still determined to solve the mystery and wrote to tell me that she had tried stirring hair from her young kittens with human amniotic fluid. That didn't work either and the origin of the seal pup's hairballs remains a mystery to this day. Nevertheless, a paper has been written and published about this, with Dr Widdowson as a co-author.

The third issue that fascinated Dr Widdowson was the small size (350g) of bear cubs at birth. Why did the mothers produce such small cubs when they were in a hibernating state, and produce them when the weather conditions were so bad? Eventually, she realised that the growth of the fetuses would put a tremendous strain on the mother's glucose metabolism, and that the importance of restricting gluconeogenesis and conserving protein meant that it was easier to give birth to small cubs and keep them in a den (pseudo-womb), until they were big enough to forage in the outside world. We have just written up this work during Dr Widdowson's recent visit to us.

The other important recollection that should be included here relates to the first time Mary Allen met Elsie Widdowson. In 1981 there were two nutritionists at US zoos—Mary was nutritionist at the Brookfield Zoo in Chicago and I was nutritionist at the National Zoo in Washington. We hardly knew each other then, but we were sent by our respective institutions to attend a symposium on captive management of giant pandas at the Zoological Society of London; afterwards we visited several zoos and nutritionists in the UK including Dr Elsie Widdowson.

I wanted to meet with Elsie to discuss neonatal nutrition, but even more significantly, Mary spoke with Elsie about the problem of calcium deficiency in zoo animals fed solely on insects. Elsie explained that insectivorous birds in the wild often obtained calcium from the gastrointestinal contents of caterpillars and worms, and gave Mary a fascinating paper she had published with LW Bilby in 1971. Mary became eager to pursue this topic, and set up a series of studies demonstrating the effects of dietary calcium on the whole body composition of crickets. This technique became the basis for her PhD thesis at Michigan State University which she completed in 1989. Another consequence of this visit to the UK was a budding romance that resulted in Mary and I getting married in 1982.

Meeting Dr Widdowson has been quite a different experience from what we had both anticipated. Because of her fame and eminence, we had imagined someone at a very different social level. We certainly didn't expect her to be 'without airs' and someone who would treat us as equals. She is sharp, considerate and kind—a unique combination of talents for a scientist.

Selected Lectures

Professor McCance and Dr Widdowson were each asked to select for facsimile reproduction two publications that presented their own thoughts about some aspect of research, that is, they should be philosophical rather than experimental. Four 'named' lectures have therefore been chosen, covering 35 years in all, and they are reproduced here in chronological order.

The first, *The Practice of experimental medicine* (1951) was written years before ethical committees were set up to oversee experiments on human beings. In this lecture, Professor McCance set out the ethics that he adopted in all his research involving human subjects, whether infants or adults.

The second paper is the first of the two Lumleian lectures that Professor McCance gave at the Royal College of Physicians of London in 1962. *Food, growth and time* has clearly impressed several contributors to this book, for many have referred to the influence it has had on their thinking.

The third paper, Dr Widdowson's University of London Sanderson-Wells Lecture, *The harmony of growth* (1970), has also elicited much appreciation, as evidenced by that from Professor Charles Brook which is reproduced with it.

The fourth paper is Dr Widdowson's EV McCollum Lecture, delivered as the finale to the 13th International Congress of Nutrition held in Brighton in 1985. *Animals in the service of human nutrition* describes the pros and cons of using experimental animals in studies relating to human nutrition.

I was present at that lecture and I always remember that Dr Widdowson thanked McCollum for treating her as an equal even though she was very much his junior. She said that she had been determined to follow in his footsteps and at that moment I could understand her own caring attitude to younger colleagues, including myself. At the end of the lecture I overheard two middle-aged men discussing Dr Widdowson and the astuteness of her comments. One said 'I hope I'll be as sharp as she is when I'm her age'. The other replied, 'I wish I was as sharp as that now!'

MA

Section of Experimental Medicine and Therapeutics

President—Professor R. A. McCANCE, M.A., M.D., F.R.C.P.Lond., F.R.S.

[*December 12, 1950*]

The Practice of Experimental Medicine

PRESIDENT'S ADDRESS

By Professor R. A. McCANCE, M.A., M.D., F.R.C.P.Lond., F.R.S.

Department of Experimental Medicine, Tennis Court Road, Cambridge

WE have most of us a picture in our minds of what we mean by medical practice, both in its broader aspects, and in its narrower fields of general practice, consulting practice and so on. Each of these phrases conjures up something very real. To most of us the doctor comes to heal and we can picture his work: we appreciate the disciplines, responsibilities and the ethical background of the life of anyone who dedicates himself to such a service. Few people have such a clear picture of what the practice of experimental medicine involves; yet broadly speaking, those who set out to advance our knowledge of disease and treatment must sooner or later have recourse to experiment, for in the biological sciences experiment is the only sure way by which any advance can be established.

Claude Bernard's writings entitle him to be regarded as the father of experimental medicine but Harvey, Jenner and John Hunter were brilliant exponents of its possibilities long before his time, and the practice was already well established by the middle of the last century. Many of Claude Bernard's writings on the subject of experimental medicine do not require to be brought up to date. They are ageless. Changing customs and the passage of time, however, have created new situations and fresh problems and it is with these that I propose to deal.

Let us start with the word experiment, which most biologists use very loosely to cover any investigation, however trifling, made to advance knowledge. The term generally implies some deliberate change of conditions without foreknowledge of the results but with subsequent observation of them. It may be used, however, even when the conditions are not being deliberately changed, when the term observation would be more correct. Many doctors would not regard the attempt to cure an individual patient as an experiment, yet it undoubtedly may be, if the results are observed and followed up, for the essence of treatment is to do something positive to a patient, i.e. alter his conditions, in the hope that the effect will be of benefit to him.

People who are sick are often apprehensive. They long for reassurance which they do not find in the word "experiment". Worse still, the word may conjure up alarming possibilities in their minds. This is partly due to the activities of the antivivisection societies, partly to the casual use of terms such as "human guinea-pigs", partly to the atrocities which were perpetrated in concentration camps, and partly to the investigators themselves. The only comment made by a member of the governing body of the hospital when our department was being formed was that the name was an unfortunate one. I hope it was not, for I think it was the correct name, and we shall certainly do our best to prove it.

There is one fundamental difference between the investigator and the physician.

MAR.—EXPER. MED. 1

A good investigator may be as full of bedside charm and therapeutic ability as a good physician, but he must primarily be interested in his problem. The physician is interested first, last and all the time in his patients, and he has little sympathy with the attitude of the man who appears from time to time in the wards with a request to be allowed to disturb in some way one of his patients who may just be turning the corner after a critical illness. It goes against the grain to allow his patients to be used for a controlled therapeutic experiment if it means deliberately withholding from half of them the treatment which he believes, albeit unjustifiably, will do them good. He forgets, indeed he may not even know, that what he would have regarded as an "unjustifiable experiment" five years ago may have become one of his standard diagnostic or therapeutic procedures. The investigator finds it equally difficult to see eye to eye with a colleague who can alter a patient's treatment in the middle of one of his experiments without even letting him know, so nullifying two or three weeks of his work. Tact and a spirit of mutual co-operation and understanding are the only solutions. Taking a little trouble to develop new micro-methods often gives the entrée to a children's department, and placing a few beds at the disposal of an investigator often allows him to organize and complete good work to everyone's satisfaction and benefit.

Patients provide the problems, and disease may produce conditions which could never have been achieved experimentally and which demand detailed investigation, but if the illness is acute and treatable it is usually unjustifiable to withhold the remedy for long enough to make all the observations desirable in a satisfactory experiment. Chronic disease offers greater opportunity, but the basis of all successful experimentation is control of the conditions, and in the wards this may be very difficult. It is often much more satisfactory to work on normal men and women. Normal men and women are ideal for all physiological experiments when the "stress" originates in the environment, and some of the metabolic disease states can be reproduced in normal people. I have never had much difficulty in obtaining the co-operation of normal subjects. It is always a great help to have made the same experiment on oneself first and to be prepared if necessary to do so again. This is certainly true of metabolism experiments. Students make good subjects for some tests and they have frequently been employed, but in my experience they are not the best subjects for most experimental work. They can seldom give the necessary time for metabolism experiments, and they are often so overcome by the sight of blood that the complication of a faint is introduced into any test involving its removal. An experienced laboratory worker, male or female, is infinitely preferable. Subjects can, I believe, be hired for experimental work in some countries, and this may be a satisfactory arrangement, but I should be sorry to see this kind of service placed upon a commercial basis in this country. In the United States the patient is expected to contribute materially towards the expenses of his stay in hospital and he is generally anxious, therefore, to make this as short as possible. The hospital, in fact, may have to be reimbursed if a patient's discharge is delayed for experimental work, or if a special admission is made for such purposes. Valuable work was done by groups of conscientious objectors during and just after the war, and this is a form of national service which might very well be encouraged if the volunteers have the necessary mental and physical balance. Service personnel are now being employed for some experimental work on the physiological effects of heat and cold, high and low atmospheric and other gas pressures, and the stresses and strains of warfare. These men volunteer for the work and for some purposes they may be excellent.

Those who practise experimental medicine are naturally most interested in human disease and physiology and, as Claude Bernard put it: "Il est bien certain que pour les questions d'application immédiate à la pratique médicale, les expériences faites sur l'homme sont toujours les plus concluantes." Nevertheless, the advantages of turning to animals are numerous, and the greater part of the work of a department of experimental medicine is often carried out on them. They can be obtained as and when required; their size is often convenient; they can be killed if necessary. Greater numbers of small animals than of human beings can be used and a better statistical result obtained. Their rapid rate of reproduction and short life span are invaluable for work on nutrition, genetics and carcinogenesis. In fact, once the investigator has posed his problem to himself he generally looks around for the most suitable animal on which to study it, and his choice often makes for success or failure. "Le choix intelligent d'un animal présentant une disposition anatomique heureuse est souvent la condition essentielle du succès d'une expérience et de la solution d'un problème physiologique très important." Claude Bernard was right but it is not always possible to reproduce in animals the set of conditions which have been under observation in man, and many since his time have forgotten that what has been proved for one species may not hold for another, and one of the attributes that makes for success in experimental medicine is the instinct which tells a man when to check his results on a second species, and above all when to turn from animals to man, or *vice versa*.

There is no difficulty about working with animals in this country, provided suitable accommodation can be found for them. One must comply with the Law relating to experiments on animals, but few people would wish to do otherwise. A licence is obtainable for any justifiable work on living animals. The investigator then has to make an annual return of his experiments and his animals are periodically inspected, but he benefits in that he is protected from unauthorized interference. The Authorities at the Home Office have always been most helpful to me. A licence is not required to kill animals, so that any of their tissues may be obtained immediately after death for chemical, metabolic or pathological work without let or hindrance.

There is no difficulty about making some kinds of experiments on one's fellow creatures, and they are the only mammals for which a vivisection licence is not required in this country, but the use of man as one's experimental material raises all kinds of issues, moral, ethical and legal which have never really been faced and which, in my opinion, should be faced. A hundred years ago the issue was clear. "On a le devoir et par conséquent le droit de pratiquer sur l'homme une expérience toutes les fois qu'elle peut lui sauver la vie, le guérir ou lui procurer un avantage personnel. La principe de moralité médicale... consiste donc à ne jamais pratiquer sur un homme une expérience qui ne pourrait que lui être nuisible à un degré quelconque, bien que le résultat pût intéresser beaucoup la science, c'est-à-dire la santé des autres."

We should, I think, for present purposes, regard anything done to a patient, which is not generally accepted as being for his direct therapeutic benefit or as contributing to the diagnosis of his disease, as constituting an experiment, and falling, therefore, within the scope of the term experimental medicine. The definition, however, should not include all those unplanned experiments which are inseparable from the admission of any child or adult to a hospital, and which are often attended with considerable physical and psychological dangers, nor should it include the administration of established prophylactic remedies, even though some of them, particularly the attenuated viruses, may involve risk. The experiment visualized may be one of omission and consist of withholding treatment from a "control", or it may be one of commission and consist of making some test on a patient for which there is no obvious and immediate need. Whatever the problem interesting the investigator, however, it is, of course, true to say that the results of such tests must always help to characterize the diseased state and when known may sometimes be of benefit to the patient on whom the tests have been made. There is a case to be made out for regarding all these tests as being "investigations" conducted in the sufferer's best interests and therefore not constituting an experiment made solely for the advancement of knowledge. Wassermann reactions are carried out on every patient admitted to some hospitals and every patient entering the Mayo Clinic is, I believe, subjected to an elaborate series of investigations. The real distinction is a subtle one and may depend upon the mental approach of the man who makes the tests. Nevertheless, I regard collecting an extra specimen of urine or taking an extra 5 c.c. of blood from a vein puncture, made purely for established diagnostic or therapeutic purposes, as falling within the range of the term "experiment". I would certainly regard weighing a baby "unnecessarily" as an experiment. Some people may think I am taking up a ridiculous attitude over this, but if an experiment is not defined in this way, where is the line to be drawn?

All experiments involve some risk. It may be an infinitesimally small one, but it is always there—you, or the nurse, may drop the baby for instance. If the experiment involves special vein punctures, or perhaps infusions, the risk is considerably enhanced, but it still remains immeasurably small in the hands of an experienced operator. Nevertheless, I have myself seen and experienced the most alarming effects from pyrogens and I think it quite likely that the virus which gave me a mild attack of jaundice in 1939 reached me through a syringe. In assessing the risks involved in any experiment and therefore the justification for doing it, there are many factors which require consideration. The skill and experience of the investigator are important ones, but so is the place where the experiment is to be performed. A procedure which would be perfectly safe in a well-equipped and well-staffed establishment might be quite unjustifiable somewhere else. A well-trained person is much less likely to make a mistake over a drug or its dosage than an untrained technician in a badly staffed hospital. I have recently given this question a good deal of thought in connexion with our work in Germany and other "field" work.

The mention of assistants brings me to another point. Many experimental workers are not qualified in medicine, and yet they take part in hospital work and experiments on normal people. Could they conceivably be regarded as "unqualified assistants", and what would be the position if an accident were found to be due to one of them? If a foreign medical man has come to this country to work in a department of experimental medicine it has, since 1947, been possible for him under the Medical Practitioners and Pharmacists Act to have his name placed temporarily on the Medical Register. This legalizes his position and if he can then join one of the Medical Defence Unions he and the department should be fully covered.

If an experiment is the first of a series it involves much more risk than one which has been made many times before by the same people out of the same bottles. I never worry at all, however, about trying out an unknown substance on man, for with a little patience one can work up the dose on oneself or other normal people so gradually that the risk can be reduced to vanishing point, but I do not think I would ever have had the temerity to carry out the first hepatic biopsy or cardiac catheterization. Our pioneer studies of renal function in newborn infants were made on babies which had been born with inoperable meningo-myelocœles. Hundreds of these experiments have now been made on normal newborn and on premature infants in other countries—yet I am still hesitating about doing so.

The risk involved in any experiment depends very much on whether the investigator knows that he will always retain control of the situation. An experiment on salt deficiency or dehydration can be pushed till the subject is showing severe effects, because the remedy is available all the time. To inoculate someone with icterogenic serum is a risk that I personally would never take, nor would I ever have cared to take it even before the risks were so well known, for once the inoculation had been made, I would have lost control. Everyone working experimentally with normal human subjects or with patients must remember not only his responsibility to the subject or patient but also his responsibility to the discipline of experimental medicine. One irresponsible experimenter can do great harm to medical science.

No experiments can be carried out on a healthy colleague without his co-operation and consent and any elaborate experiment should be preceded by a medical examination; the same thing applies to a healthy child. It would also, I believe, be regarded as an offence under common law to make any investigation upon a child which involved the removal of hair, skin or blood without its parents' consent. In consequence of this, school children are so well protected by their teachers and other officials that it is often a very elaborate affair arranging for an experiment on a group of them. When a person comes into hospital, however, many investigations are made, and necessarily made, for direct diagnostic or therapeutic purposes, and patients expect a certain number of "tests". These are part of the hospital routine, and although patients have the right to refuse, it is extremely rare in this country for anyone to do so, and, as a matter of fact, many appreciate the attention. Hence, many experiments, even quite elaborate ones, can be made on patients, within the therapeutic routine of the hospital so to speak, without anyone thinking anything of it. Many experiments are made on this basis, and all help to define the effects of disease on function but the results seldom get recorded on the patients' notes. If the experiment is more elaborate and demands considerable co-operation, the investigator may feel it desirable to ask the patient for his "permission". It is often difficult for an investigator to explain the nature and object of his work to a non-scientific colleague and generally quite impossible to a patient. The investigator can only tell the patient in very general terms what his experiment will involve, explain the nature of the risks and ask for his co-operation. Experiments on children and infants are carried out on exactly the same basis except that parents have to be approached for permission, and the whole procedure becomes much more formal and tricky, for it is generally possible to size up a prospective subject before asking him for his co-operation, whereas it is a very different matter to go up to an unknown parent on visiting day and make your request. It is still more difficult to approach a newly delivered mother about an experiment on her baby, even if this only involves a study of how it breathes, and the inclination to make the experiment without doing so is very great. Patients and parents, however, rarely refuse, and in my experience opposition to experimental work in hospital generally comes from colleagues under whom the patients have been admitted, and from the nursing staff who are, in general, antagonistic to research, especially on children, unless maybe it is being carried out by their own particular "chief". An experimental study always involves them in extra work the reason for which they do not fully understand and which often appears to them to run counter to their ideas about the comfort and care of the patient. They are on the whole satisfied with the knowledge of to-day. They forget that nothing in this world is static and that knowledge can be lost as well as gained. Research has made our knowledge great and can make it greater, but without research knowledge would fall away as it did in the Middle Ages. All our triumphs of to-day would be forgotten —they may be anyway—but without continuous research there would be nothing to take their place. Those who educate medical students and nurses should therefore emphasize to them the value of the experimental approach, and encourage them at some point in their careers to do something for the medical science of to-day and to-morrow by taking an active interest in experimental work.

No doubt the practice differs from one hospital to another, but the principles just outlined about "permission" seem to hold generally throughout this country. In some continental countries the position is rather different and the co-operation of the patient or parent is seldom sought and in some places it is generally assumed that it would be refused. This is an unfortunate state of affairs. A little thought shows that the whole position in this country depends upon trust. The patient trusts the staff of the hospital, and the investigator, knowing this, usually dispenses with the formality of asking for "permission", when his experiments simply involve procedures which are the commonplaces of clinical practice, but he generally prefers to take the patient or parent into his confidence over anything more elaborate, and this is where his conscience and judgment become so important.

This seems a happy arrangement and one which we are fortunate to have evolved. Some other nations have not been so successful. The whole atmosphere of trust would be destroyed if patients had to be asked to fill in a printed form of consent for experiment as they are as a rule for an operation. I would feel happier, however, for the future, if patients could be made more aware that at some hospitals—the best hospitals—experimental work is carried out not only for the benefit of the immediate sufferers, but also for the benefit of mankind, and that they themselves owe incalculable advantages to work of this kind which has already been done on others; furthermore, that if they or their children are privileged to be admitted to these hospitals, they may be expected to co-operate. In the form given to patients on admission to one hospital I know, there is a small paragraph and the addition of a few words to it illustrates the sort of thing I have in mind. The additions proposed are in italics. "The hospital staff seeks your assistance in carrying out the hospital's duty to the community in the *investigation of disease and in the* training of doctors and nurses; if a member of the staff wishes to *make a special study of your condition or to* explain it to a medical student, doctor or nurse, it is hoped that we may have your co-operation."

Although it is legal to kill an animal without any vivisection licence and tissues can be taken immediately after death without any formalities whatever, it is extremely difficult to obtain fresh human tissues for experimental work unless they have been removed by a biopsy, for once a person has died a post-mortem examination may only be made with the permission of the next of kin or the person in lawful possession of the body (unless of course the coroner or the official referee under the Cremation Acts orders a post-mortem to be carried out to ascertain the cause of death). These manœuvres all take time during which the chemistry of the cells becomes completely disorganized, but, the law being as it is, it would, I feel sure, be unlawful to remove any part of the body for purposes of research immediately after the death of the patient without the previous consent of the nearest relative. This makes it very difficult to carry out many desirable investigations, and even the gross composition of the human body is still only known to us in very vague terms because of the legal obstacles which prevent a *bona fide* investigator from obtaining the complete body of a human being for analysis. With the co-operation of an anatomy school it can be done, and we have ourselves done it, but the removal for examination must not take place until forty-eight hours after death, and it is necessary to comply with other legal formalities. There is much more work to be carried out on the metabolism of fresh human tissues and on the chemical composition of the organs of whole bodies by people with the necessary interests and opportunities.

A great deal more might be said about the practice of experimental medicine, and its place in medical practice as a whole. Almost every statement I have made could have been greatly enlarged but it would be better for others to do this in the light of their own experiences. As I see it, however, the medical profession has a responsibility not only for the cure of the sick and for the prevention of disease but for the advancement of knowledge upon which both depend. This third responsibility can only be met by investigation and experiment, and from the nature of things it is always likely to remain the task of a few men and women specially gifted and/or trained for the purpose. Some of these people have in the past sacrificed considerable wealth for the mental satisfaction of their work. This may not have to be so in the future but all such practitioners have a right to expect the fullest co-operation from their medical colleagues, from nurses and other assistants, from hospital managements, from patients and relatives and from the community at large.

FOOD, GROWTH, AND TIME *

R. A. McCance

C.B.E., M.A., M.D., Ph.D. Cantab., F.R.C.P., F.R.S.

PROFESSOR OF EXPERIMENTAL MEDICINE
IN THE UNIVERSITY OF CAMBRIDGE

LECTURE I.

LIFE, whether of the cell or the whole animal, abounds with rhythmical functions. Some of these have no value as chronometers because their timing depends upon the activities of other, non-rhythmical, functions. The pulse-rate is a good example. Others, however, are closely linked with chronological time. There is, for example, a small crayfish which lives in the river Styx in the Mammoth Cave in Kentucky. The animals have inhabited the cave for more than a million years, during which time they have never seen the light of day, or known what it is to feel hot or cold; yet they have a regular rhythm of diurnal activity, and breed only in the winter (Brown 1961). The causes of such rhythms and their timing are still very obscure (Harker 1958, Webb and Brown 1959).

Although not strictly a rhythmical function, in that nobody has ever been given the chance of repeating it, life as we know it has many of the properties of one, and as the generations follow one another each man's journey through life tends to be very like the man's before. Consider how predictable the time-keeping is. The baby will be born about 10 lunar months after conception. It will weigh about 7 lb. The usual gains in weight and height thereafter have all been documented. If the baby is a girl she may be expected to menstruate 13 to 14 years after birth and stop growing at a roughly predictable height a few years later. She will normally remain sexually mature till she is 45 or 50. By threescore years and ten the great events are over and the journey must end soon; but few clocks would have kept such good time for so long. We shall not know all that makes life run to time before mine ends, but it is possible to put forward partial explanations now and to suggest some experimental possibilities for others to explore.

The Food of the Fœtus

In earlier phases of development the embryo derives its nourishment from the trophoblast, and the nature of

* The Lumleian lectures for 1962 delivered before the Royal College of Physicians of London on April 30 and May 2.

the food at that time is not yet known. In later gestation the food-supplies of the fœtus are blood-borne. The nature of these nutrients has been investigated by Popják (1954a and b) and others, and consists of aminoacids, glucose, a limited amount of protein, but apparently no fat. Fat may be taken up by the placenta, but if so it is then broken down to smaller molecules which pass on to the fœtal soma for synthesis in the appropriate way. It is not yet known, however, how the fœtus acquires its " essential " fatty acids (Zöllner and Wolfram 1962). The aminoacids and many minerals seem to reach the fœtal blood-stream by active transport across the placenta (Hagerman and Villee 1960, Huggett 1961, McCance and Widdowson 1961, Widdas 1961). It follows that the amount of food reaching the fœtus depends upon the quantities of available nutrients in the maternal blood flowing through the placenta and the size, age, and other parameters of this organ which together go to make up its " efficiency ". Until such time as we have perfected an artificial placenta (Lawn and McCance 1961, 1962) it will not be possible to investigate the food intake of a fœtus directly and make balance studies upon it as we can upon an infant after birth, but a certain amount can be found out indirectly by studying growth-rates in utero.

Development in Utero

Before relating rate of growth to supplies of food it is necessary to exclude possible interferences. Environmental temperature, which is so important for mammals after birth, need not be considered; and hereditary influences, which may affect so strikingly the mature size of an animal, can also almost be disregarded, as Walton and Hammond (1938) and Joubert and Hammond (1954, 1958) have demonstrated in horses and cattle, Hunter (1957) in sheep, Brumby (1960) in mice, and Robb (1929), rather less convincingly, in rabbits. If Shire horses, for example, are crossed with Shetland ponies, the size of the young at birth conforms much more closely with the size of the mother than with that of the father or the ultimate stature of the cross. The same is true in a more limited way of man (Cawley et al. 1954a, McKeown and Record 1954, Walker 1954) and has been taken to mean that the size attained in utero depends upon the services which the mother is able to supply. These are mainly food and accommodation. In the earlier stages of gestation both are always ample. The embryos in a litter all gain weight equally fast at first whatever their genetic background, their number, or their position in the uterus. In the later stages of gestation, however, the number and position of the fœtuses can have a profound effect upon their sizes at birth. The nutritional status of the mother is also important. Fat women tend to have large babies (Widdowson 1955, McKeown and Record 1957), and in some species lowering the mother's plane of nutrition towards the end of gestation can materially reduce the size of the newborn. The weights of twin lambs can be halved in this way without any reduction in the length of gestation (Wallace 1948a, b, and c, Thomson and Thomson 1948–49), and this must be due to less food having reached the placental area in the maternal blood. Effects of this magnitude are perhaps unusual except in a sheep carrying twin lambs. Singleton lambs are less affected, piglets may not be affected at all, and babies' weights are reduced only by a very small amount (Dean 1951, Thomson 1951, 1959) even in seriously undernourished communities. Smoking, which probably leads to constriction of the uterine vessels and so reduces the delivery of food-supplies to the fœtus, may make almost as much difference (Lowe 1959, Herriot et al. 1962).

It is a matter of common knowledge among obstetricians and stockbreeders that the size of a baby or an animal at birth depends upon the number of young in the litter (Minot 1891, Kopéc 1924, Gates 1924–25, Angulo y Gonzalez 1932, Eaton 1932, Watts 1935, Venge 1950, McKeown and Record 1952). As a rule the birthweight falls as the numbers go up, but in cats Hall and Pierce (1934) found there was an optimum number of five and in pigs Lush et al. (1934) one of four. In animals like the rat or the pig in which the length of gestation is not reduced by an increase in litter size, the fall in birthweight which accompanies it must be attributed to less food being available for each fœtus. The limit may be in the supply of blood for the uterus and/or in the nutrients which can be made available for that supply.

The nutrition and growth of the individual fœtuses in a litter of mice depend upon the location of their placentæ both in the uterus and with reference to their neighbours (McLaren and Michie 1960). It has often been held to depend greatly on placental size, but this is less certain. The placenta at first grows more rapidly than the fœtus (Huggett 1946–47, Huggett and Hammond 1952, Walker 1954) and it may greatly exceed the weight of the fœtal body for a time (Ibsen 1928, Barcroft 1946). Thereafter the placenta loses its priority of growth, and its weight increases more and more slowly towards term (Hosemann 1948–49b). Most investigators have found a correlation between fœtal weight and placental weight (Calkins 1937,

Dow and Torpin 1939, McKeown and Record 1957, Joubert and Hammond 1958), but it is not necessarily very close (Campbell et al. 1953, McKeown and Record 1953), and remarkable exceptions have been demonstrated (Ramsey 1954).

Time operates in all pregnancies. The fœtus can spend only a limited period in utero, and even the growth of a singleton human fœtus begins to falter towards the end of its normal time there (Hosemann 1948–49a, McKeown and Record 1952), because of the ageing of the placenta, which may become so inefficient after full term that the postmature fœtus may show signs of undernutrition and actually lose weight (Hammond 1934, Flexner et al. 1948, McKeown and Record 1952, Clifford 1954, 1957, Smith 1959, McCance and Widdowson 1961). In some animals, however—notably in the guineapig and in man—length of gestation is progressively reduced by an increase in litter size (Minot 1891, McKeown and Record 1952, Eckstein and McKeown 1955) and this further limits the weight which multiple fœtuses can attain in utero, by curtailing the length of time they can spend there (Kopéc 1924). The duration of pregnancy depends upon the amount of distention which the uterus will tolerate, and in some species fœtuses are often forced to enter the world before they are fully grown, or before their placentæ have begun to " age ", because their mother can no longer provide accommodation for them. In man fœtal weight is independent of fœtal numbers before the 26th week of gestation, but quadruplets begin to grow more slowly than singletons then, triplets a week later, and twins from the 30th week. The " tolerance " of the uterus to distention falls towards term, and is less in first than second human pregnancies (McKeown and Record 1952). Guineapig mothers behave like human ones in these respects (Ibsen 1928, Eaton 1932, Eckstein and McKeown 1955, Eckstein et al. 1955).

Maturity and Size

To a large extent the size of an animal at birth determines its functional maturity and ability to survive. Given a similar period of gestation, size is largely a matter of food and is determined by the position of the fœtus in the uterus, the number in the litter, and the maternal plane of nutrition. On the other hand a small reduction in the total time spent in utero can make a large difference to the size of a fœtus and the extent of its functional development at birth, because the gain in weight is very rapid shortly before term. Food and time both operate together in multiple human or guineapig pregnancies to reduce the size at birth and this is why the birthweight of twins and particularly of triplets is often so small.

There is, however, a further point. Although a high plane of nutrition promotes rapid growth and development, and a small animal of the same age is always less mature than a bigger one, if one animal reaches a given size more slowly than another it will in some respects be more mature by the time it does so. This applies throughout the whole period of growth. It was shown by Appleton (1929) to apply to the bony development of the fœtus, but it holds also after birth (Outhouse and Mendel 1932–33, Moment 1933) and will be discussed more fully in that connection. It follows, therefore, that a newborn baby which has a small birthweight after a normal gestation period will be more mature than one of the same weight born prematurely. Cort's (1962) work on the morbidity of premature infants suggests that this has clinical application.

The Food-supply of the Newborn

Birth means the end of the bloodborne supply of food from the placenta, and, although triglycerides and fatty materials generally form no part of this food (Popják 1954a and b), they certainly participate in the nutrition of the newborn animal. All milks contain fat, some nearly 50%, and this most probably reaches the blood-stream partly as triglycerides (Senn and McNamara 1937, Rafstedt 1955); but how it is metabolised, in the rat at any rate, is by no means clear (Hahn et al. 1961). The milk of this species contains very little carbohydrate—not enough to meet a tenth of the newborn's energy requirements— and glycogen accumulates in the liver if olive oil is given by mouth. Milk is the only source of protein for nearly all newborn animals, and the milk of cows, sheep, pigs, dogs, rats, and other animals contains γ-globulins which are absorbed unchanged, expand the volume of circulating blood (Bangham et al. 1958, McCance and Widdowson 1959), and provide the newborn animals with passive immunity to many potentially lethal infections until such time as they develop their own active immunity (Hemmings and Brambell 1961). In rabbits and in man, this passive immunity is acquired before birth by other routes. In Nature the whole future of the young depends upon an adequate supply of milk, and the only way to ensure this is to provide a satisfactory plane of nutrition for the mother (Wallace 1948a, b, and c, Dean 1951). Even so she may not be able to provide enough for a large litter, for lactation is a much greater nutritional strain on the mother than pregnancy.

Development after Birth

Owing to the interactions of food, growth, and time during fœtal development, young may be born which differ considerably in size and maturity. The future for these animals is a matter of considerable importance both to medicine and animal husbandry. The large offspring presents no problems once it has been safely delivered. The large baby tends to become the large child and often an obese one (Widdowson 1955), but the prospects for the small and immature animal are not good in Nature. It is naturally weaker and less robust. It has a worse chance of maintaining a normal body temperature and requires more food to do so. The handicaps vary to some extent with the species (Wallace 1948a, b, and c, Pomeroy 1960), and for one reason or another many of these animals die soon after birth. Those which survive continue their development, and differences in size which are present at birth become modified by time and the new environment. Differences may disappear or decrease (Eaton 1932, Hammond 1932, Huggett 1946–47, Cawley et al. 1954b) but they often become exaggerated, for a time at any rate. A piglet, for example, which is less than 0·5 kg. lighter than one of its littermates at birth may appear to be growing reasonably well and yet be 15 kg. lighter a few months later. The small animal may take weeks or months longer than its larger littermate to reach bacon weight, even if it has always had access to plenty of food, and this makes it a very uneconomical proposition. A baby which is small at birth often remains a small child until puberty (Illingworth 1939, 1950, Illingworth et al. 1949, 1950), and the outlook for the very small premature infant is not good at present (Capper 1928, Drillien 1958a and b, 1960, Lubchenco et al. 1961). Nutrition cannot be held to account for the whole of this, and King (1916–17) showed that even if the "runts" in a few litters of albino rats were given special attention and unlimited food they did not weigh quite so much as their littermates even as adults. The ultimate fate of the animal which enters the world too small is important theoretically and practically, but little is known about it because few runts in the world of animal husbandry are allowed to reach maturity and children tend to get lost among the general population after a certain age.

There is no evidence that newborn babies in 1962 are appreciably larger than they were in 1862 (Abolins 1962); yet in most of the well-documented parts of the world children of school age are taller and heavier today than they were 10, 20, 50 years ago (Tanner 1955, Falkner 1958, Cone 1961, Hagen and Paschlau 1961). Hence they must

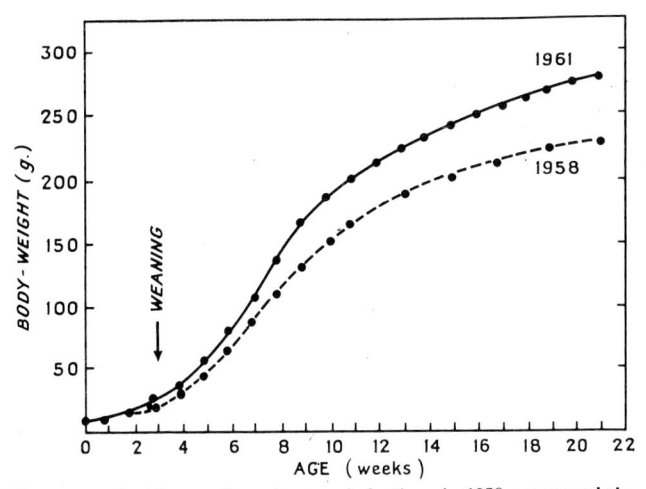

The greater incidence of respiratory infections in 1958 prevented the rats growing so fast as they did in an identical experiment 3 years later.

be growing faster after birth, setting up new times as it were. Adults are taller also (Boyne and Leitch 1954, Boyne 1960, *British Medical Journal* 1961) and many have regarded this as due to improvements in nutrition. There have been improvements in nutrition, particularly in some populations, but this is not the whole story. Tanner has suggested that the changes are the result of outbreeding. Hybrid vigour is a well-documented phenomenon (Haines 1931, Mather et al. 1955–56) and may well have contributed to the new timing, but there is evidence now that a reduced incidence of infections has had something to do with it. It is well established, for instance, that the growth-rates of animals can be improved by the addition of antibiotics to their food (Barber et al. 1957, Lucas and Calder 1957, Taylor and Rowell 1957, Bunch et al. 1961, Taylor 1962). 10 to 15 years ago, moreover, Large White pigs reached 200 to 210 lb. live weight in 200 to 220 days. In the virus-free herds which it is now possible to establish, pigs make so much better use of their food that they are expected to attain the above weight in 160–170 days, and some may do so in an even shorter time (Goodwin 1961).

We have, moreover, recently carried out identical growth experiments on two large groups of rats. In the first one in 1958 a number of the rats had an unmistakeable upper respiratory infection. Some died but the others seemed little if at all upset, although slight checks were noted in their growth curves. Fewer infections marred the early part of the 1961 experiment and the figure shows the growth-rates of male rats in 1958 and 1961.

McGregor et al. (1961) have compared the growth-rates of children in Gambia and Great Britain. The former begin to fall behind when the children are about 20 weeks old, although their diets are reasonably satisfactory by tropical standards, and by a year old their growth-rate is no more than that of a British child of 2 or 3 years of age. This is probably due to the parasitic and other less obvious infections from which all suffer and many die. Those who survive till they are two or three grow at much the same rate as British children thereafter, and the curves for the heights and weights of the two populations taken together resemble many of the pairs of curves which have been published over the past 50 years by writers interested in secular trends. There is no reason why both undernutrition and infections should not act cumulatively (Acheson 1960), and this work in Gambia and the experience of Mellbin (1962) in Lapland suggest that they very well may. Experimental results will be quoted later which support this.

External Temperature

Most adult animals maintain a stable internal temperature by rapid variations in their rate of heat loss. The immediate reaction of a rat or a mouse, however, to a change of environmental temperature is to vary its rate of heat production, and this is the only mechanism of importance available to many animals in early life. It is, moreover, often poorly developed at birth. Consequently the newborn animal is at a serious disadvantage when the environmental temperature is low; for, if it makes any response, it catabolises food materials which might have been used for growth. At best the young animal will grow more slowly, and if there is not enough food available it may become helpless and immobile because of a fall in body temperature (McCance 1959). Prematurity or (and) a small size accentuate these handicaps. Continuous exposure to extreme temperatures from birth may alter the form and structure of an animal. Mice reared at $-3°C$ reduce their loss of heat by developing short tails and longer hair, but their food requirements remain relatively enormous (Barnett 1959, Barnett et al. 1959). A hot environment makes for long tails (Harrison et al. 1959). It also accelerates growth in early life, as one might expect, but delays it later. Very unfavourable high temperatures may interfere with human development (Mills 1950).

Nutrition and Development

Growth is a complicated and highly integrated process, and it has been known for centuries that all parts of the body do not develop equally fast or at the same time. Bones —some in particular—have relatively high " priorities ", and it was known to Xenophon (B.C. 400), for instance, and reported by Markham (1617), that one could predict the ultimate size of a horse from the measurement of its shin bone (the fused metatarsals) at birth. Some reference has already been made to these " priorities " in describing the comparative growth-rates of the placenta and the fœtus. Similar ones can be demonstrated in all the phases of growth and have been well documented (Jackson 1909, 1926, Jackson and Lowey 1912, Morgulis 1923, Hamilton et al. 1945). " Priorities " also exist within the cell and have been explored.

Davison and Dobbing (1961) have offered some explanation for these well-known anatomical facts in terms of molecular stability. They point out that everything in the body is not in the free dynamic state suggested by the first isotope studies. There is probably an infinite range in the permanence of the cellular framework and the turnover rates of its constituents. Some molecular structures—D.N.A. for instance—must be relatively stable and break up very slowly once they are formed. In the neurone, moreover, which is not normally renewed during life, there is likely to be relatively complete stability at the cell level.

Structural stability, possibly maintained by thyroid hormones (Tata et al. 1962), must be important in determining relative growth-rates; for tissues which incorporate labelled molecules into stable structures after single injections and hold them there are likely to be ones that grow fast, and such experiments measure incorporation rates rather than " turnover " rates, which may be much higher in another tissue which is not growing at all. Collagen in some parts of the body may appear to have a low incorporation rate if it is being formed relatively slowly in a phase of rapid cellular development in a skeletal muscle; but it may yet have great structural stability at the molecular level once it has been formed. An example of structural stability of a pathological nature is provided by the accumulations of glycogen in the glycogen-storage diseases, and the way in which hormones operate on the enzymes involved in glycogen metabolism give us an inkling about how growth priorities may be induced by the activation or inhibition of key enzymes (Field 1960).

Undernutrition reduces the rate of growth. This must have been known for thousands of years: the literature on the subject is enormous, and has been surveyed from time to time (Morgulis 1923, Smith 1931, Keys et al. 1950, McCance 1951). Undernutrition, however, does more than this. By limiting the supply of nutrients and growth materials it accentuates the development of those parts which have at the time in question greater structural stability and perhaps mitotic activity (Bullough 1962) than the rest. Thus, it alters the whole form and shape of the animal as well as its rate of growth, particularly if the animals are all compared at a fixed weight (Pomeroy 1941). Since bones have relatively high priorities, growth in height is interfered with less than growth in weight, which results from muscular development and the accumulation of fat, and consequently the animal is tall and thin (Waters 1908, 1909, Aron 1911a and b, Moulton et al. 1921, 1922a and b, McMeekan 1940a, b, and c, 1941a and b, Bonnier and Hansson 1945–46, Wallace 1948a, b, and c, Hammond 1952, Crichton et al. 1959, 1960a and b).

A very high plane of nutrition, by saturating the growth requirements of an animal, accelerates the development of all tissues, but particularly, and certainly relatively, those with little structural stability and therefore low priorities. Fat is one of these, certainly in early life; and this is why children who eat enough to become very fat—conspicuously so in fact—do not become giants, but merely tend to be somewhat taller than their fellows who have lived at a more " usual " plane of nutrition (Mossberg 1948, Wolff 1955, Carter 1961, Lloyd et al. 1961). If a high plane of nutrition follows a low one, most observers have found that a relatively normal form is the ultimate outcome (Lucas et al. 1959, McCance and Widdowson 1962). McMeekan (1940a, b, and c, 1941a and b) and Hammond (1952), however, found that it produced very fat pigs when they were slaughtered at a weight of about 200 lb. or at maturity (McMeekan and Hammond 1940), and they considered that imposing this high plane of nutrition " late " had emphasised the development of those parts which normally only began to develop rapidly at that chronological age. This influence of chronological time—i.e., of age on the pattern of development—is an important thought and will be discussed later. Curiously enough, the observations which led to it have not been easy to confirm in pigs or other animals (McCance and Widdowson 1962) and must have been due to the particular conditions involved (Lucas et al. 1959).

If development receives a setback for some reason in utero, an animal has little chance of making up the lost ground by the time of birth; but after birth it has more time at its disposal (Hammond 1932, Cawley et al. 1954b), and long delays due to undernutrition can sometimes be made good before the end of the growing period (Moulton et al. 1921, Crichton et al. 1960a). Many of the experiments, however (Clarke and Smith 1938), particularly those on large animals, have not been continued long enough to make sure (Hammond 1952, Hammond and Marshall 1958), and, in some of those that have, recovery has been incomplete (Aron 1911b, Bonnier and Hansson 1945–46). Environments in which growth has been slow but continuous may not be so prejudicial to the attainment of full body size as those in which the body-weight has been held almost constant for long periods of time and full nutrition restored thereafter (Hogan 1928, Bohman 1955). The rats in the experiments of Hatai (1907) and of Osborne and Mendel (1914, 1915) attained their expected size even after prolonged growth restriction, but this has not been the experience of others with rats (Jackson and Stewart. 1920, Smith 1931, Jackson 1937, Schultze 1955), although the animals may grow with the vigour of youth when a high plane of nutrition is first restored. Brody (1928) pointed out in this connection that the velocity of an animal's growth on a high plane of nutrition depends upon the amount of growth remaining to be made—i.e., on the size of the animal at the time—and that it is only when growth has been uniformly good that its rate appears to be a function of age.

Nutrition and Life Expectancy

In the race against time which characterises the whole period of growth, from conception to maturity, undernutrition is always a disadvantage. The prolongation of life, on the other hand, may be thought of as a feat of endurance rather than a race against time, and in it undernutrition curiously enough may be advantageous. McCay et al. (1939) showed that, if rats were subjected to prolonged and severe undernutrition from the time of weaning, many of them fell by the wayside from the hazards involved, but the remainder lived up to three times as long as the normal rat. This was discussed by McCance (1953) and has been confirmed (Silberberg and Silberberg 1955, Ross 1959, Berg and Simms 1960, Comfort 1960).

However beneficial a high plane of nutrition may be during growth, if it leads to obesity in an adult man it shortens the length of time he is likely to live to enjoy it (Strange 1959). Life-assurance statistics demonstrate this, and experiments prove it for animals (McCance 1953). In some species the cause is known (Kennedy

1957) and genetically obese animals can be protected against themselves by controlling their food intake (Lane and Dickie 1958).

REFERENCES

Abolins, J. A. (1962) *Acta pædiat., Stockh.* **51**, suppl. **135**, 8.
Acheson, R. M. (1960) Effects of nutrition and disease on human growth. *In* Symposia of the Society for the Study of Human Biology, vol. 3: Human Growth (edited by J. M. Tanner). London.
Angulo y González, A. W. (1932) The prenatal growth of the albino rat. *Anat. Rec.* **52**, 117.
Appleton, A. B. (1929) The relation between the rate of growth and the rate of ossification in the fœtus of the rabbit. *C.R. Ass. Anat.* 24th meeting, Bordeaux, pp. 3–25.
Aron, H. (1911a) Wachstum und Ernährung. *Biochem. Z.* **30**, 207.
— (1911b) Nutrition and growth. *Philipp. J. Sci. B. (Med. Sci.)* **6**, 1.
Bangham, D. R., Ingram, P. L., Roy, J. H. B., Shillam, K. W. G., Terry, R. J. (1958) The absorption of ^{131}I-labelled serum and colostral proteins from the gut of the young calf. *Proc. roy. Soc. B*, **149**, 184.
Barber, R. S., Braude, R., Mitchell, K. G., Rook, J. A. F. (1957) Further studies on antibiotic and copper supplements for fattening pigs. *Brit. J. Nutr.* **11**, 70.
Barcroft, J. (1946) Researches on Pre-natal Life. Oxford.
Barnett, S. A. (1959) The skin and hair of mice living at a low environmental temperature. *Quart. J. exp. Physiol.* **44**, 35.
— Coleman, E. M., Manly, B. M. (1959) Oxygen consumption and body fat in mice living at $-3°C$. *ibid.* p. 43.
Berg, B. N., Simms, H. S. (1960) Nutrition and longevity in the rat: II. Longevity and onset of disease with different levels of food intake. *J. Nutr.* **71**, 255.
Bohman, V. R. (1955) Compensatory growth of beef cattle: the effect of hay maturity. *J. Anim. Sci.* **14**, 249.
Bonnier, G., Hansson, A. (1945–46) Studies on monozygous cattle twins: V. The effect of different planes of nutrition on growth and development of dairy heifers. *Acta agric. succ.* **1**, 172.
Boyne, A. W. (1960) Secular changes in the stature of adults and the growth of children, with special reference to changes in intelligence of 11-year-olds. *In* Symposia of the Society for the Study of Human Biology, vol. 3: Human Growth (edited by J. M. Tanner). London.
— Leitch, I. (1954) Secular change in the height of British adults. *Nutr. Abstr. Rev.* **24**, 255.
British Medical Journal (1961) ii, 502.
Brody, S. (1928) An analysis of the course of growth and senescence. *In* Growth. New Haven.
Brown, F. A. (1961) Diurnal rhythm in cave crayfish. *Nature, Lond.* **191**, 929.
Brumby, P. J. (1960) The influence of the maternal environment on growth in mice. *Heredity*, **14**, 1.
Bullough, W. S. (1962) Growth control in mammalian skin. *Nature, Lond.* **193**, 520.
Bunch, R. J., Speer, V. C., Hays, N. W., Hawbaker, J. H., Catrow, D. V. (1961) Effect of copper sulphate, copper oxide, and chlortetracycline on baby pig performance. *J. Anim. Sci.* **20**, 723.
Calkins, L. A. (1937) Placental variation: an analytical determination of its clinical importance. *Amer. J. Obstet. Gynec.* **33**, 280.
Campbell, R. M., Innes, I. R., Kosterlitz, H. W. (1953) Some dietary and hormonal effects on maternal fœtal and placental weights in the rat. *J. Endocr.* **9**, 68.
Capper, A. (1928) The fate and development of the immature and of the premature child. *Amer. J. Dis. Child.* **35**, 443.
Carter, C. O. (1961) The Englishman's height. *Brit. med. J.* ii, 518.
Cawley, R. H., McKeown, T., Record, R. G. (1954a) Parental stature and birth weight. *Amer. J. hum. Genet.* **6**, 448.
— — — (1954b) Influence of the pre-natal environment on post-natal growth. *Brit. J. prev. soc. Med.* **8**, 66.
Clarke, M. F., Smith, A. H. (1938) Recovery following suppression of growth in the rat. *J. Nutr.* **15**, 245.
Clifford, S. H. (1954) Postmaturity—with placental dysfunction. Clinical syndrome and pathologic findings. *J. Pediat.* **44**, 1.
— (1957) Postmaturity. *Advanc. Pediat.* **9**, 1.
Comfort, A. (1960) Nutrition and longevity in animals. *Proc. nutr. Soc.* **19**, 125.
Cone, T. E. (1961) Secular acceleration of height and biologic maturation in children during the past century. *Pediatrics*, **59**, 736.

Cort, R. L. (1962) Clinical observations in newborn premature infants. *Arch. Dis. Childh.* **37**, 53.
Crichton, J. A., Aitken, J. N., Boyne, A. W. (1959) The effect of plane of nutrition during rearing on growth, production, reproduction and health of dairy cattle: I. Growth to 24 months. *Animal Production*, **1**, 145.
— — — (1960a) II. Growth to maturity. *ibid.* **2**, 45.
— — — (1960b) III. Milk production during the first 3 lactations. *ibid.* p. 159.
Davison, A. N., Dobbing, J. (1961) Metabolic stability of body constituents. *Nature, Lond.* **191**, 844.
Dean, R. F. A. (1951) The size of the baby at birth and the yield of breast milk. Studies of Undernutrition, Wuppertal 1946–49. *Spec. Rep. Ser. med. Res. Coun., Lond.* no. 275, p. 346.
Dow, P., Torpin, R. (1939) Placentation studies: correlations between size of sac, area of placenta, weight of placenta, and weight of baby. *Human Biol.* **11**, 248.
Drillien, C. M. (1958a) Growth and development in a group of children of very low birth weight. *Arch. Dis. Childh.* **33**, 10.
— (1958b) A longitudinal study of the growth and development of prematurely and maturely born children: 2. Physical development. *ibid.* p. 423.
— (1960) A longitudinal study of the growth and development of prematurely and maturely born children: 7. Mental development, 2–5 years. *ibid.* **36**, 233.
Eaton, O. N. (1932) Correlation of hereditary and other factors affecting growth in guineapigs. *U.S. Dept. Agric. Tech. Bull.* **279**.
Eckstein, P., McKeown, T. (1955) Effect of transection of one horn of the guineapig's uterus on fœtal growth in the other horn. *J. Endocr.* **12**, 97.
— McKeown, T., Record, R. G. (1955) Variation in placental weight according to litter size in the guineapig. *ibid.* p. 108.
Falkner, F. (1958) Some physical measurements in the first three years of life. *Arch. Dis. Childh.* **33**, 1.
Field, R. A. (1960) Glycogen deposition diseases. In The Metabolic Basis of Inherited Disease (edited by J. B. Stanbury, J. B. Wyngaarden, and D. S. Fredrickson). New York.
Flexner, L. B., Cowie, D. B., Hellman, L. M., Wilde, W. S., Vosburgh, G. J. (1948) The permeability of the human placenta to sodium in normal and abnormal pregnancies and the supply of sodium to the human fetus as determined with radioactive sodium. *Amer. J. Obstet. Gynec.* **55**, 469.
Gates, W. H. (1924–25) Litter size, birth weight, and early growth rate of mice (*Mus musculus*). *Anat. Rec.* **29**, 183.
Goodwin, R. F. W. (1961) Growth rates of pigs in virus-free herds. Personal communication.
Hagen, W., Paschlau, G.v.R. (1961) Wachstum und Gestalt. Stuttgart.
Hagerman, D. D., Villee, C. A. (1960) Transport functions of the placenta. *Physiol. Rev.* **40**, 313.
Hahn, P., Koldovsky, O., Melechar, V., Novák, M. (1961) Interrelationship between fat and sugar metabolism in infant rats. *Nature, Lond.* **192**, 1296.
Haines, G. (1931) A statistical study of the relation between various expressions of fertility and vigor in the guineapig. *J. agric. Res.* **42**, 123.
Hall, V. E., Pierce, G. N. (1934) Litter size, birth weight, and growth to weaning in the cat. *Anat. Rec.* **60**, 111.
Hammond, J. (1932) Growth and Development of Mutton Qualities in the Sheep. London.
— (1934) The fertilisation of rabbit ova in relation to time. *J. exp. Biol.* **11**, 140.
— (1952) Farm Animals: Their Breeding, Growth and Inheritance. London.
— Marshall, F. H. A. (1958) The life-cycle. In Marshall's Physiology of Reproduction (edited by A. S. Parkes). London.
Hamilton, W. J., Boyd, J. D., Mossman, H. W. (1945) Human Embryology (prenatal development of form and function). Cambridge.
Harker, J. E. (1958) Diurnal rhythms in the animal kingdom. *Biol. Rev.* **33**, 1.
Harrison, G. A., Morton, R. J., Weiner, J. S. (1959) The growth in weight and tail length of inbred and hybrid mice reared at two different temperatures. *Philos. Trans., B*, **242**, 479.
Hatai, S. (1907) Effect of partial starvation followed by a return to normal diets on the growth of the body and central nervous system of albino rats. *Amer. J. Physiol.* **18**, 309.
Hemmings, W. A., Brambell, F. W. R. (1961) Protein transfer across fœtal membranes. *Brit. med. Bull.* **17**, 96.
Herriot, A., Billewicz, W. Z., Hytten, F. E. (1962) Cigarette smoking in pregnancy. *Lancet*, i, 771.
Hogan, A. G. (1928) Some relations between growth and nutrition. In Growth. New Haven.
Hosemann, H. (1948–49a) Schwangerschaftsdauer und Kopfumfang des Neugeborenen. *Arch. Gynæk.* **176**, 443.
— (1948–49b) Schwangerschaft und Gewicht der Placenta. *ibid.* p. 453.

Huggett, A. St.G. (1946–47) Some applications of prenatal nutrition to infant development. *Brit. med. Bull.* **4**, 196.
— (1961) Carbohydrate metabolism in the placenta and fœtus. *ibid.* **17**, 122.
— Hammond, J. (1952) Physiology of the placenta. *In* Marshall's Physiology of Reproduction, vol. 2 (edited by A. S. Parkes). London.
Hunter, G. L. (1957) The maternal influence on size in sheep. *J. agric. Sci.* **48**, 36.
Ibsen, H. L. (1928) Prenatal growth in guineapigs with special reference to environmental factors affecting weight at birth. *J. exp. Zool.* **51**, 51.
Illingworth, R. S. (1939) The after-history of premature infants, with special reference to the effect of the birth weight on the weight chart. *Arch. Dis. Childh.* **14**, 121.
— (1950) Birth weight and subsequent weight. *Brit. med. J.* i, 96.
— Harvey, C. C., Gin, S. Y. (1949) Relation of birth weight to physical development in children. *Lancet*, ii, 598.
— — Jowett, G. H. (1950) The relation of birth weight to physical growth. *Arch. Dis. Childh.* **25**, 380.
Jackson, C. M. (1909) On the prenatal growth of the human body and the relative growth of the various organs and parts. *Amer. J. Anat.* **9**, 119.
— (1926) Some aspects of form and growth. *In* Growth. New Haven.
— (1937) Recovery of rats upon refeeding after prolonged suppression of growth by underfeeding. *Anat. Rec.* **68**, 371.
— Lowrey, L. G. (1912) On the relative growth of the component parts (head, trunk, and extremities) and systems (skin, skeleton, musculature and viscera) of the albino rat. *ibid.* **6**, 449.
— Stewart, C. A. (1920) The effects of inanition in the young upon the ultimate size of the body and of the various organs in the albino rat. *J. exp. Zool.* **30**, 97.
Joubert, D. M., Hammond, J. (1954) Maternal effect on birth weight in South Devon x Dexter cattle crosses. *Nature, Lond.* **174**, 647.
— — (1958) A crossbreeding experiment with cattle, with special reference to the maternal effect in South Devon-Dexter crosses. *J. agric. Sci.* **51**, 325.
Kennedy, G. C. (1957) Effects of old age and over-nutrition on the kidney. *Brit. med. Bull.* **13**, 67.
Keys, A., Brožek, J., Henschel, A., Mickelsen, O., Taylor, H. L. (1950) The Biology of Human Starvation. Minneapolis.
King, H. D. (1916–17) On the postnatal growth of the body and of the central nervous system in albino rats that are undersized at birth. *Anat. Rec.* **11**, 41.
Kopéc, S. (1924) On the influence exerted by certain inheritance factors on the birth weight of rabbits. *Anat. Rec.* **27**, 95.
Lane, P. W., Dickie, M. M. (1958) The effect of restricted food intake on the life span of genetically obese mice. *J. Nutr.* **64**, 549.
Lawn, L., McCance, R. A. (1961) An artificial placenta. *J. Physiol.* **158**, 2P.
— — (1962) Ventures with an artificial placenta: 1. Principles and preliminary results. *Proc. roy. Soc. B.* **155**, 500.
Lloyd, J. K., Wolff, O. H., Whelan, W. S. (1961) Childhood obesity: a long-term study of height and weight. *Brit. med. J.* ii, 145.
Lowe, C. R. (1959) Effect of mother's smoking habits on birth weight of their children. *ibid.* ii, 673.
Lubchenco, L. O., Horner, F. A., Metcalf, D., Hassel, L., Cohig, R., Elliott, H. (1961) Development of premature infants of low birth weights. *Amer. J. Dis. Child.* **102**, 752.
Lucas, I. A. M., Calder, A. F. C. (1957) Antibiotics and a high level of copper sulphate in rations for growing bacon pigs. *J. agric. Sci.* **49**, 184.
— — Smith, H. (1959) The early weaning of pigs: 6. The effects of early weaning and of various growth curves before 50 lb. weight upon subsequent performance and carcass quality. *ibid.* **53**, 136.
Lush, J. L., Hetzer, H. O., Culbertson, C C. (1934) Factors affecting birth weights of swine. *Genetics*, **19**, 329.
McCance, R. A. (1951) The history, significance and ætiology of hunger œdema. Studies of Undernutrition, Wuppertal 1946–49. *Spec. Rep. Ser. med. Res. Coun., Lond.* no. 275, p. 21.
— (1953) Overnutrition and undernutrition. *Lancet*, ii, 685, 739.
— (1959) Maintenance of stability in the newly born. *Arch. Dis. Childh.* **34**, 361.
— Widdowson, E. M. (1959) The effect of colostrum on the composition and volume of the plasma of new-born piglets. *J. Physiol.* **145**, 547.
— — (1961) Mineral metabolism of the fœtus and new-born. *Brit. med. Bull.* **17**, 132.
— — (1962) Nutrition and growth. *Proc. roy. Soc. B.* **156**, 326.
McCay, C. M., Maynard, L. A., Sperling, G., Barnes, L. L. (1939) Retarded growth, life span, ultimate body size, and age changes in the albino rat after feeding diets restricted in calories. *J. Nutr.* **18**, 1.
McGregor, I. A., Billewicz, W. Z., Thomson, A. M. (1961) Growth and mortality in children in an African village. *Brit. med. J.* ii, 1661.

McKeown, T., Record, R. G. (1952) Observations on fœtal growth in multiple pregnancy in man. *J. Endocr.* **8**, 386.
— — (1953) The influence of placental size on fœtal growth in man, with special reference to multiple pregnancy. *ibid.* **9**, 418.
— — (1954) Influence of prenatal environment on correlation between birth weight and parental height. *Amer. J. hum. Genet.* **6**, 457.
— — (1957) The influence of body weight on reproductive function in women. *J. Endocr.* **15**, 410.
McLaren, A., Michie, D. (1960) Control of prenatal growth in mammals. *Nature, Lond.* **187**, 363.
McMeekan, C. P. (1940a) Growth and development in the pig, with special reference to carcass quality characters. *J. agric. Sci.* **30**, 276.
— (1940b) Growth and development in the pig, with special reference to carcass quality characters: II. The influence of the plane of nutrition on growth and development. *ibid.* p. 387.
— (1940c) III. Effect of the plane of nutrition on the form and composition of the bacon pig. *ibid.* p. 511.
— (1941a) IV. The use of sample joints and of carcass measurements as indices of the composition of the bacon pig. *ibid.* **31**, 1.
— (1941b) V. The bearing of the main principles emerging upon the many problems of animal production and human development. *ibid.* p. 17.
— Hammond, J. (1940) The relation of environmental conditions to breeding and selection for commercial types in pigs. *Emp. J. exp. Agric.* **8**, 6.
Markham, G. (1617) *Cavalarice*; book 1, chap. 14.
Mather, K., and others (1955–56) A discussion on hybrid vigour. *Proc. roy. Soc. B.* **144**, 143.
Mellbin, T. (1962) The children of Swedish nomad Lapps: A study of their health, growth, and development. *Acta pædiat., Stockh.* **51**, suppl. 131.
Mills, C. A. (1950) Temperature influence over human growth and development. *Human Biol.* **22**, 71.
Minot, C. S. (1891) Senescence and rejuvenation. *J. Physiol.* **12**, 97.
Moment, G. B. (1933) The effects of rate of growth on the postnatal development of the white rat. *J. exp. Zool.* **65**, 359.
Morgulis, S. (1923) *Fasting and Undernutrition*. New York.
Mossberg, H. O. (1948) Obesity in children. *Acta pædiat., Stockh.* **35**, suppl. 2.
Moulton, C. R., Trowbridge, P. F., Haigh, L. D. (1921) Studies in animal nutrition: 1. Changes in form and weight on different planes of nutrition. *Univ. Mo. agric. exp. Sta. Res. Bull.* **43**.
— — — (1922a) 2. Changes in proportions of carcass and offal on different planes of nutrition. *ibid.* **54**.
— — — (1922b) 3. Changes in chemical composition on different planes of nutrition. *ibid.* **55**.
Osborne, T. B., Mendel, L. B. (1914) The suppression of growth and the capacity to grow. *J. biol. Chem.* **18**, 95.
— — (1915) The resumption of growth after long continued failure to grow. *ibid.* **23**, 439.
Outhouse, J., Mendel, L. B. (1932–33) The rate of growth: 1. Its influence on the skeletal development of the albino rat. *J. exp. Zool.* **64**, 257.
Pomeroy, R. W. (1941) The effect of a submaintenance diet on the composition of the pig. *J. agric. Sci.* **31**, 50.
— (1960) Infertility and neonatal mortality in the sow: 3. Neonatal mortality and fœtal development. *ibid.* **54**, 31.
Popják, G. (1954a) The origin of fetal lipids. *Cold Spr. Harb. Symp. quant. Biol.* **19**, 200.
— (1954b) Placental impermeability to fetal lipids. *In* Mechanisms of Congenital Malformation. Second Science Conference, Association for the Aid of Crippled Children; p. 56.
Rafstedt, S. (1955) Studies on serum lipids and lipoproteins in infancy and childhood. *Acta pædiat., Stockh.* **44**, suppl. 102.
Ramsey, E. (1954) Relation between fœtal and placental size. *Cold Spr. Harb. Symp. quant. Biol.* **19**, 40.
Robb, R. C. (1929) On the nature of hereditary size limitation: 1. Body growth in giant and pigmy rabbits. *Brit. J. exp. Biol.* **6**, 293.
Ross, M. H. (1959) Proteins, calories and life expectancy. *Fed. Proc.* **18**, 1190.
Schultze, M. O. (1955) Effects of malnutrition in early life on subsequent growth and reproduction of rats. *J. Nutr.* **56**, 25.
Senn, M. J. E., McNamara, H. (1937) The lipids of the blood plasma in the neonatal period. *Amer. J. Dis. Child.* **53**, 445.
Silberberg, M., Silberberg, R. (1955) Diet and life span. *Physiol. Rev.* **35**, 347.
Smith, A. H. (1931) Phenomena of retarded growth. *J. Nutr.* **4**, 427.
Smith, C. A. (1959) *The Physiology of the Newborn Infant*. Springfield, Ill.
Strange, J. M. (1959) Obesity. *In* Diseases of Metabolism (edited by G. G. Duncan); p. 529. Philadelphia and London.
Tanner, J. M. (1955) *Growth at Adolescence*. Oxford.

Tata, J. R., Ernster, L., Lindberg, O. (1962) Control of metabolic rate by thyroid hormones and cellular function. *Nature, Lond.* **193**, 1058.
Taylor, J. H. (1962) Antibiotics and other growth promoting substances. *Proc. Nutr. Soc.* **21**, 73.
— Rowell, J. G. (1957) The effect of various levels of penicillin and chlortetracycline in the diet of fattening pigs. *Brit. J. Nutr.* **11**, 111.
Thomson, A. M. (1951) Human fœtal growth. *ibid.* **5**, 158.
— (1959) Diet in pregnancy: 3. Diet in relation to the course and outcome of pregnancy. *ibid.* **13**, 509.
— Thomson, W. (1948–49) Lambing in relation to the diet of the pregnant ewe. *ibid.* **2**, 290.
Venge, O. (1950) Studies of the maternal influence on the birth weight in rabbits. *Acta zool., Stockh.* **31**, 1.
Walker, J. (1954) Weight of the human fetus and of its placenta. *Cold Spr. Harb. Symp. quant. Biol.* **19**, 39.
Wallace, L. R. (1948a) The growth of lambs and afterbirth in relation to the level of nutrition; I. *J. agric. Sci.* **38**, 93.
— (1948b) II. *ibid.* p. 243.
— (1948c) III. *ibid.* p. 367.
Walton, A., Hammond, J. (1938) The maternal effects on growth and conformation in Shire horse–Shetland pony crosses. *Proc. roy. Soc. B.* **125**, 311.
Waters, H. J. (1908) The capacity of animals to grow under adverse conditions. *Proc. Soc. Prom. agric. Sci. N.Y.* **29**, 71.
— (1909) The influence of nutrition upon the animal form. *ibid.* **30**, 70.
Watts, R. M. (1935) The effect of administration of preparations of growth hormone of the anterior lobe of the pituitary upon gestation and the weight of the newborn (albino rats). *Amer. J. Obstet. Gynec.* **30**, 174.
Webb, H. M., Brown, F. A. (1959) Timing long cycle physiological rhythms. *Physiol. Rev.* **39**, 127.
Widdas, W. F. (1961) Transport mechanisms in the fœtus. *Brit. med. Bull.* **17**, 107.
Widdowson, E. M. (1955) Reproduction and obesity. *Voeding*, **16**, 94.
Wolff, O. H. (1955) Obesity in childhood. *Quart. J. Med.* **24**, 109.
Xenophon (B.C. 400) *In* Xenophon: scripta minora. Loeb Text, translated by E. C. Marchant (1925) London.
Zöllner, N., Wolfram, G. (1962) *Klin. Wschr.* **40**, 267.

HARMONY OF GROWTH*

ELSIE M. WIDDOWSON

*Dunn Nutritional Laboratory,
Infant Nutrition Research Division,
University of Cambridge and Medical Research Council*

THE growth of living organisms is a highly complex affair, involving a multitude of different processes working together in harmony, each cutting in and cutting out again at the appropriate time. A beautiful example of this is the way in which the teeth appear and grow at the precise moment the jaw has reached the stage when it is ready to accommodate them. Except in unicellular organisms the full-grown animal is vastly different from the cell from which it came. The chicken bears no resemblance to the egg, nor does the newborn baby to the human ovum. Most of the differentiation takes place during the early stages, when the developing organism is hidden from our view, and it is for this reason that it is especially exciting to find ways of studying the growth and development of mammals before birth.

Increasing Body-weight

The general principles about growth apply to all species, but species vary very much among themselves, most obviously perhaps in the rate at which the body grows and the ultimate size that it becomes. Table I

TABLE I—RATE OF GROWTH OF TEN SPECIES BEFORE BIRTH

Species	Length of gestation days	Weight at birth (g.)	Mean growth-rate (g. per day)
Mouse	21	2	0·09
Rat	21	5	0·24
Cat	63	100	1·6
Dog	63	200	3·2
Pig	120	1500	4·2
Man	280	3500	12·5
Calf	280	35,000	125
Elephant	600	114,000	190
Hippopotamus	240	50,000	210
Blue whale	330	3,000,000	9000

* Based on the Sanderson-Wells lecture delivered at the Senate House, University of London, on March 12, 1970.

TABLE II—RATE OF GROWTH OF NINE SPECIES DURING SUCKLING

Species	Weight at birth (g.)	Length of suckling (days)	Weight at weaning (g.)	Mean growth-rate (g. per day)
Mouse	2	15	9	0·47
Rat	5	21	40	1·7
Cat	100	35	600	14.
Dog	200	35	1200	29
Pig	1500	56	18,000	295
Man	3500	180	8000	25
Calf	35,000	60	70,000	580
Elephant	114,000	1460	600,000	335
Blue whale	3,000,000	210	21,000,000	86,000

illustrates this. It shows the average gain in bodyweight per day of ten mammalian species before birth. All these animals started life as a single cell, but the growth in weight of the embryo and fetus during the whole of its gestation may be 100,000 times as great in one as in another. The mouse grows at a mean rate of 0·09 g. a day, the blue whale at a mean rate of 9 kg. Man comes in between, and 12·5 g. a day may seem rather a mediocre performance but, even so, during prenatal life his weight increases several billion times.

Table II carries growth a stage farther and shows what happens while the animal is living on mother's milk. The young gain more weight per day during suckling than they did before birth, but the rate at which the bodies multiply their starting weight is far greater before birth because the weight of the ovum is so very small relative to the birth-weight of the animal it is going to become.

The rate of growth before and after birth depends primarily upon the supply of food and the ability of the animal to make use of it. The blood of the mother supplies the fetus with all its nutrients, and one might suppose that its composition would be one of the things which determined the fetal rate of growth. This is not so, however, for the composition of the plasma is much the same throughout the mammalian world, and the mouse's plasma is very similar to the whale's. The nutrients provided for the fetal whale must clearly be many times greater than those provided for the fetal mouse, but the vast quantity of blood reaching the fetal whale is what enables it to grow so big. There is no magic whatever in its composition.

After birth, milk is the natural food for all mammals, and although all milks have the same general characteristics they are by no means as constant in composition as the maternal plasma. Table III shows that after birth quality as well as quantity begins to determine the rate of growth, and each milk satisfies exactly the

TABLE III—COMPOSITION OF MILKS OF NINE SPECIES (PER 100 g.)

Species	Protein (g.)	Fat (g.)	Carbohydrate (g.)	Calories
Rat	9	9	3	134
Cat	11	11	3	159
Dog	8	9	4	134
Pig	6	9	5	129
Man	1	4	7	70
Calf	3	4	5	70
Elephant	5	9	4	121
Hippopotamus	7	18	2	205
Blue whale	12	40	1	426

genetic growth potential of the animal for which is was designed.

The rate at which the animal gains weight is not linear, either before birth or after it. The growth curve of all species is sigmoid, rising slowly at first then more rapidly around the time of birth, only to slow off again later. In man birth takes place on the steepest part of the growth curve, but in rodents and carnivores, which are born much earlier in their developmental life, birth takes place before the growth curve reaches its steepest part. The same is true of the pig, although this animal is relatively mature when it is born.

Number and Size of Cells

Of all the processes concerned with growth protein synthesis is probably the most fundamental. It begins at the moment the ovum is fertilised, but the first divisions of the ovum are not preceded by any significant increase in size, so the individual cells become successively smaller. (This is characteristic of undernutrition later on, and it makes one wonder whether the embryo in its earliest days may not be a little undernourished.) By the time the blastocyst has become implanted in the wall of the uterus, synthesis of protein from the aminoacids, and the water and inorganic substances that reach it begin to enlarge the cells before they divide. There is a change, too, in the timing of the divisions. The first few occur almost simultaneously, but after a few days cell division becomes staggered so that only a small proportion of the cells are dividing at the same time. Yet co-ordination is never lost and harmonious growth goes on.

Protein synthesis is the responsibility of the nucleic acids. D.N.A. is almost entirely confined to the cell nucleus, where it is the chief component of the chromosomes. The amount of D.N.A. in a diploid nucleus is rather constant at about 6·2 pg., so if we measure the amount of D.N.A. in an organ which has mononuclear cells and which is known to have only diploid nuclei within them we can calculate the number of cells in that organ. This measurement and

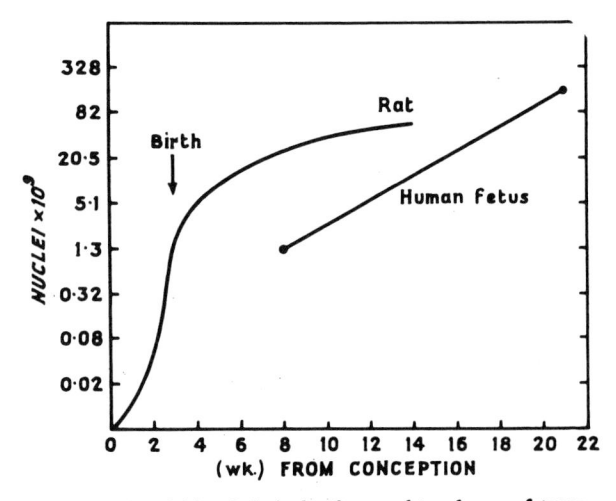

Number of nuclei in whole body of rat and two human fetuses.

calculation have been applied to the whole body of the rat at various ages from 10 days after conception to 14 weeks after birth,[1] and to the bodies of two human fetuses of 8 and 21 weeks gestation.[2] There are snags here in that some cells are multinucleate, others have polyploid nuclei, and yet others, the erythrocytes and thrombocytes, have no nuclei at all, but if these complications are neglected, the rate of cell division appears to be more rapid in the body of the rat before birth than it ever is in the human fetus (see figure). This may seem to contradict table I which showed that the mean daily gain in weight of the human fetus is greater than that of the rat; but this is not so. By going on for 9 months instead of 3 weeks the human fetus doubles and redoubles its starting weight many more times, and therefore becomes much larger than the rat before it is born. If we compare the two on the same time scale, as in the figure, then the rat's ovum multiplies itself two to three thousand million times during the 3 weeks gestation, whereas the human fetus only achieves half that number of cells in its first 8 weeks. This is evident in the total weight of the body too, for the human embryo 3 weeks after fertilisation weighs much less than the 5 g. of the newborn rat. This 8-week human fetus weighed only 3·7 g.

We can get more accurate information about different parts of the body by determining the amount of D.N.A. in individual organs at different ages before and after birth. Winick and Noble [1] have done this systematically in the rat, and they used the protein/D.N.A. ratio, or the amount of protein per nucleus as a measure of the size of the cell. From their results they concluded that from conception until about 15 days after birth liver, kidney, heart, brain, and lung cells divide frequently. Some organs continued to grow in this way 40–50 days after birth, in others cell division slowed down after 15 days, but eventually it ceased in all of them. At a particular time for each organ—15 days after conception for the heart, at about the time of birth for the brain, and about 14 days after birth for the kidney—the protein per nucleus began to increase rapidly, indicating that division was now being accompanied by an increase in the size of the cells. When this process also came to an end growth of the organ was over. Not only do organs start to grow at different ages after conception but they also cease to grow at their own appointed time, and this is essential for the harmonious growth of the body as a whole.

The amount of D.N.A. and the number of nuclei in the skeletal muscle of the rat goes on increasing for at least 14 weeks, which is long after cell division in the internal organs has stopped.[3] Cheek[3] added a further point that males have more nuclei in their muscles than females at all ages after 3 weeks. Cheek has also used D.N.A. as an index of cellular development in a study of muscle growth after birth in man.[3] He measured D.N.A. levels in biopsy samples of gluteal muscles, assumed that this was representative of all the muscles in the body, and calculated the amount of D.N.A. in the whole muscle mass. He estimated the muscle mass from the creatinine excretion, and his results on 33 boys and 19 girls suggested that there was an increase in the number of muscle nuclei right through human childhood, and that in boys there was a spurt in the rate of increase of nuclei at the time of puberty, which doubled the number of nuclei between 10 and 16 years. There was a fourteen-fold increase in the number of nuclei in the muscle of boys after birth. In girls the increase was smaller.

The cells, more usually called fibres, in skeletal muscle are multinucleate, so the amount of D.N.A. in a muscle tells us nothing about the number of fibres in it; nor does the ratio protein/D.N.A. or protein per nucleus tell us anything about the size of the muscle cell. It does give us information, however, about the amount of cytoplasm associated with each nucleus, and this ratio rises in human muscle as it does in other organs during growth after birth until the correct functional relationship has been achieved. Table IV shows how far the ratio protein/D.N.A. has progressed in the muscle of the rat, pig, and human baby at the time of birth.[4] This table also gives the ratios for adult muscle of the same three species. The muscle of the newborn baby has a more mature protein/D.N.A. ratio than the muscle of the rat or pig, and this is in line with the stage of development reached by the muscles of these three species at birth as judged in other ways. The similarity between the adults

TABLE IV—AMOUNT OF PROTEIN (mg.) ASSOCIATED WITH EACH mg. OF D.N.A. IN SKELETAL MUSCLE

Species	Newborn	Adult
Rat	15	400
Pig	33	380
Man	175	300

of the three species with such very different body sizes suggests that 300–400 mg. of protein per mg. of D.N.A., or 2·0 to 2·5 µg. protein per nucleus may be the approximate ratio for all adult mammalian striated muscle, and be an index of the desirable amount of muscle cytoplasm for one nucleus to control.

The only human fetal organ which has been analysed systematically for D.N.A. is the brain.[5,6] Increase in D.N.A. in the human brain is almost over by 3 months after birth, but the brain is such a complicated organ, with many different kinds of cells, that it is difficult to be precise about the types of cell which are developing in the brain from an analysis of D.N.A. in it. There are big species differences too, for the brain of the guineapig has already acquired its full complement of D.N.A. by the time the animal is born.[7] The mouse gets to this stage about 14 days after birth, and the rat by 17 days.[5] In the pig the full amount of D.N.A. is reached only after 3 years.[8]

The weight of the human brain increases linearly from birth to 13 months, and it goes on increasing till it reaches its adult weight of about 1300 g. at 6 years. Deposition of myelin follows the peak rate of cell division and accounts for much of the increase in weight of the brain in the later phase of its development in all species, and this must be regarded as an important aspect of the growth in weight of the brain. Myelination, as determined chemically, takes place at characteristic ages in different parts of the nervous system. In the pig, for example, myelin accumulates more rapidly in the cerebellum than in the forebrain.[8]

Deposition of Fat

During the first half of gestation the body of the human fetus contains a mere 0·5% of fat, but by the 28th week from conception, when the fetus weighs about 1200 g., it may have about 3·5% fat in it (i.e., some 42 g.). During the last 2 months of gestation the fat in the body increases rapidly; a premature baby weighing 2·2 kg. at 34 weeks may contain about 165 g., and a full-term baby weighing 3·5 kg. about 560 g. or 16% of its body-weight.[9] The amount of fat in the body varies from one baby to another, just as it does later in life, and in fetal life, as later, the deposition of fat is a sign of the plane of nutrition which at that time depends primarily upon the mother. It takes place, moreover, just at the time when the lean parts of the body are also gaining weight rapidly, and this is why it is such a delicate index of a satisfactory pregnancy.

Rats, cats, dogs, and pigs, and other species too, are born before the deposition of fat really begins, and these animals only start to deposit fat during the first weeks after birth.[10] The percentage of fat in the body of the rat may rise from less than 1% to 16% in the first 2 weeks after birth, and here again the fat is deposited just when the body as a whole is growing very rapidly. Even if animals are born without fat, they have fat cells waiting to be filled, but we know that in both rats and man, and probably in other species too, the number of fat cells in the body goes on increasing for some long time after birth—in the rat for about 15 weeks and in man throughout the whole growth period and possibly longer.

The number of fat cells can be affected by undernutrition early in life. If rats are undernourished during the first 3 weeks after birth by being suckled in large numbers on one mother they never have as many fat cells as others suckled in small groups and fed plentifully over the same early period in their lives.[11] Can the number of fat cells in the body be increased by overnutrition or do some individuals have more fat cells than others, so that they tend to become obese? Knittle[12] took subcutaneous fat from normal and obese individuals from 2 years old and upwards, counted the number of fat cells, and measured the amount of fat in them. He also measured the total amount of fat in the body. He found that the obese people had more fat in each cell, but much more important was the fact that they had three times as many fat cells, and it was clear that the large size of their fat depots was due primarily to an increase in number of cells and to a lesser extent to an increase in lipid content of each cell. This applied with equal force to both children and adults, but we have no idea when these obese individuals acquired their extra fat cells—whether they were born with them or whether they developed them later—perhaps in response to an increased demand for storage accommodation due to overeating. One thing we suspect is that the number of nuclei and hence the number of fat cells, like all other cells, cannot be reduced later in life, for once a nucleus has been made it is never destroyed by any physiological process until the cell dies. Indeed Knittle found that patients had just as many fat cells after their weight had been reduced, but each cell contained a little less fat. This explains why an obese person so easily puts fat on again after a brave attempt at slimming. The large number of well-filled fat cells may be a disadvantage to him æsthetically and physically, but if they are produced in response to an intake of food too large for all reasonable requirements they must surely be regarded as the acme of harmonious growth.

Increased Functional Demand and Liver Cells

Since the cells of each organ stop dividing at a fairly circumscribed age, and since there is also an upper limit to the size these cells can attain, it follows that the maximum size of an organ depends on the number of cells it had in it when cell division stopped—unless cell division can start up again. In some parts of the body this can undoubtedly happen, but only in those organs which retain the power of nuclear and cell division in response to an increased physiological demand. The liver is particularly endowed in this way.[13] Kennedy and Pearce [14] showed that if three-fifths of the liver of the rat were excised, for example, there was an almost immediate onset of cell division throughout the remainder of the organ, and the amount of D.N.A. in it might double within a week. After 12 weeks the number of cells was almost back to the original one. A large increase in the intake of calories, moreover, which takes place normally during lactation in the rat, was followed by enlargement of the liver, due again to an increase in the number of its cells.[15] If the functional demand on the liver is reduced—at the end of lactation for example—the liver becomes smaller, not because there is a reduction in the number of cells, but because the amount of cytoplasmic protein in each cell gets less.

Cells and Undernutrition

The effect of undernutrition on the number of cells in an organ varies with the stage of development it has reached when the undernutrition is imposed. If the cells have already ceased to divide the organs lose weight, as the liver does after lactation, by a decrease in the size of each cell, but not a reduction in their number.[16] Functional equilibrium has been restored at the cost of an anatomical change in the size of the adult cells. If the undernutrition is imposed while cell division is still going on this process slows down and may ultimately stop before the full complement for the organ has been attained. If this happens the number of cells in the organ will always be too few, except perhaps in the liver where cell division is possible at any age in response to functional demand.

I have been investigating the effect of undernutrition before birth, for this has an application to the baby that is small for its gestational age. A baby or animal may be small at term for a variety of reasons and the mother may be well nourished or malnourished. I am using runt pigs, weighing only a third to a half as much as their littermates

TABLE V—WEIGHTS OF ORGANS (g.) OF PIGS

Organ	Fetus	Runt pig	Large littermate of runt
Body-weight	576	578	1586
Liver	15·3 (2·65%)	12.8 (2·20%)	45·6 (2·90%)
Heart	3·9 (0·68%)	4·7 (0·81%)	11·4 (0·72%)
2 kidneys	3·8 (0·66%)	4·0 (0·69%)	10·8 (0·68%)
Brain	20·1 (3·50%)	27·6 (4·80%)	34·5 (2·20%)
2 quadriceps muscles	6·1 (1·06%)	4·4 (0·76%)	14·8 (0·93%)

because they had been badly sited in the uterus, to serve as the model for small babies born to well-nourished mothers at term. I have used two types of control—animals of the same gestational age (i.e. large littermates, born with the runts, at term at 120 days) and animals of the same size (i.e. well-grown fetuses of about 90 days gestation).

Table V gives the average weights of the liver, heart, kidney, brain, and quadriceps muscles in the smallest and largest piglets in 6 full term litters, and the same information about 6 fetuses 90–95 days after conception. The full-term runts had small livers and quadriceps muscles, smaller even than those of the fetuses, and much smaller than those of their big littermates of 120 days gestational age. Their hearts were a little larger for their body-weights than those of the other two groups, and their kidneys were about the right size. Their brains weighed more than those of the well-grown fetal pigs, but less than those of their well-grown littermates. They were larger than either as a percentage of the body-weight. Undernutrition has introduced a note of disharmony, by disturbing its coordination. One organ goes on growing, another stops. The development of muscle is severely retarded, that of the brain much less so.

Table VI shows the total amount of D.N.A. in these tissues. Cell division was clearly hindered by undernutrition before birth, but it was not entirely stopped, and the amount of D.N.A. in the heart, kidneys, and brain of the runt piglets that were small for dates lay between those for the well-grown 90–95 day fetuses which were the same size and the larger full-term littermates which were, of course, exactly the same age. Not so the muscle. In this tissue nuclear division had been held up at a stage of development

TABLE VI—TOTAL D.N.A. IN ORGANS OF PIGS (mg.)

Organ	Fetus	Runt pig	Large littermate of runt
Heart	16·1	30·0	46·3
2 kidneys	28·5	37·7	65·8
Brain	25·5	35·2	48·3
2 quadriceps muscles	22·0	15·9	31·0

TABLE VII—PROTEIN/D.N.A. RATIO (mg.) IN PIGS

Organ	Fetus	Runt pig	Large littermate of runt
Heart	16·7	16·1	21·8
Kidneys	9·9	8·4	12·7
Brain	34·0	39·4	42·3
Quadriceps muscles	18·7	19·7	38·0

which well-nourished 90–95 day fetuses had already reached and passed.

Table VII shows the ratio of protein to D.N.A. in these same tissues. The cells of the heart and kidneys of the runt were about the same size, as judged by this ratio, as those of the younger fetus of the same weight, and smaller than those of the heavier littermate. In the runt's muscle too, the amount of cytoplasm associated with each nucleus was the same as in the fetus, but far less than in the muscle of its large littermate. In the runt's brain, however, the protein/D.N.A. ratio was intermediate between the other two.

Table VIII shows some values for the muscle of newborn guineapigs, undernourished before birth by severe undernutrition of the mother all through pregnancy. The controls were the newborn young of well-nourished mothers, and they weighed twice as much on the average as the others, 112 g. against 56 g. The total D.N.A. and the ratio protein/D.N.A. were both low in the muscle of the undernourished newborn guineapigs, as they were in the muscle of the runt pigs. We have counted the number of fibres in a section across the belly of the quadriceps muscles of these undernourished newborn guineapigs and their controls and the table shows that there were only half as many fibres in the small muscles of the undernourished animals. The cross-sectional area of each fibre was the same. Similarly the fibres of the runt pig are of approximately the same diameter as those of the large littermates, but we have not yet made full fibre-counts across the whole muscle.

TABLE VIII—PROTEIN, D.N.A., AND NUMBER OF FIBRES IN QUADRICEPS MUSCLE OF NEWBORN GUINEAPIGS

—	Mothers under-nourished	Mothers well nourished
Weight 2 whole quadriceps muscles (mg.)	418	900
Protein (mg.)	71	132
D.N.A. mg.	1·08	1·40
Protein/D.N.A.	65·5	94·0
Area of section across belly of lateral quadriceps muscle (sq. mm.)	9·45	20·77
Number of fibres in cross-section	58,360	130,430
Area of cross-section of one fibre sq. mm $\times 10^{-4}$)	1·62	1·59

Body Size and Recovery from Undernutrition

The size that animals undernourished at different stages of development can be expected to attain when they are rehabilitated depends upon the stage of development they were at when they were undernourished. If they are undernourished as adults, at a time when their cells have already reached their full number, then they catch up their well-nourished fellows without any trouble.[16,17] If they are undernourished early, while the cells are still dividing, they may never catch up, for their tissues never have as many cells as they should. We see this in rats undernourished from birth to 3 weeks of age, and then rehabilitated.[16,18] We see it in the runt pig versus its big littermate. Both grow well, but the runt never quite catches up. Just the same is true of guineapigs born of undernourished mothers and themselves small at birth. They always remain small, and these animals too have fewer cells in their internal organs and fewer muscle fibres.

Skeletal development, like the development of the soft tissues, can be hindered by undernutrition before or soon after birth. The bone development of 3-week-old rats that have been undernourished since birth is behind that of well-grown animals of the same age, though it is farther advanced than that of well-grown animals of the same weight but only 10 days old.[19] Similarly, the runt pig has smaller bones and fewer ossification centres than its large littermate. The bones of these animals that are undernourished during the early part of their lives never grow as long as the bones of those that grew well in the early stages.[19,20] Closure of the epiphyses is not the explanation, for rat's epiphyses never close, and those of the pig not until $3^{1}/_{2}$–4 years—long after the bones have ceased to grow in length. If the bones do not grow as long, it is difficult to see how the skeletal muscles can do so. And by how much is the growth of the brain limited by the smaller skull?

Normal skeletal development before birth is characteristically different for each species, and beautifully adapted to the life the animal will have to lead in the world outside the uterus. Some animals are born with very short limbs—the rat, the kitten, and the human baby for example. These short-limbed animals are all helpless at birth, their mothers care for them and bring them their food. Their short limbs make for a small surface area and therefore a small heat loss, which makes it easier for these immature newborn animals to maintain their body temperature. Other species, which are much more mature when they are born, the lamb, the calf, the foal, the giraffe, and the camel for example, have long limbs with highly calcified bones in them. These animals are by nature wanderers, sometimes travelling long distances to water and in search of food, and the young need their long legs to keep up with their mothers for protection and food, which is sometimes quite high up. The limbs of the newborn kangaroo have differential rates of development. At birth the forelimbs are far better developed than the hind limbs; which enables the tiny animal to crawl up its mother's abdomen into her pouch to reach her teat, but by adult life they have become much smaller than the long and immensely powerful back legs. Thus within each species the growth and development of the bones is in perfect harmony with that of the rest of the body, and is exactly attuned at each age to the function they have to perform.

" Differing in size, in note, in weight,
Yet, small or great,
We harmonise."

So runs the inscription on the bells of Colchester Town Hall: one could say the same of animal growth.

REFERENCES

1. Winick, M., Noble, A. *Devl Biol.* 1965, **12**, 451.
2. Osgood, E. E. *Pediatrics, Springfield*, 1965, **15**, 733.
3. Cheek, D. B. Human Growth. Philadelphia 1968.
4. Widdowson, E. M. in The Physiology and Biochemistry of Muscle as a Food (edited by E. J. Briskey and R. G. Cassens); vol. II. (In the press.)
5. Winick, M. *Pediat. Res.* 1968, **2**, 352.
6. Howard, E., Granoff, D. M., Bujnovszky, P. *Brain Res.* 1969, **14**, 697.
7. Dobbing, J., Sands, J. *ibid.* 1970, **17**, 115.
8. Dickerson, J. W. T., Dobbing, J. *Proc. R. Soc. B*, 1967, **166**, 384.
9. Widdowson, E. M., Spray, C. M. *Archs Dis. Childh.* 1951, **26**, 205.
10. Widdowson, E. M. *Nature, Lond.* 1950, **166**, 626.
11. Knittle, J. L., Hirsch, J. *J. clin. Invest.* 1968, **47**, 2091.
12. Knittle, J. L. in Problems of Nutrition in the Perinatal Period: report of the sixtieth Ross conference on Pediatric Research; p. 203. Ross Laboratories, Columbus, Ohio.
13. Harkness, R. D. *Br. med. Bull.* 1957, **13**, 87.
14. Kennedy, G. C., Pearce, W. M. *J. Endocr.* 1958, **17**, 149.
15. Kennedy, G. C., Pearce, W. M., Parrott, D. M. V. *ibid.* p. 158.
16. Winick, M., Noble, A. *J. Nutr.* 1966, **89**, 300.
17. Widdowson, E. M., McCance, R. A. *Proc. R. Soc. B*, 1963, **158**, 329.
18. Widdowson, E. M., Kennedy, G. C. *ibid.* 1962, **156**, 96.
19. Dickerson, J. W. T., Widdowson, E. M. *Proc. R. Soc. B*, 1960, **152**, 207.
20. Lister, D., McCance, R. A. *Br. J. Nutr.* 1967, **21**, 787.

The Lancet Office,
7 Adam Street, Adelphi, London W.C.2

A PAPER THAT CHANGED MY PRACTICE

The harmony of growth

With her inimitable and succinct style Elsie Widdowson strode through the world of biology in her 1970 Sanderson-Wells University of London lecture, and the *Lancet* published her paper on 2 May. It set out to show how perfectly a multitude of different processes working together in harmony resulted in the complex growth of living organisms. There were plenty of data in the paper, but what struck me was the breadth of knowledge of the author and the thread she sought to demonstrate running across the species.

I was struggling at the time to make sense of that experiment of man called obesity, specifically obesity in childhood, and from this time I began to see a logic in the work I was doing. Dr Widdowson's own experiments (with Professor McCance) on animal (and human) growth have been amply confirmed in the studies with which I have since been concerned on the control of human growth in infancy, childhood, and puberty, but it was the lateral thinking in the paper which changed things for me.

Medical students and young doctors receive a more or less constant input of sensory information and you try to make the best of what comes out. When you start in research the future stretches indefinitely and busy clinicians (who often hide the paucity of creation behind their business) have suddenly to generate their own stimulation. The desk is void until you fill it—and everybody else around you seems so clever and busy. Many clinicians find such sensory deprivation hard to bear and the time that has to elapse between the starting of the collection of data and the pleasure in analysing it deeply depressing. This is one reason why research is such hard work but ultimately so rewarding. Dr Widdowson's paper showed me how wide could be the appreciation of such a set of data, how infinite the elegance of nature in the control of biological processes.

Her paper ended with the inscription on the bells of Colchester town hall:

> Differing in size, in note, in weight,
> Yet, small or great,
> We harmonize.

That is what has illumined my clinical practice.—C G D BROOK, *professor of paediatric endocrinology, University College London, and consultant paediatrician, Middlesex Hospital*

Widdowson E.M. Harmony of growth. *Lancet* 1970;i:901-5.

1985 E.V. McCOLLUM INTERNATIONAL LECTURESHIP IN NUTRITION

Animals in the Service of Human Nutrition

Elsie M. Widdowson, FRS, DSc, PhD

I feel extremely honored to have been invited to give the McCollum Lecture at this Congress, especially as Professor McCollum has been one of my heroes for the past 50 years. I only saw him once, in 1936, when, as a young and inexperienced research worker, I went to the United States for the first time. I knew of his work and I very much wanted to meet him, so I wrote him and told him so. He invited me to visit him in his laboratory at Johns Hopkins, which I did. He was a great man and I was a nobody, yet he treated me with courtesy and kindness, shared his sandwich lunch with me, and made me feel as though I was someone who mattered. I have never forgotten his lesson and example.

When I was given the title of my lecture by the organizers of the Congress, I realized that it could be interpreted in more than one way. Therefore, I want to make it clear at the outset that I am not going to talk about the nutritional value of meat or milk. What I propose to do is, first, to say something about the history of the use of animals in research on human nutrition; second, to refer to the application of the results of studies on animals to human beings; and third, to say a few words about the use of animals in research on nutrition in relation to the difficulties many are experiencing in doing such research at the present time.

Some Historical Highlights

Nutrition is a subject that lends itself to experimental work with animals. Thousands of experiments have been performed on numerous species in which the diet has been unusual in one respect or another, and the effect on the animals has been followed in various ways. Many of the early studies, however, were made on animals fed supposedly adequate diets, and their metabolism of energy and protein was measured. England and France led the way in nutritional work with animals. The era of energy metabolism may be said to have opened with Priestley, Crawford, and Lavoisier in the latter part of the 18th century. These men were not employed to do this work. Priestley, for example, was a clergyman, and Lavoisier was supposed to be concerned with agriculture. Crawford wrote a book in 1778 entitled *Experiments and Observations on Animal Heat*,[1] two years before the publication of the classic paper of Lavoisier and Laplace.[2] Crawford and Lavoisier both used guinea pigs. Lavoisier and Laplace put a guinea pig inside a bell jar surrounded by ice and left it there for 10 hours. They commented that they chose this animal because it is docile and will go for a long time without food and water. After the ice melted, they measured the water from it and calculated the amount of heat given out by the guinea pig which melted the ice. The carbon

---

Dr Widdowson is Professor, Department of Medicine, Addenbrooke's Hospital, Hills Road, Cambridge CB2 2QQ, England. Her McCollum Lecture was delivered during the XIII International Congress of Nutrition at Brighton, England, in August, 1985.

Dr Widdowson's lecture was the fifth presentation in the E.V. McCollum International Lectureship Series. This lectureship was established in honor of Dr McCollum to encourage and recognize advances in nutrition science and their sound application.

dioxide in the expired air was also measured.

Lavoisier also studied his own respiratory exchanges and those of his friends. Among other things, he showed that oxygen uptake and carbon dioxide output were raised by a fall in environmental temperature, by exercise, and by the process of digestion after a meal. Sadly, these were among Lavoisier's last experiments, for in May 1794, at the age of 51, Lavoisier was guillotined. The results were never published in full, but they were described in a letter written in November 1790 to Joseph Black, discoverer of carbon dioxide.[3]

The principle Lavoisier initiated — making parallel studies on human beings and animals — was handed down to his French pupils, who passed it on to those who came to France from Germany over the next 50 years. Liebig studied in Paris around 1822, and when he returned to Germany he trained Voit who trained Rubner, Pettenkoffer, Bischoff, and others. Throughout their work we can see the influence of Lavoisier. These German investigators used experimental animals, particularly dogs, side by side with human beings, in their studies of energy and protein metabolism. Rubner built an animal calorimeter, and Voit and Rubner made a great many studies on the basal metabolism of human beings and animals. Rubner formulated his surface area law, which stated that the basal metabolism is proportional to the surface area of the animal, provided that measurements of different species are made at the same environmental temperature.

Some of the German work was undoubtedly inspired by the famines that had periodically devastated Europe, and the effects of starvation on the metabolism of protein, fat, and carbohydrate were carefully worked out on dogs. Professional fasters were also studied to compare the physiologic effects of human and animal starvation. Such comparisons brought out the important fact that a fasting dog can obtain adequate water from the catabolism of its own tissues, whereas a man would die of dehydration if he had no water, long before he would succumb to starvation if water were supplied. This is because dogs do not lose water by sweating, and their kidneys can produce a more concentrated urine than human kidneys.[4]

While the dog was the experimental animal chosen by German investigators before the start of the 20th century, the rat was undoubtedly the animal that contributed most to the discovery of vitamins from 1900 through the 1920s, although chickens, pigeons, guinea pigs, mice, and dogs also played their part. What we now know to be vitamin deficiency diseases had long been familiar in various parts of the world, but no one understood their cause until Eijkman, a prison medical officer in the Dutch East Indies, noticed that chickens fed polished rice developed a paralysis similar to that characteristic of prisoners suffering from beri-beri. Eijkman discovered that when he gave the birds unmilled rice or a water extract of rice polishings, they did not develop the paralysis. His findings were published in 1897.[5]

In the days of long sailing voyages, there were often outbreaks of disease among sailors, who lived on dry foods. Japanese sailors, like prisoners, ate polished rice, and they also got beri-beri, but it was found that the disease could be prevented with fresh food. The Norwegian navy was also ill. After the turn of the century, Hölst, working at the University of Christiania (now Oslo), supposed the Norwegian sailors had beri-beri, too. He repeated Eijkman's studies on chickens, but he used pigeons because "these animals are cheaper than chickens and do not take up so much room." He got a similar result.[6] Then, for some unknown reason, Hölst and his colleague Frölich gave a cereal diet to guinea pigs, expecting them to develop the paralysis of beri-beri, but they became ill in a different way.[7] This illness was, of course, scurvy, which affected Norwegian sailors as it did the British sailors in Captain Cook's day. Captain Cook had successfully treated scurvy by giving his crew fresh food. When the Norwegian guinea pigs were given fresh cabbage or potatoes along with their cereal, the disease did not occur. Hölst and Frölich made the further observation that the "nutriment" they postulated the cabbage contained was partially lost by boiling it in water for half an hour.

Hopkins knew nothing of all this when he embarked on his famous studies using rats. In fact, his work on vitamins was rather a sideline for him. Among biochemists, he is far more famous for his isolation of tryptophan and glutathione than for his work with vitamins. His studies on tryptophan,[8] in which he used mice as experimental animals, seemed to have given him the idea that "no animal can live upon a mixture of pure protein, fat, and carbohydrate, and even when the necessary inorganic material is carefully supplied the animal still cannot flourish. The animal body is adjusted to live either upon plant tissues or the tissues of other animals, and these contain countless substances other than proteins, carbohydrates, and fat."[9] Hopkins began to experiment around 1906, but the paper describing his main experiment was not published until 1912.[10] When he later discovered that he was not the first to suggest that unknown nutrients were essential, or to conduct animal experiments, he was anxious to make amends, which he did in his 1929 Nobel lecture. He shared the 1929 Nobel prize with Eijkman.

Hopkins used groups of 4 to 6 animals weighing 30 to 50 g, housed two to a cage for, as he said, "Rats progress more normally when they have a companion than when kept singly." He fed them a diet consisting of casein, raw potato starch, cane sugar, lard, and mineral salts, produced by incinerating equal parts of oatmeal and dog biscuits. He stated specifically that he provided no roughage. To one group of animals in each experiment he gave fresh milk — 1, 2, or 3 ml per rat per day. Those consuming milk grew, while the others ate less food, failed to grow, and soon began to lose weight, so that after about 20 days the experiment had to be terminated. When after 18 days, the treatment was reversed, those recently given milk started to grow, while those newly deprived of milk lost weight. Hopkins postulated that the milk contained something that was essential for growth and health of the animals. Unfortunately, no one could repeat these experiments and achieve identical results, because Hopkins did not describe in his original paper every experimental detail of his procedure. In fact, Hopkins found this out himself when he repeated his original experiments 30 years later.[11] But Hopkins' original paper inspired a large amount of work. Even though his Nobel prize seems to have been awarded for his concept, rather than the publication of his single, somewhat sketchy paper, the honor met with general approbation because it was recognized that he was responsible for opening up a new field of discovery which largely depended on the use of the rat.

In 1906, when Hopkins' thoughts were turning to those "countless substances other than proteins, fats and carbohydrates," E.V. McCollum obtained his PhD degree at Yale. In 1907, McCollum obtained a post in the Department of Agricultural Chemistry at the University of Wisconsin. Unlike Hopkins, McCollum was a great reader of the literature, and he soon found that a number of investigations had been made between 1873 and 1906 in which small animals, usually mice, had been fed restricted diets of isolated proteins, fats, and carbohydrates. In every instance, he wrote, "they promptly failed in health, rapidly deteriorated physically, and lived only a few weeks." He concluded that the most important problem in nutrition was to discover what was lacking in such diets.

McCollum reasoned that he must use small experimental animals with a short life span and, like Hopkins, he decided to use rats. Rats did not seem to be available at the University of Wisconsin, and McCollum did not get much encouragement from the Dean of the College of Agriculture, who refused to provide any money, so he had to get the rats himself. He described how he did this in a 1948 letter to Dr Salmon of the Alabama Polytechnic Institute (Dr Prebluda kindly sent me a copy of this letter.) Even in 1907, McCollum was evidently aware of Hopkins' early experiments and ideas, for he wrote, "In the autumn of 1907 I decided to try to take up studies of the effects of purified food mixtures where Professor F.G. Hopkins had left off the preceding year. Because of total lack of comprehension of what such studies meant in the way of experimental management of animals, I decided upon using wild grey rats. Accordingly, I caught 17 one afternoon in the horse barn at the Wisconsin Experiment Station Farm and set out to feed them experimental rations. They were so terrified and ferocious when I tried to do anything to them that I soon gave it up and chloroformed them. I then bought a dozen "albino" rats from an animal dealer in Chicago. He was a pet stock man. I do not remember his name. I began with this stock, and soon had sufficient experimental young animals for my small resources." He subsequently acquired other rats which he interbred with his own, and so set up his hybrid colony. What McCollum doesn't say in this letter is that he had to buy his first 12 rats from the pet stock man with $6 of his own money, and then pay for their cages. Later, Professor Hart, head of the Department of Agricultural Chemistry, allowed him to spend $50 for two animal units. The carpenter, who was sorry for him, made him three units for the price of two.

In January, 1908, McCollum was ready to start. He believed the rats did not do well on purified diets because these diets were unpalatable. This notion led him nowhere, but it was not until 1911 that he gave up the idea. He devoted much of his time to his rat colony during those early years, caring for them himself, but he badly needed help. Assistance came providentially in the shape of Marguerite Davis, a graduate student who wanted to study biochemistry with McCollum. When she learned about his rat colony and how he was doing everything himself, she volunteered to look after the animals for him. This she did for 5 years without pay; it was only in the sixth year that Dr McCollum managed to get a small salary for her. Her practical help led to a fruitful collaboration, and the publication of 11 joint papers. Among their important discoveries was that the substance present in whole cereals that prevents polyneuritis in chickens and pigeons was also necessary for rats.[12,13] Further, even when the diet contained whole cereals, young rats needed something else, which was apparently contained in butterfat, but not in lard or olive oil.[14-16] Thus, McCollum and Davis discovered that two factors, fat-soluble vitamin A and water-soluble vitamin B, were necessary for the growth of rats. One outcome of this work was that the colony of rats, which had been barely tolerated in the Wisconsin College of Agriculture, now became important because they had been used to prove that butter was superior to olive oil and lard. This was great news for the dairy farmers of Wisconsin.

When Miss Davis left in 1916 she was replaced by Nina Simmonds. Together, McCollum and Simmonds discovered that green leaves had activity similar to that of fat-soluble vitamin A,[17] and that vitamin A had functions other than promoting growth. Its deficiency produced eye lesions, and McCollum and Simmonds[18] used the word xerophthalmia to describe the condition.

Now we come back to England, to Mellanby. Mellanby studied in Cambridge, and in 1906 he spent a year working under Hopkins. He then went to London to qualify in medicine, and in 1913 he was appointed Professor of Physiology at Kings College for Women in Kensington, London. In 1914 the Medical Research Committee, which later became the Medical Research Council, held a meeting at which Hopkins was present. Rickets was still a great scourge in Britain, and Hopkins suggested that the nature and cause of rickets would be a suitable subject for investigation. He recommended that Mellanby be invited to undertake the work.

Mellanby knew that puppies got rickets, so he chose them as his experimental animals. There was no place at the college to keep the puppies, so they were housed in Cambridge, while the histological and biochemical investigations were done at Kings College for Women. At that time, rickets was believed to be due to lack of exercise or to an infection. After a long series of experiments, however, Mellanby was able to prove that a dietary deficiency was the cause, and that the essential nutrient was present in animal fat, especially in cod liver oil, but was lacking in vegetable oil. It therefore seemed to correspond with McCollum's fat-soluble A factor. However, in 1920 Mellanby showed that two unknown factors must exist, because some fats cured the eye lesions that McCollum called xerophthalmia, and others cured rickets. Cod liver oil would cure both. Mellanby made some preliminary communications,[19,20] and his full publication "Experimental Rickets" appeared in 1921.[21]

In 1917 McCollum moved to Johns Hopkins, taking 50 female and 10 male rats with him. The following year he noticed that rats developed a rachitic condition if they were fed cereals and the diet had an abnormal calcium: phosphorus ratio. This condition could be prevented by giving small amounts of cod liver oil. McCollum devised a line test — a line of calcification in the bone of a deficient rat when it was given a source of vitamin D.[22]

So McCollum and Mellanby, between them, separated the two fat-soluble vitamins A and D. Thanks to their studies on animals, and those of Dame Harriette Chick and her colleagues, on Viennese children after the first World War,[23] rickets virtually disappeared. Not so xerophthalmia and blindness due to vitamin A deficiency. In spite of the 70-year-old work of McCollum, vitamin A deficiency is still with us. It is a sad reflection on the world today that 5 million children every year suffer xerophthalmia, of whom 250,000 become blind.[24]

The work of Hopkins, McCollum, Mellanby, and other pioneers was followed by many studies using rats, some very good, some less so. In the 1930s about 3,000 papers a year were published on some aspect of vitamin research, generally involving the use of rats as experimental animals.

New and important work on trace elements was opening up at this time. Those with the longest history of study are iodine and iron, and in both instances the original observations were made in human beings. By 1928 Hart, in Wisconsin, was himself using rats, presumably from McCollum's colony. With colleagues, he mastered the technique of feeding rats purified diets containing all the essential mineral elements apart from the trace element they were studying. They discovered that copper and iron are necessary for blood formation,[25] that manganese is essential for normal ovarian function,[26] and that zinc is essential for growth and development.[27]

McCollum had been interested in inorganic nutrients since 1909. His early studies concerned the role of inorganic phosphorus in animal nutrition.[28] In the 1930s, he and his student Elsa Orent began investigating the effects of magnesium deficiency on young rats and puppies.[29,30] They also showed that manganese deficiency causes degeneration of the testes and sterility in male rats. Manganese-deficient females produce their young normally but do not suckle or care for them.[31] The newspapers got hold of this and reported that manganese is necessary for the maternal instinct.

So much for the use of animals in the discoveries of vitamins and trace elements. In 1939 came the second World War, and the war years and those following them saw a revival of interest in deficiencies of energy and protein. The description by Cicely Williams, working in the Gold Coast in the 1930s, of a protein deficiency disease which she called kwashiorkor[32] sparked a large amount of postwar work with children and with experimental animals. The Medical Research Council set up units in Uganda and Jamaica for studying children, and research centers were established by the United States, Sweden, and other countries. Investigations were also made in many countries in the 1950s and 1960s on the effects of energy and protein deficiencies on rats, pigs, dogs, primates, and other species. We made some ourselves, but I think the important, fundamental observations were made, and are still being made, on children and their mothers in Africa, Jamaica, India, and Central America.

In western countries, obesity, cardiovascular disease, and the importance of dietary fiber are now the aspects of human nutrition of most concern. Are animals helping us with this knowledge? So far as cardiovascular disease and dietary fiber are concerned, the important observations are being made in human beings. Obesity and regulation of energy balance is being studied in humans and experimental animals with calorimeters and by other means, just as the German investigators were doing 100 years ago.

I think the heyday of animals in the service of human nutrition was in the first two decades of this century, and that is why I have devoted much of my lecture to this period. New techniques have now made it possible to conduct human studies that would hitherto have been out of the question.

The Applicability of Results in Animals to Human Nutrition

There are, of course, important differences between human beings and animals, and for those of us who are interested in comparative nutrition, these provide the fun. However, if our concern is primarily with human nutrition, there are certain things we must bear in mind. There are a few species differences in metabolism —

for example, all animals except humans and guinea pigs can synthesize vitamin C, and feline metabolism of fatty acids and amino acids is distinctive. But most species differences are quantitative, due to differences in size, rate of metabolism, growth, maturation, and reproduction, and hence, nutrient requirements. These can be an advantage or a disadvantage, as the case may be. The rapid growth of small animals like the rat, with their correspondingly high requirement for nutrients, was vital in the identification of various accessory food factors. In using animals as human models, whether at birth, during childhood, as adults, or in old age, it is important to know the characteristics of the chosen species. Claude Bernard was so right when he wrote, in 1865, in his *Introduction to the Study of Experimental Medicine,* "The solution of a physiological or pathological problem often depends solely on the appropriate choice of the animal for the experiment."[33]

Current Problems

Investigators in many countries are very troubled at the present time about how long their experimental work with animals will be allowed to continue. Don't despair. Scientists had the same problems in Britain in 1890 when Thomas Henry Huxley wrote about them,[34] and in France in 1865 when Claude Bernard did the same thing.[33] Animal experiments must go on, for who knows what discoveries lie ahead? I have used many species, including the human one, in my investigations. In fact, I have to confess that for the first 20 years of my research life I never touched an experimental animal at all.

Professor McCance and I worked entirely with human beings, ourselves included, studying the response to salt deficiency; the absorption and excretion of calcium, magnesium, iron, and other elements under various conditions; the voluntary intake of food; the expenditure of energy; the response to undernutrition; and, the nutritive value of different kinds of bread for undernourished children. It was only after we returned to Cambridge from Germany in the early 1950s that we started work with animals. Since then, pigs, cats, dogs, rats, mice, guinea pigs, rabbits, elephants, seals, eels, and trout, not to speak of blackbirds and thrushes, have been used by us to investigate aspects of nutrition and growth. It always seemed strange when I was busy with studies on human beings in the 1930s and 1940s that, while all animal experiments in the United Kingdom were strictly controlled, there were no regulations about human experiments. Now human experiments are under the supervision of ethical committees, but this is a recent development. I think Professor McCance's 1951 paper "The Practice of Experimental Medicine" was one of the first to draw attention to this matter.[35] Yet as long ago as 1876, the British Cruelty to Animals Act was passed. I always think this is rather an unfortunate title. The Home Office not only licenses every institution in which experiments are done and supervises them by inspection, but issues licenses and certificates to individual investigators, all of whom have to be approved beforehand as competent and responsible persons. The types of experiments they are permitted to perform, and the conditions they must fulfill, are all clearly described, and all experiments have to be reported to the Home Office. No experiment that is likely to cause pain is permitted unless the animal is anesthetized. Legislation is soon to be introduced to even more tightly control the use of experimental animals. Not only the scientists, but each of their projects will have to be approved beforehand. I have never resented the Home Office Regulations concerning animal experiments. In fact I have welcomed them as providing a form of protection and help. I do not know the situation in other countries, so I must leave you to compare our way of dealing with the supervision of animal experiments with your own.

Animals have served human nutrition well over the past century. Many critical discoveries, particularly concerning vitamins and trace elements, could not have been made without them. They are still of great service in human nutrition and may be more essential in the future as proper animal models for human disorders are discovered. Nonetheless, I think human beings are becoming more important as subjects of study. It seems as though we are rediscovering the philosophy of Alexander Pope, from early in the 18th century, that "the proper study of mankind is man." □

Honours

Robert A McCance

born 9th December 1898; died 5th March 1993

1922	Bachelor of Arts (BA) (University of Cambridge)
1927	Bachelor of Medicine (MB) (University of Cambridge)
1929	Doctor of Medicine (MD) (University of Cambridge)
1935	Fellow of the Royal College of Physicians (FRCP)
1936	Goulstonian Lecturer (Royal College of Physicians)
1938	Fellow of Sidney Sussex College (University of Cambridge)
1945	Personal Chair: Professor of Experimental Medicine (Medical Research Council and University of Cambridge)
1948	Fellow of the Royal Society (FRS)
1949	Triennial Gold Medal (West London Medico-Chirurgical Society)
1953	Commander of the Order of the British Empire (CBE)
1953	Humphrey Rolleston Lecturer (Royal College of Physicians)
1959	Leonard Parsons Lecturer (Birmingham University)
1960	Conway Evans Prize (Royal College of Physicians and The Royal Society)
1961	James Spence Medal (British Paediatric Association)
1962	Lumleian Lecturer (Royal College of Physicians)
1964	Honorary Doctor of Science (DSc) (Queen's University, Belfast)
1966	Fellow *Ad eundem* of the Royal College of Obstetricians and Gynaecologists (FRCOG)
1971	First Annual Lecturer for the British Nutrition Foundation

Honorary offices held:

1950 to 1952	President, Section of Experimental Medicine & Therapeutics, The Royal Society of Medicine
1959 to 1965	President, The Neonatal Society

SELECTED LECTURES

Honours
Elsie M Widdowson

born 21st October 1906

1928	Bachelor of Science (BSc) (University of London)
1931	Doctor of Philosophy (PhD) (University of London)
1948	Doctor of Science (DSc) (University of London)
1970	Sanderson-Wells Lecturer (University of London)
1975	Honorary Doctor of Science (DSc) (University of Manchester)
1976	Fellow of the Royal Society (FRS)
1979	Commander of the Order of the British Empire (CBE)
1981	James Spence Medal (British Paediatric Association)
1982	Second Bristol Myers Award for Distinguished Achievement in Nutrition Research
1982	Annual Lecturer for the British Nutrition Foundation
1983	First European Nutrition Award (Federation of European Nutrition Societies)
1983	Boyd Orr Memorial Lecturer (The Nutrition Society)
1984	Rank Prize Funds Prize for Nutrition
1985	EV McCollum International Lecturer in Nutrition and Award
1986	Atwater Lecturer and Award
1988	Nutricia International Award
1989	Muriel Bell Lecturer (Nutrition Society of New Zealand)
1992	First Edna and Robert Langholz International Nutrition Award (American Dietetic Association Foundation)

Honorary Offices held:

1977 to 1980	President, The Nutrition Society
1978 to 1981	President, The Neonatal Society
1986 to present	President, The British Nutrition Foundation

McCance & Widdowson
A Scientific Partnership of 60 Years

Index

Abrahams, Margery 33, 58
Adams, Georgian 34
Addenbrooke's Hospital,
    Cambridge 17, 40 162, 172, 206
Alington, Barbara 148
Allen, Mary 211
Amino acids 31, 72, 74, 123
Apples 13, 14, 70, 149, 150, 157, 161, 176
Archbold, Helen 31, 58
Atwater 34, 70, 71, 258

Balance experiments 24, 35, 101, 134, 150, 165
Barcroft, Sir Joseph 58, 158
Barrington, Cambridgeshire 17, 139, 148, 156, 175, 192, 197
Bartlow, Cambridgeshire 38, 157, 161, 175, 176, 181
Bart's, see
    St. Bartholomew's Hospital
Bears 42, 118, 210
Bedford College, London 158, 161, 163
Belfast 19, 178, 193, 195, 196, 200, 257
Bernard, Claude 40, 59, 79, 91, 154, 197
Black, Douglas 23, 79, 156
Body composition 37, 40, 56, 87, 104, 113, 182, 192
Bone calcification 94
Boyd Orr Memorial Lecture 258
Boylan, John 43, 179
Brain, composition 41, 95
Bread 24, 35, 56, 138, 139, 140, 148, 149, 150, 156, 157, 161, 162, 163, 165, 166, 170, 175, 195

Bristol Myers Award 209, 258
British Medical Association 36
British Nutrition Foundation 7, 15, 40, 61, 67, 257, 258
Brook, Charles 213, 249

CAB International 18
Cadmium 101
Calcium 24, 25, 35, 84, 94, 103, 146, 150, 151, 156
Carbohydrates 19, 31, 70
Carbohydrate, unavailable 33, 70, 84, 202
Cathcart, Professor 20, 25, 35
Chatfield, Charlotte 34
Chick, Dame Harriette 26, 35
Chickens, poultry 91, 92, 114, 115, 116
Children, undernourished 28, 36
Conway Evans Prize 257
Copper 39. 193
Cowen, Terry 15, 114, 176, 181
Cowley, John 193
Czechoslovakia 191

Dauncey, Joy 203
Dean, Rex 28, 29, 36, 39, 43, 106, 112, 121, 164, 166, 174
Department of Experimental
    Medicine, Cambridge 15, 17, 43, 70, 73, 87, 111, 118, 141, 146, 154, 161, 166, 172, 174, 178, 184, 193, 200
Department of Health 7, 100
Department of Investigative
    Medicine, Cambridge 17, 40, 206

INDEX

Department of Medicine,
  Cambridge 17, 35, 148, 156, 161
De Valera 36
Diabetics 20
Dickerson, John 30, 37, 87, 182, 184, 200
Dietary survey 34, 35, 64, 134
Dietetics 32, 33
Dobbing, John 95, 96, 104, 182
Dodds, EC 32
Dublin 35, 36
Duisburg 36, 162
Dunn Nutrition Laboratory,
  Unit or Centre, Cambridge 15, 17, 40, 74, 90, 176, 184, 201, 203, 208

Edholm, Otto 37
Edna and Robert Langholz Award 16, 258
Elkinton, J Russell 186
Elneil, Hamad 194, 198
EV McCollum International Lecture 91, 213, 251, 258

Fat, body 37, 40, 89, 105, 154, 155, 205
Fiorotto, Marta 208
Flour 25, 35, 36, 84, 148
Food, composition 32, 35, 69, 71, 72, 74, 99, 201, 202
Food industry 61
Food tables 15, 33, 34, 58, 69, 71, 134, 202

Gell, Philip 26
Germany 25, 28, 35, 37, 39, 57, 60, 66, 112, 121, 162, 168, 169, 170, 173, 175
Glaser, Eric 27, 43, 152, 170
Goulstonian lectures 80, 86, 137, 152, 156, 257
Group of European Nutritionists 75
Growth, normal 22, 30, 111, 96, 104, 159
Growth, retarded 30, 119, 114, 123
Guinea pigs 37, 40, 89, 112, 116, 117, 159

Gunther, Mavis 26
Gurr, Michael 206

Haldane, JBS 20
Harland, Erasmus 123
Harris, Isaac 25, 156
Harrison, Marion 90, 174, 179
Haynes, Alec 21, 149
Hervey, Romaine 27, 28, 30, 151, 179, 187
Himsworth, Sir Harold 28, 29, 39, 124
Holman, Ian 43, 179
Hopkins, Sir Frederick Gowland 16, 19
Howarth, Sheila 26
Hume, Dr EM 26
Humphrey Rolleston lecture 257
Hungary 158
Huxley, Andrew 23, 24, 139, 143

Imperial College, London 31, 58
Individual intakes 35, 134
Infant nutrition 99, 100, 146, 159, 203, 204, 209
Infantile Malnutrition Research Unit, Kampala, Uganda 17, 39, 121
Infant Nutrition Research Division, Cambridge 17, 25, 40, 74, 202
Intestine 41, 102, 210
Iron 21, 39, 72, 101, 168

James Spence Medal 257, 258
John, Peter 181, 184, 187
Jonxis, Jan 146, 205

Keatinge, Bill 27, 187
Kennedy, Gordon 38, 43, 112, 154, 179, 187, 194
King's College Hospital, London 17, 19, 20, 21, 32, 99, 134, 136
Kittens, cats 22, 37, 89, 94
Kodicek, Egon 202, 203, 204
Kwashiorkor 91, 112, 121, 122, 123, 126, 127

INDEX

Lake District 23, 139, 143
Lawrence, RD 19
Learmouth, Daphne 172, 178, 184, 187, 201, 202
Leonard Parsons Lecture 257
Life rafts and boats 28, 30, 147, 152
Lister, David 30, 111, 194, 198
London, University 258
Lumleian lectures 111, 213, 221, 257

McCance, Colin 24, 139, 144
McCance, Mary (Mollie) 19, 175
McCance, Robert
 too numerous to list!
McCracken, Kelvin 200
McCullagh, Keith 29, 202
Manchester, University 258
Manganese 101
Marasmus 123, 127
Medical Research Council 7, 19, 20, 21, 24, 25, 26, 33, 39, 70, 112, 122, 140, 145, 164, 190
Mellanby, Sir Edward 25, 36
Melland, Amicia 149
Menstruation 189, 191
Milk composition 40, 100, 209, 210
Mineral metabolism 21, 73, 79, 101
Ministry of Agriculture, Fisheries and Food 7, 74, 201
Morrison, Ashton B (Archie) 30, 178
Mottram VH 32, 58
MRC, see Medical Research Council
Muriel Bell lecture 176, 258
Muscle, composition 90, 91, 92, 93

National Institute for Medical Research, London 112, 154
Neonatal physiology 58, 99, 111, 146, 158, 186
Neonatal Society 99, 158, 160, 199, 257, 258
Netherlands, The 146, 148
New Zealand 23, 138, 174, 176, 258
Nichols, Buford 208
Nutrition databases 69, 73
Nutrition Society 18, 159, 206, 258

Oedema 26, 103, 165, 168
Oftedal, Olav 42, 209

Pařísková, Jana 191
Parsons, Sir Leonard 21, 105
Paul, Alison 16, 37, 74, 201
Pickles, Vernon 189
Pigs, newborn, developing 22, 37, 38, 89, 102, 103, 106, 177, 185, 194, 198
Pigs, runt 40, 116, 117
Pigs, undernourished 28, 38, 39, 91, 92, 114, 115, 116, 128, 180, 202
Protein-energy malnutrition 92, 95, 122, 125
Protein 31, 72, 121, 163
Puppies and dogs 22, 180

Rabbits 22, 37, 89, 100
Rank Prize Funds 258
Rationing, experimental study of 23, 24, 139, 145, 159
Rats 22, 30, 37, 38, 89, 91, 104, 112, 113, 161, 174, 179, 180, 187, 189, 193, 194, 195, 196, 200
Renal function 21, 65, 128, 140, 180
Richards, Audrey 35
Robinson, James 23, 138, 144, 174, 179, 187
Rosenbaum, Dorothy 25, 26, 164, 168
Royal College of Physicians 80, 111, 156, 213, 257
Royal Naval Committee 26, 151
Royal Society, The 57, 143, 257, 258
Royal Society of Medicine 142, 213
Rutishauser, Ingrid 125
Ryle, JA 21, 23, 138, 143

Salt deficiency 20, 80, 136
Sanderson-Wells Lecture 159, 213, 237, 258
Sandhurst 37, 38
Science Citation Index 53
Seals 37, 42, 209, 210
Sea sickness 28, 153

INDEX

Seawater, danger of drinking 26, 30, 84, 153, 179
Self-experimentation 22, 58, 152
Sherlock, Sheila 26
Shipp, HL 20
Sidney Sussex College, Cambridge 7, 15, 18, 107, 157, 161, 183, 194, 206, 257
Skin, composition 92, 93
Skeleton 94
Sodium 21, 79, 103, 105, 126
South London 31, 168
Southgate, David 30, 37, 69, 200, 201
Spence, Sir James 26
St. Bartholomew's Hospital, London 33, 134, 148
St. Bees, Cumbria 19, 196
Strangeways, Brian 164, 179
Strontium 22, 23, 101
Sudan 57, 129, 198
Survival at sea 26, 140, 151, 180, 195

Temperature control 57, 126, 129, 152, 198
The Composition of Foods 33, 37, 56, 71, 72, 99, 201
Third World nutrition 121

Thrussell, Lois 26, 164, 169, 172

Uganda 17, 38, 99, 121, 124
United States of America 16, 34, 41, 60, 75, 208, 209

Verdon-Roe, Monica 35, 134

Walsham, Christine 161
Water deprivation 82, 151, 156
Waterlow, John 95
Watt, Bernice 75
Wharton, Brian 29, 99, 125
Whitehead, Roger 29, 39, 106, 121
Whitteridge, David 136
Widdowson, Elsie
  too numerous to list!
Widdowson, Eva 27, 189
Wilkinson, Betty 163
Wilson, Dagmar 35
Wuppertal 17, 25, 36, 161, 164, 168, 170

Young, Maureen 158, 161
Young, Winifred 21, 43, 105

Zinc 39, 101

The British Nutrition Foundation (BNF) was established in 1967, and its Founder Members included a number of eminent scientists and such well known company names as Rank Hovis McDougall, Beechams, Heinz, Marks and Spencer, Schweppes, Tate and Lyle and Unilever. Today, its Member Companies continue to share common concerns with the scientific community about nutritional problems which affect consumers.

The BNF is an impartial scientific organisation which sets out to provide reliable information and scientifically based advice on nutrition and related health matters, with the ultimate objective of helping individuals to understand how they may best match their diet with their lifestyle: its principal functions fall under the headings of information, education and research.

The BNF is a non-profit making organisation, registered as a charity. Its work is principally funded by donations from its membership. The Foundation draws upon the expert knowledge and extensive experience of the eminent members of its Council and committees: their support underpins and underwrites the Foundation's integrity and reputation.